# Contributions to
# Developmental Neuropsychiatry

# Contributions to
# Developmental Neuropsychiatry

By PAUL SCHILDER, M.D.
(1886–1940)

Edited by LAURETTA BENDER, M.D.

INTERNATIONAL UNIVERSITIES PRESS, INC.
New York

To

Michael, Peter, and Jane

# Contents

# Preface

Two months before the death of Paul Schilder, M.D., Ph.D., his "Vita" was published. He had written it himself although using the third person pronoun. The last part is appropriately quoted here (Schilder, 1940):

"Coming to Bellevue Hospital in 1930, Schilder found himself confronted with many new practical problems. He found that psychiatry in America was in closer contact with social realities than psychiatry in Europe. The problem of constructive psychology, in its relation to gestalt, took a more definite form. He planned to write a treatise on psychology in several volumes to embrace first the body image [*Image and Appearance of the Human Body*, 1935], second, perception and thought [*Mind: Perception and Thought in Their Constructive Aspects*, 1942], third, goals and desires [*Goals and Desires of Man*, 1942a], and fourth, psychotherapy [*Psychotherapy*, 1938c].[1] In addition he had planned further volumes on art[2] and sociology.[3]

"Since Schilder believes that theory must lead to action, he has worked out methods of group psychotherapy [Schilder, 1939, 1940b]. In addition, the problems of ideologies [Schilder, 1936a] has loomed as a problem of great importance without which human life cannot be understood.

"A great part of this work has been done in close conjunction with Lauretta Bender, his wife. This is particularly true of his work

---

[1] The second and third of these volumes were published posthumously (1942).

[2] A volume on *The Art of the Emotionally Disturbed Child* was written, with Bender as coauthor, in the early 1930's, but never published as a whole. Several chapters have appeared in Bender's four volumes of Bellevue Studies in Child Psychiatry (Bender, 1952, 1953, 1954, 1955).

[3] The volume on sociological papers was not completed by Schilder, but a collection of his sociological papers was published (1951).

with children. Whereas Schilder had been previously skeptical of the possibility of understanding children and had felt that there was a danger of projecting insights gained with adults into children, he now feels that the principles of constructive psychology can help in the deeper understanding of the child. The behavior of the child can only be understood as a continuous process of trial and error, which leads to construction and configuration as a basis for action. He now feels that behavior difficulties and neuroses are interruptions in this constructive psychological process. Only when an individual strives in his environment and in the world will he have full emotional experience and a full life as a personality. An individual is truly alive as long as he errs and tries. Human beings drive into the future by trial and error, and thereby find their happiness. Schilder finds the final proof for the irresistible drive into the future in his two sons, Michael, aged three and Peter, aged two." (His daughter, Jane, was born shortly after this writing.)

Schilder's contributions to the psychology, psychopathology, psychiatry, and neurology of childhood, in terms of the child himself, his development, and the adult which the child ultimately becomes, have had tremendous influence on American psychiatry. They were written in the last ten years of his life and first published in scientific journals; some have been reprinted, especially in the four volumes of the Bellevue Studies in Child Psychiatry (Bender, 1952, 1953, 1954, 1955). They are collected here in a more complete form and represent a comprehensive view of the field.

Here will be found many examples of Schilder's inimitable verbal interviews and case histories; many examples of his unique capacity to observe and describe motility and behavior; several special test procedures which he developed to explore perception, thought processes, and other psychological phenomena; and, finally, his capacity to accumulate such data, analyze it, and develop his own point of view into a "constructive psychology."

Often, these observations, and their analysis and conclusions were shared with co-workers, such as Walter Bromberg, Frank J. Curran, David Wechsler, and the editor.

His early writings (in German) on Encephalitis Periaxialis Diffusa or Schilder's disease (Schilder, 1912, 1912a, 1913, 1914), on motility in chorea affecting children (Schilder, 1911), and on the psychology of the epidemic of encephalitis of 1920, as it affected children (Schilder, 1921), are not included. However, it will be noted that he takes occasion to refer to some of these early studies in his later writings.

Permission to republish has always been requested of former publishers and always granted; sources are indicated where appropriate.

The content of this book is entirely in the words of Schilder. The editor has only arranged the material. Any necessary editorial comments have been made in footnotes. Footnotes have also been used for follow-up reports on the children interviewed, examined, and discussed by Schilder.

My personal thanks are due to Gloria Faretra for her encouraging and faithful help with editorial problems.

For the editor, this has been a work of love.

LAURETTA BENDER

New York City
April, 1960

# I

# Primitive Perception and the Construction of the Object

## A Constructive Approach to Childhood Problems[1]

This approach to childhood problems is a definite dynamic and constructive one. The child is seen as a growing organism with definite problems of maturation, as has been particularly emphasized, in American literature, by Gesell (1939, 1940; Gesell and Thompson, 1934). Great stress, however, should be placed on living situations and the emotional problems of childhood life, as these are continually modifying the developmental process. The development of the child is viewed, in accordance with the general principles of psychoanalysis, as an emotional interdependence between the parents, the surroundings of the child, and the child himself. Furthermore, human beings, in general, are considered as having social connections and therefore we place particular emphasis on the psychology of the group.

Thus, one observes that the development of the child is not seen merely as a maturation process, but also as a continuous process of social experimentation by which, after trial and error, final construction is reached. This final construction is dependent on basic principles of psychophysiological organization, which, in the form of configurations and gestalten, determine the beginning, continuation, and end of the experimental process.

[1] From Curran and Schilder (1940-1941).

1

## OPTIC PERCEPTION[2]

The earliest experiences of the child certainly do not consist of simple sensations. The primitive experience seems to be much more complex and diffuse than does the completely developed perception. Experience is not only something going on in the body but also something occurring in the world. Perceptions or impressions mean that something is going on in space. Primitive experience is an experience of movement which is definite, yet which fills the whole field of experience. This is particularly clear in the optic field.

In primitive optic perception, we find spirals, glittering waves, and vortices. Points are not perceived as such in primitive optic experience. The loop, circle, and even the star, seem to be more primitive than the point. The straight line is not as primitive as the curved line and the angle is also a later development.

The prevalence of curves, circles, ellipses, and whorls in primitive perception corresponds to the fact that similar movements prevail in primitive motor action.

Even these primitive optic experiences have some kind of shape and size. We do not know under what condition the angle is definitely differentiated from primitive forms. Children are not able to draw a diamond before the seventh year. One may, of course, say this is due to motor incapacity of the child. However, a sharp division between motility and perception is not justified. The prevalence of the curve over the straight line has been justly emphasized by gestalt psychologists. In our experiment in optic imagination (Kanner and Schilder, 1930; Bender, 1938) the prevalence of the curved line is clearly revealed. At some time, however, the curved line flattens out into a straight line and there is also a tendency for indentations to flatten out. One has the impression that forms and shapes which have distinct sharp angles are maintained in the imagination only by effort. The size of a primitive optic perception remains rather indefinite. As long as it is of primitive character, a picture may become smaller or larger. We have no definite knowledge about the limits of these size variations in perception. Children are somewhat insensitive to the size of a reproduc-

---

[2] The material for this section appeared in Schilder (1942), unless otherwise specified.

tion. In general, in primitive perception and imagination, size is not definite; it becomes so only with further development.

W. Stern (1924) found that children may perceive objects rotated 90° to 180° from their position. Children, more readily than adults, recognize objects which are turned around, upside down, or from left to right. P. Meyer (1913) also found that children make more mistakes concerning position than adults. Mistakes in right and left are much more common than mistakes in above and below. Figures which were not symmetrical were reproduced as symmetrical. The investigations of Bender (1938) on gestalt figures (which will be discussed later in detail) offer further material illustrating these points. Le Maitre (1910) reports an adolescent who had attacks, twice a month, in which he had the impression that he had experienced the present situation in dreams in which everything was upside down, so that human beings had their feet up and their heads down.

Jaensch (1930) has tried to show that perception of depth is, in great measure, dependent upon the influence of attention and that eidetic images show this phenomenon particularly clearly. He also emphasizes the influence of emotions on localization in depth. He says that relative constancy in depth values is secondary and is built up later, whereas, in the earliest stages of development, there is a great plasticity in depth values. Even if the experimental proofs of Jaensch, concerning the depth perception of juveniles and children, should be reliable, there is still a question as to why we find, in adults, a relative constancy comparatively little influenced by attention.

The following observations of anxiety states in children are pertinent: one patient was afraid, as a child, that life-size lions might jump out of a toilet bowl; another child was afraid of being sucked into the drain of the bathtub and washed away. In these fears, the infantile disregard of size is evident. A four-year-old girl could not distinguish between a cube and a sphere; it is even doubtful whether she saw them differently.

## AUDITORY PERCEPTION

The nature of primitive hearing is difficult to understand. Most of the experimental evidence brought forward in this field concerns

3

tones, whereas our world of hearing consists chiefly of noises of all kinds. To a great extent, speech also belongs in this category. Judging from the motor performance of children as they sing, it is improbable that tone, as such, plays a very important part in a child's life. Pleasure derived from noises of various kinds, especially rhythmic noises, is at least as great as the pleasure of singing. Buehler (1929) writes that a child enjoys the terrible screeching of an unoiled carriage axle as much as the most beautiful lullaby. Buehler also emphasizes the importance of rhythm. Both Buehler and Gross (1933) describe vividly the pleasure children have in the production of noises. It is difficult to imagine what are the outstanding factors in this acoustic world. Noises certainly have the qualities of brightness and darkness, even if the character of pitch is not clearly expressed.

## Vestibular Sensation

It is important, for the understanding of vestibular phenomena, to realize that the child gets pleasure out of every vestibular sensation. The child likes to be rocked, tossed in the air and swung. These excitations of the vestibular apparatus are undoubtedly connected with some more-or-less pronounced sexual feelings. Every quick movement downward provides sensations, as everyone who has been on a scenic railway will recognize. The phenomenology of these sensations is not yet known and we do not know anything about the underlying finer mechanisms. A great number of phenomena are allied to the function and dysfunction of the vestibular apparatus, such as dizziness and acute awareness of heights. We know that there is a natural tendency to get into a position which is in a proper relation to the optic surroundings.

The close relation between motor tendencies and inner perceptual motion is particularly emphasized in vestibular disturbances which prove that we deal with an apparatus which can act exclusively on one side of the body. The vestibular apparatus has a threefold influence: on the perceptual experience directly; on the inner motion in perception; and on tonus (which again influences perception and its inner motion). The unifying tendencies of the vestibular apparatus influence all these. Gelb and Goldstein (1918,

4

1919) believe that the tonic influences upon perception take place outside the psychic sphere, and they are inclined to feel that psychological factors do not play any part in distortions. Jaensch (1930), who has seen similar phenomena in eidetic images, stresses the factor of attention. Attention is a direction of an individual toward a stimulus. This direction is psychic as well as physiological. It may originate in the psychic sphere, it may originate in the physiological sphere, but there is always something in common between the psychological and physiological direction of the organism.

Through studying the vestibular apparatus, we may most closely approach problems of intersensory relations. We have learned that the vestibular apparatus is responsible for the phenomena which occur after turning and for the perception of accelerations. It consists of two different parts, each with a different function. The semicircular canals are organs which help us in the perception of movements. There is some question as to whether they serve for perception of circular movement only or of progressive movement also. Disease of the vestibular organ provokes dizziness. In the labyrinth, there is evidently another organ which helps us to perceive gravity. We are not quite sure whether this is the sacculus-utriculus, but there are many facts which point in this direction. There is little doubt that the labyrinth is not the only graviceptor; skin and muscle sensitivity also play a part in the perception of gravity. The semicircular canals are the organ for the perception of the circular movement and, probably, they also help in the perception of progressive movements of the body. However, the otoliths are the most important organs for this function.

The vestibular apparatus is not only an organ of perception; it is an organ which gives rise to very important reflexes which are caused in part by the semicircular canals. These are reflexes to turning and progressive movement. There are also reflexes which are determined by the position of the labyrinth in space. These are postural reflexes, probably related to the function of the otoliths. The labyrinth is, therefore, an organ which influences the muscle tone of the body. Certainly it is only one of the many organs responsible for tone, motor attitude, and posture. The vestibular apparatus is the means for bringing into clearest focus the sensory impulses which influence our system of attitude and tone. It is a great system for orienting ourselves in the world. This system is, of course, not isolated, but cooperates with the other systems of orientation, especially that of the optic perceptions. It is more closely related to primitive motility than is vision. We no longer believe that there are isolated senses. Impressions of the tactile and auditory sphere are always connected with our optic impressions; synesthesia is not an exceptional occurrence but is, rather, one of the basic principles of perception. After all, we never have optic impressions alone, but perceive objects by seeing, hearing, or touch. These visual objects are also objects for all the senses.

## TACTILE PERCEPTION

Little is known about tactile perception, especially in children. Tactile sensation is more purely subjective than any other sensory experience; it immediately points to something going on in our own body. To a much greater extent, hearing, seeing, smelling, and taste are directed toward the outer world.

We think that these phenomena are very often the basis for psychic elaboration in hallucinations. In order to show this, we will give here the protocols of a boy who was hypnotized. In the after-effects, he sometimes felt as if dust were coming out of his skin. When directed, instead of imagining a cross on his hand, he felt a circle in one of the quadrants.

M. A., a boy aged thirteen, had a history of fainting spells. He had become quarrelsome and was somewhat of a disciplinary problem at home. The past history was essentially negative. The falling seizures were described as occurring most often at night, when the patient would fall out of bed. He rarely hurt himself. He would become unconscious, but had no clonic or tonic movements. In the hospital, the seizures were observed and considered to be psychogenic in nature. Physical findings were negative. During residence in the hospital, hypnosis was tried for its therapeutic effect, and it was at this time that the experiments detailed below were done. While under light hypnosis, the patient was given the commands without further suggestion, except where noted:

A cross was drawn on the left hand. "I feel the cross. It feels as if something were coming out of my hand. Now only the left upper corner is left. I feel something coming out of my hand, like when the room is darkened and sunshine comes through a crack in the window. Now I feel a tickling over the whole hand, over the wrist, like a strip."

6

A line was drawn on patient's hand. "It feels like a 'J' and the turn of the 'J' is all gone. Now it is starting to chip away at the top and now it is all gone."

M. A. was asked to imagine a cross on his hand. "I feel it well. Now it has gone away. My hand itches and I feel an incomplete circle in the upper right corner quadrant of the cross. Now the cross and the circle fade away, but I feel all kinds of things mixed up where the cross was—squares, circles, and all of them are moving into each other very fast. (The suggestion was made that the patient pick out the square and feel it.) I only feel two sides of the square but not the angle. Now the ends of the line chip off and everything is very faint, and it all goes away."

## OBJECT CONSTRUCTION[3]

Final elaboration of the world of perception is dependent upon the motor impulses. The tone of the postural and righting reflexes —"induced tone," in Goldstein's (1934) terminology—is only a small sector of the motor possibilities of the organism. Besides these mass reactions, which usually involve at least one half of the body, there are more specific ones which are based upon these more primitive functions. To this class belong the reactions of groping, grasping, and incorporating into the body, which especially appear in the primitive grasp reflexes. Here too, belongs the sucking reflex which reappears after certain lesions of the brain. Many primitive defense reactions also belong to this group. One is entitled to say that with every perception a double series of kinetic and motor phenomena is coordinated; the tonic phenomena seem more primitive. Tonic and phasic influences affect perception. In one patient, who showed the syndrome of spontaneously turning around on his longitudinal axis with an increase in postural and righting reflexes,

[3] This concept, "construction of the object," is a basic tenet of Schilder's. D. Rapaport has used the term "intending the object" in his 1953 translation of Schilder's (1924) *Medical Psychology*. However, Schilder, in his own translation of the same or similar material, always used "construction of the object" or some equivalent. He felt that a "constructive psychology" best described his point of view, meaning that each individual is always actively constructing his own psychic experiences, including the objective world. Note his titles: *Mind: Perception and Thought in Their Constructive Aspects* (1942), "A Constructive Approach to the Problems of Childhood and Adolescence" (Curran and Schilder, 1940-1941), "Language and the Constructive Energies of the Psyche" (1936), and *Image and Appearance of the Human Body: Studies in the Constructive Energies of the Psyche* (1935).

a macroscopia and polyopsia occurred probably due to the effect of the motor impulse on optic perception.[4]

In discussing the vestibular apparatus, I emphasized the influence of vestibular tonic impulses on perception. There exists a formative influence of the motility on perception. It is difficult to determine how inner motion in perception, and the motor impulses elicited by perception, work together. Stein (1927) hypothesizes that the inner motion of perception, which he calls "sensory movement," is the factor which creates sensation and perception. But this point of view is difficult to justify. I have tried to show that primitive perception is a state of motion. Motion is not something independent and separate from perception, but is of its very essence. The inner motion of the perception is not created, but is a part of the primary experience. Development is in the direction of the elimination of the inner motion of the perception. Motility is one of the important factors in this process of the stabilization of perception. On the other hand, we know that moving objects have a particular influence on motility; they are, so to speak, the prime movers of action. The consolidation of perception therefore depends on motility. By this very fact, the impression gets its spatial localization.

The unified object which gives a specific orientation for action is not an isolated experience, but is related to the attitudes and actions of the individual. Primitive optic experience consists of colors, movements, spirals, and vortices that are only incompletely differentiated from the background. Whenever the beginning of figure-background differentiation appears, the differentiation is increased by factors involving the organism as a whole. The figure becomes a rallying point in a background composed of all other sense perceptions and of vegetative influences. This is followed by tonic and phasic impulses which lead to the development of clearer perception. Clearer articulation prepares the way for directed organismic action resulting in even clearer definition and articulation of an object and its properties, and is, therefore, a new unification which involves the perceptual data of other senses and creates a synesthesia, which may be considered a concordance of senses in the second

[4] Some of this discussion involves data obtained from adults, as well as children, with reference to "primitive experiences." Its evident pertinence to the problems of psychological development justifies its inclusion here, in order to round out the discussion in the words of Paul Schilder himself.

degree. Further manipulation of objects reveals new properties in the optic and tactile sphere, gives a more distinct form to the spatial relations, and may lead, by bringing the object to the mouth, to new data concerning the olfactory and gustatory qualities of the object, adding in this way to the completeness of perceptual data concerning the object. It is, therefore, of special significance that groping, grasping, sucking, and bringing the object to the mouth belong to the most primitive organic reactions.

I have emphasized that rhythmic qualities are important in primitive perception. Optic images and optic afterimages come and go. Sound and tactile impressions have definite rhythmic qualities. In smell and taste, however, there is no definite hint of rhythmic tendencies. Rhythm is ingrained in the motor structure of the organism. The experiments of Sherrington (1911) have shown rhythmic qualities in simple spinal reflexes, like the scratch reflex. Brown (1911) has shown that the rhythm of gait is a central rhythm independent of outside influences. Proprioceptive and exteroceptive stimuli merely modify the rhythm of the central nervous system. Physiologically it seems, therefore, that the rhythmic influences become definite isolated impulses under the influence of closer relations with the object. The same condition which increases postural and righting reflexes, also increases the tendency to rhythmic movements. In a case of decerebrate rigidity in an idiot child, turning of the head provoked rhythmic gait movements. It is interesting that stimuli applied to the sole of the foot may provoke rhythmic movements of crawling and creeping, as was observed by Bauer (1925) in a normal suckling and by Zingerle (1927) in his cases of automatosis (increased postural and righting reflexes). Fischer and Wodak (1924) have shown that vestibular phenomena of the motor type, as well as of the sensory type, show an exquisite rhythmic character. In the sensory field, in the development from primitive perception to organized perception, it seems that rhythm becomes subordinated to the impression of a stabilized object. The suppression of rhythm in perceptual development is as important a step as the suppression of motion.

We always speak of unchanging objects. However, objects are continually changing—and still they remain the same objects (Boring, 1933). Not only do objects change, but there is a continuous change in the sensory impulse which is the basis for the perceptual object. The static object is a product of late development. The primitive object is in motion internally and externally. In pathological cases, the tendency of change inherent in all our experiences comes out in an intensified form. When, because of the inner structure of the perception and because of tonic and kinetic influences, the experience of motion is not sufficient to disrupt the object completely or to move it as a whole, distortion takes place, which is experienced as change. In some cases, the change seems to be independent of the movement, while in other cases, movement and change are present at the same time. In an atropine delirium, changes can be produced in the optic hallucination by vestibular irritation. The experience of change is closely related to the primitive experience of motion and is exaggerated by the dissociation of motor impulses. The impression of a static object is dependent on the suppression of the inner motion of the perception and on the coordination of motor impulses. This does not remove the question of how we reach the perception of a stabilized object. I do not believe that primitive perception does not point to an objective world. With the exception of tactile experiences, which belong decisively to the sphere of the body, every sensation points not only to the body, but also, predominantly, to the outside world; this primitive outside world has more motion, more rhythm, more color, and less sharply distinguished spatial relations than has the developed perceptual world. Its synesthetic character is different from that met in the fully developed experience. Some definite characteristics belong to this primitive world, such as the tendency against sharp angles; the preference for curves, vortices, and circles; the prevalence of movement and rhythm; the tonic mass reaction; and the rhythmic phasic reaction. This problem must be exemplified in the important field of gestalt and its developments.

## Gestalt Function[5]

We cannot understand the development of the primitive perception without acquiring better insight into the problem of configuration.

[5] From Curran and Schilder (1940-1941).

In children with behavior problems, as well as in normal children, the organic pattern formations have to be continually considered. From this point of view, studies in gestalt perception are of particular importance. By letting subjects copy Wertheimer's (1923) gestalt figures, Bender has given a complete picture of the developmental processes of gestalt formation.[6]

Gestalt psychology, as developed by the work of Wertheimer, Köhler (1929), and Koffka (1928, 1935), has given a new impetus to psychology. It has given a new insight into the relation between the whole and its parts and has shown that perception cannot be understood as the summation of single sensations. Sensory fields are replete with qualities and properties which cannot be understood if one takes the individual sensations as the units of understanding. The organism does not react to local stimuli by local events; it reacts to constellations of stimuli by a total process which is the response of the whole organism to the total situation. Such a process regulates itself and distributes itself dynamically. Gestalt psychology has stressed the dynamic inner factor, self-regulation in perception. Previous experience cannot, in itself, explain the existence of segregated units in experience as the grouping of points and lines, for instance, in the configurations of stars. Furthermore, it cannot determine what will be in the foreground and what will be in the background of one's perceptual experience. This is determined by the total situation. Simple connotations like figure, whole, foreground, background, group, open, closed, circle, complete and incomplete, starting, beginning, end, and good gestalt or bad gestalt, gain a new significance. Children would not learn how to organize a visual field even after years of trial and error.

Organization gets its final meaning only in relation to concrete situations of life which adapt the patterns to the actions and experimentations of individuals. In the field of perception, gestalt psychology has deepened our insight considerably, is a new definite proof of the validity of a dynamic psychology, and complements the fundamental ideas of American psychiatry.

The method which Bender has developed—copying of gestalt forms—immediately broadens the field of observation. Her method

[6] Schilder wrote the Introduction to Bender's Monograph (1938), from which these paragraphs are quoted.

does not merely answer the question of what the individual perceives, but also the question of what the individual uses his perception for. Her method allows, therefore, a much more direct expression of the biological factors than do the experiments in which the subjects merely describe their experiences. Psychological experimentation often artificially disrupts perception and motility. This is avoided here by the simple expedient of having the individual draw what he perceives.

Bender's work approaches the fundamental problems of perception and action from a new angle. It shows the primitive forms of experience and the maturation process in the course of development. It shows the continuous interplay between motor and sensory factors. A new world of primitive perception opens up. It has even been possible to standardize the development of the visual motor gestalt function. Bender's investigations show, furthermore, the close relation of the development of optic form to visual imagination. It is of particular interest that the primitive forms of visual motor experience also make their appearance when the time of perception is shortened (with tachistoscope). One obtains the impression that every individual, in almost every experience, passes through the whole maturation process, through which the individual developed during his childhood.

The Berlin gestalt psychologists, Wertheimer, Koffka, and Köhler, claim that a structuralized configuration is immediately perceived in such a way that it corresponds with the external stimulating world. The pattern is the result of a dynamic interaction between the sensory field (internal organizing forces) and the stimulus (external organizing forces); or, as Köhler puts it, the sensory field is organized by the relative properties of stimulation. Wertheimer used figures (see Figure 1) [7] for visual perception, asking normal persons what they experienced as they perceived them. From this data, he derived his laws of good gestalten, namely, that we tend to perceive things in certain patterns because of the proximity of their parts, continuity of the structure, similarity of the parts, inclusiveness of the structure, and in natural geometrical figures. Koffka has emphasized that the first law of gestalt is the relation of the figure or structure to the background. He also em-

[7] See Bender's Monograph (1938), Plates I and II.

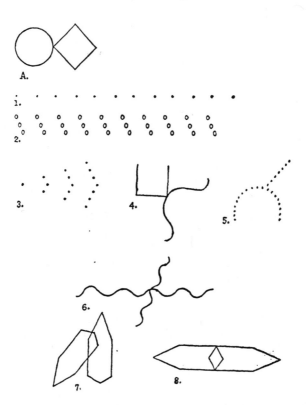

FIGURE 1. The Visual Motor Gestalt Test Figures.

phasizes the principle of inclusiveness and closure. These are the fundamental principles of optically perceived organized form according to the Berlin school of gestalt psychology. Wertheimer and the gestalt school asked their subjects to describe their experiences. It was an important step forward when Bender asked the individuals to copy these figures, because it is then possible to use the text on individuals who do not have the language capacity to describe their perceptual experience; as for example, small children, mental defectives, individuals with organic brain disease (including aphasia), and schizophrenics. In this way, it represents an integrated perceptual motor experience. This leads immediately back to one of the fundamental points of this discussion. We do not have the right to separate motility from perception. Bender's procedure is, therefore, apt to lead deeper into the fundamental problem.

13

We know that the first drawings of children are scribblings which seem to represent pure motor play. They are done for the pleasure of motor expression. The scribbled picture is a by-product, it has no meaning. It is performed by large arm movement in dextral, clockwise whirls, or pendulum waves, if the child uses his right hand, and in sinistral, counter-clockwise whirls if the left hand is used. There is no obvious picture in the mind of the child when he scribbles in the way described. But I do not doubt that even this seemingly purely motor activity must be connected with perceptual elements of primitive character. Quite in the same way as there is no perception without motility, there is no motility without perception. It is difficult to determine what kind of perception this may be. There is a relation between these primitive scribblings and the primitive spatial perceptions. The primitive wave and the primitive vortex make their appearance in the perceptual area as they do in the motor sphere. Baldwin (1903) observed, in a twenty-seven-month-old child, that his productions in drawing consisted of loops in a clockwise direction with emphasis on the horizontal plane. In her studies, Bender[8] reached the opinion that the visual motor gestalt patterns

arise from movement, probably vortical, and that internally organized gestalten evolve genetically by a progressive organization in connection with the integrated intellectual functions. It thus appears that the more primitive sensory motor patterns are dependent upon the principles of constant motion of a whirling or vortical type, with an associated radiating directional component and with a tendency to emphasize the horizontal plane. Fixed points are difficult and straight lines are not accomplished as the shortest distance between two fixed points, but as an expression of radiating tendencies. Crossed lines and angulated forms present great difficulties. The first evidence of expressed form was shown at the second year level as little units of whorls or loops which perseverated most freely in the horizontal plane in a dextral direction. Some tendencies for gestalten were seen in the third year level as rectangular forms either near each other or inside each other. But some of the gestalt principles are functions of the more highly elaborated perceptual motor capacities and only appear at the higher intellectual levels. Above three years, we find the tend-

[8] Quoted by Schilder (1942) from Bender (1938).

ency to accentuate the horizontal base line, to control perseveration and to produce wavy lines instead of broken ones for the representation of straight ones, and there is some effort to cross lines. At the five year level there is some tendency to reduce the primitive loops to points and to make straighter lines and better recognized gestalten. At the seven year level there is a capacity for many vertical and geometrical gestalten on the principle of internal organization and crossing of forms. At the eight year level nearly all gestalten are possible, slanting forms are recognized but their relation to the whole figure presents difficulties. Pairing as determined by slight differences is not accomplished. The major difficulties at this level seem to be in relationships of parts to wholes. These things are satisfactorily accomplished above the ten year level. At all levels all of the original principles are in evidence and tendencies to revert to them are always present.

Bender writes elsewhere in the same monograph (1938):

Visual motor gestalten may be tested by the copying or drawing of figures. They arise from motor behavior that first finds its expression in scribbling. The scribbling is modified by inhibition into loops or parts of loops that tend to take on significance as they correspond with the forms which are perceived by the optic field. I have previously pointed out that movement is the basis for the organization of the optic field. The two- to three-year-old child can imitate motor activity to produce new forms more readily than it can copy new optically perceived forms. Thus dots, dashes, and zigzags may be experienced first as motor behavior pattern and then either utilized more freely in response to optic stimuli that suggest them or again forgotten, while the primitive loop is resorted to in order to express relationship in all gestalten. A simple enclosed loop on a background, loops in concentric relationship, or loops in horizontal dextral direction are the first laws of gestalten. New principles may arise either from motor experience, dots, dashes, or zigzags in series or masses, or they may arise from enclosed forms built from parts of loops or, by inhibition, from partially closed or open loops. Crossed forms are difficult, and even more difficult are all slanting and oblique relationships. The niceties of actual sizes, distances, and perfection of motor control are added after the age of seven years, but most of the gestalt principles are established before that age [see Figure 2].[9]

[9] See Bender (1938), Plates I and II.

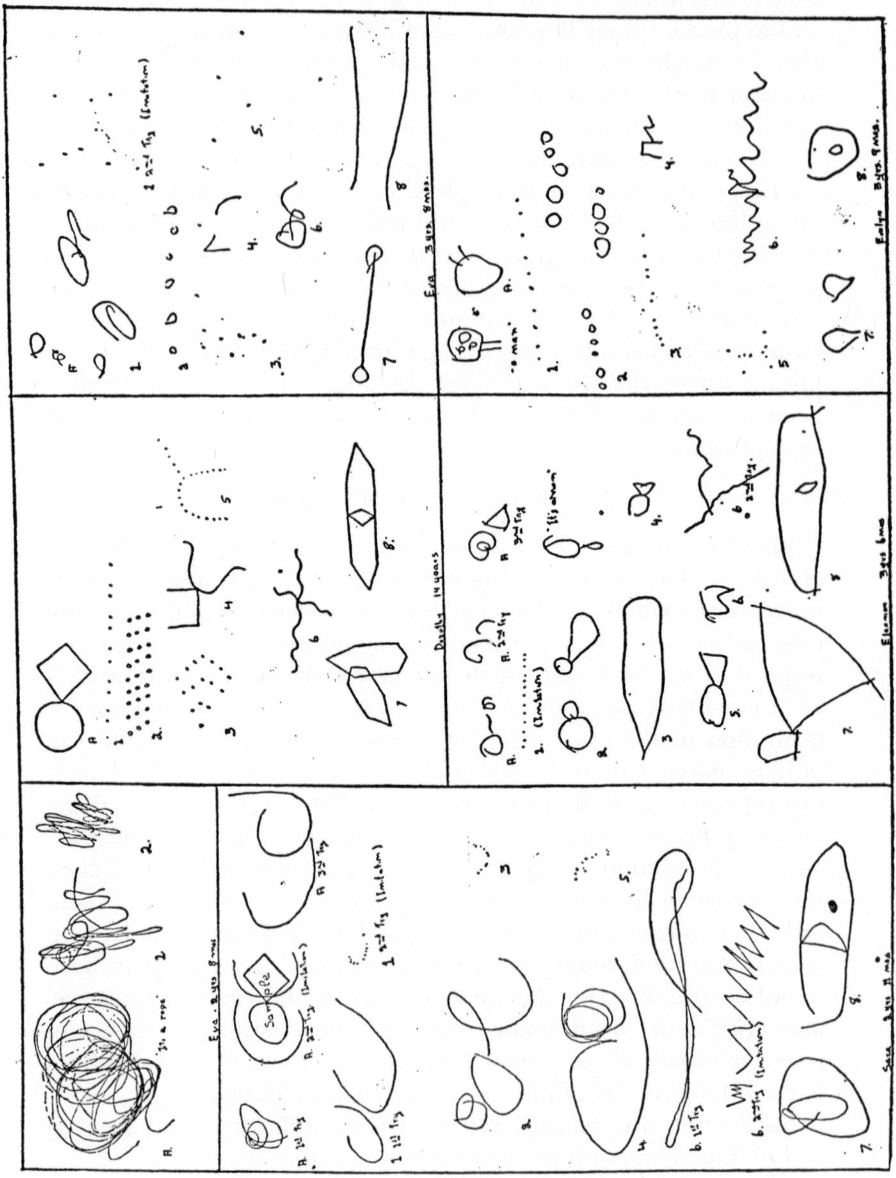

FIGURE 2. Gestalt Drawings by Children.

In psychological terms, we may say that the goal in children's drawings is to establish an equilibrium between the mental symbols, as determined by the biological background of the perceptual motor pattern at the different stages of the maturation of the organism as a whole, and the reality of the world as it is perceived. The traces that are used must correspond not alone to the stimuli that produce them but also to the organization characteristics of the sensory field.

We may conclude that there are gestalt principles which extend at first over the whole field. Under the guidance of actual experience, more definite gestalten are created. Further elaboration of the gestalten takes place by a maturation process that is continually influenced by experiences. These tendencies also appear in the sidewalk drawings of children. There is a continuous interrelation between the motility which leads to the general pattern and beyond it to more specific and elaborate forms in connection with previous experiences. New experiences are continually modifying the primitive perceptual patterns and the primitive motility. But there is another important fact that one can read from Bender's figures. The child does not change the primitive pattern when once it has been created in the early stages of development, as, for instance, in the pictures drawn by a child of three years. It seems that once created, the gestalt behaves in a more or less tyrannical way, neglecting many parts of the immediate perception.

There are some other important principles which can be derived from these figures. The gestalt principles are very often enormously simplified and at the same time exaggerated. On the other hand, gestalten which are typical for the adult may be more or less completely disrupted. When a number of points are copied, the subject reproduces the number of points rather freely. It is as if the important thing were not the exact number but "numerous points." In the adult, the direction is insignificant; in the primitive stages, the difference between the original and the copy concerning the number of points can be very considerable. Reversals from right to left and from below to above are also not uncommon.

It has already been mentioned that a slanting series is very often transformed to a vertical one. Rotations of 90° are also observed. It is of very great importance that in organic brain diseases associated with sensory aphasia, one finds a disintegration of the more integrated internal detailed organization of the gestalten; but there is a perseverance of the outstanding gestalt principle by use of the primitive loop as the unit symbol. The fundamental principles of gestalt thus appear in a primitive form. In disintegrating cerebral lesions, the gestalten tend to revert to more primitive levels and, as the brain recovers from its injury, they tend to follow the laws of developmental maturation in returning to the higher integrating responses.

We again perceive that the problem of gestalt is not only perceptual, but is also a motor problem. Gestalten are sensory motor units, although either the motor or the sensory factor may be more in the foreground. On the most primitive level, the field is in the foreground and no single construction emerges from this field. In the next step, primitive gestalten contrast against this field; experience and a continual constructive process are necessary to adapt the configuration to the reality and to the object.

On the next level, the object has been more clearly defined by continuous touch with reality (reality testing) and with more elaborated motor function. The differentiation of figure and background becomes comparatively clear.

This primitive perception provokes primitive motor answers, which finally lead to a crystallization of configurations of a more definite character. Whereas the primitive perception is, in large part, streamlike, continually moving, and "intransitive," coexistent attempts at construction lead to clear-cut configurations of the primitive type. There are always attempts to bring this moving world to a standstill and to make it a world which can be grasped in a simpler way. I have, therefore, emphasized that gestalten of a rather rigid character are coexistent with and follow the stage of the vortex. It is the first crystallization and this first one is comparatively rigid. Motility and especially the vestibular apparatus are of outstanding importance in the genesis of this first configuration. With the configuration, the seemingly objectless stream and movement become crystallized; but such a configuration is only one point in development and cannot last. In the play of children and in their spontaneous sidewalk drawings (Bender, 1932), one very often sees that the seemingly objectless movement is the starting point of the configuration. The scribblings of children are sooner or later related to objects of the outer world, become adapted to them, and more and more mark the beginning of pictorial drawing. When one studies drawings of the human figure (Goodenough, 1926) one sees how the primitive configuration crystallizations are at first used as approximations of the human figure and, finally, are integrated into the complete figure. A continuous process of construction is going on, in which the primitive gestalt is a transition point.

I offer the thesis that perception and sensation are in space and that spatial characteristics are necessarily inherent in every perception and sensation, even the most primitive. The world of colors and seen movements is before us. Even with closed eyes, black is perceived in a close relation. It is true that this space is necessarily a primitive one, since no action is possible in it. Whatever we may see is seen in space. At the same time this means that there are distinct relations between experiences and our actions. The optic space is never fully independent, since an isolated perception or imagination does not exist. It is always related to the self and the body. As we will see (Chapter II), the body image is an image in space. There are no human experiences without the experience of one's own body, and perceptions are outside one's own body. One's own body always has an extension in space.

Certain sensations, such as pain, occur only within the body space. But even in these sensations there are elements which extend beyond it. Every tactile perception has distinct spatial qualities relating to the body and to the outside world.

It is erroneous for Gelb and Goldstein (1919) to assert that there are no primary spatial qualities or primary space perceptions in the tactile sphere. According to Bromberg and myself (1932), there is a distinct spatial quality in olfactory and gustatory experiences. Even when smell, which is experienced as a substance, is spread in the air and in the nose, it is distinctly outside the body and separated from the sensation in the mucous membrane. There is no need to stress the spatial qualities of hearing. It has been frequently emphasized that primitive perception shows motion in most sense modalities and this inner motion is another spatial quality; also, this inner motion is eliminated during the process of building up the object.

When a moving object is grasped it becomes firm and acquires definite spatial qualities and characteristics. Kinesthetic sensations are important for final elaborations of space. However, one should not overrate the importance of kinesthetic sensations, because optic and tactile sensations provoke motor reaction. Groping and grasping bring new qualities into experience, which is finally formed with the help of kinesthetic sensations. Primitive space perceptions of the various senses also originate in connection with various openings of the body and of the face. In this respect, the eye is considered an opening.

These diverse spaces of the various senses have comparatively little inner contact. Only by the action of the vestibular apparatus and by active motility is the final confluence of unified space created. It is probable that a vague concept of a general space is present in the primitive spaces of the senses. Acoustic and optic spaces are indeed difficult to separate, and the olfactory space is also closely related to them. The space of taste and the space of touch have more separate qualities.

If our general idea is correct, the primitive sensation is more synesthetic than the developed one, but when the object is finally created, it again is an object for all the senses and we deal with synesthesia of a higher order. In the development of space, the tendency for unification becomes stronger. Tonic and phasic motility play the leading part in the final elaboration of space. They guarantee the final combination of the spaces of different units.

Certainly, all senses participate in these primitive experiences of space. To perceive means to have a body from which the objects are separated in space.

All experience takes place in space. I do not think that space is merely the social aspect of experience. There is a deep inner unity, of a social kind, in every phase of experience and the spatial quality of experience is merely one side of the total experience. Activity is basic in all parts of perception and is also basic for space perception. Activity is also directed toward the outside world and other human beings. Activity is therefore the primary factor in the creation of the object, but is, in its essence, a social factor. Activity is, of course, not only a motor factor; it includes drives and instincts.

Philosophers and psychologists have not given sufficient attention to the fact that there is not only a space outside of the body but also a space which is filled by the body. The image of the body extends in space and implies space perception. Without an outward space, body space is strictly senseless. When we speak of narcissism we should not forget that an outward space and the space of the body are the necessary basis for the unfolding of narcissistic tendencies.

This primitive space is probably less unified than developed space. Primitive space is centered around the openings of the body and so has several centers. Psychological factors are at work in building up the perception of space. There is first an undifferentiated relation between an incompletely developed body image and the outside space. Clearer differentiation takes place around the openings of the body. There is a zone of indifference, between the body and the outside world, which makes distortions of body space and outside space by projection and appersonation possible. These distortions are corrected by a continuous process of testing by action (reality testing). Aggressiveness may draw objects closer to the body. Generally, space develops around erogenous zones, in close connection with drives of the individual. This space is not unified and has separate parts. Under the influence of genitality, the separate space units are unified. When space distortions take place on the genital level they mean either genitals or persons as units. The final appreciation of space is dependent on our appreciation of personalities. Space is, therefore, decidedly a social phenomenon. Space is not an independent entity as Kant states, but is in functional relation to instincts, drives, emotions, and actions, with their tonic and phasic components.

## TIME PERCEPTION

Time experiences cannot be isolated from our aims in life nor from our relations to the future. We live in the present and are directed toward the future. We have aims and goals which must be understood. Spielrein (1923) has shown that the child lives chiefly in the present and immediate future. David Wechsler and I (Schilder and Wechsler, 1934) have confirmed this observation. In mental defectives, interest in the future remains limited, as confirmed by many observers (Rossel, 1925).

When one studies the ideas and attitudes of children concerning life and death and the general problems of human experience, and afterwards compares these to similar ideas in adults, one is astonished to see that the uneducated adult has thoughts neither more profuse nor more clear than those of the child. The experience of the future lies in the more or less present strivings of the individual. Again we see that we experience time as an expression of our strivings and that every change in the libidinal situation changes the time experience.

## PSYCHOPATHOLOGY OF SPACE AND TIME

One must be aware that we never deal with a mere change in space or time perception; we deal with the fundamental fact that human existence expresses itself in space and time and that it is impossible to separate the existential problems of humanity from space and time perception in this sense. A discussion of the analysis of a neurotic sixteen-year-old girl may be of further help.

Alma, sixteen years old, a well-developed girl of German descent, was the youngest of five living siblings. Two others had died, one with epilepsy and the other after an operation for cleft palate. She was an intelligent girl and successful in her high school studies. During her thirteenth year she had an attack in which she got dizzy and shook all over. In June, 1933, she had a second seizure, which was followed by several others. She was easily upset by noises, and cried a great deal. She stayed at home, never made friends, spent the day reading and helping around the house, and was often sad and depressed. On examination, she said: "I can't bear to be around people. I get frightened when anybody comes close to me. Noises drive me crazy. They make me jumpy. I am afraid of falling things. At times my eyes feel funny and I can't move them. I get strange feelings; my legs, eyes, and body get heavy. The people in school laugh at me. I want to die but I make myself stop from suicide because it would worry my mother. At times I feel as if I would like to choke people. At times I sink into black depths. I feel that I want to have pain. I like the injections I got in the other hospital. I like to be stuck. I stick my bobby pin into my hands and arms. It is not sharp enough. I try to choke my neck and see how it feels. My thoughts get mixed up and confused."

The patient submitted readily to pinpricks and other painful stimuli, and stated that she enjoyed them. She did not move at all, even when strong pain stimuli were applied, and did not even react to strong faradic currents. She never withdrew her hand and it was impossible to condition her to pain stimuli. In marked contrast, however, she reacted very strongly to sudden noises and became jumpy whenever an unexpected sound occurred. Pain never provoked any marked changes in the psycho-galvanic reflex, whereas other stimuli and noise provoked approximately normal reactions.

During the first examination she often clasped her hands as if under a great tension and wanting to suppress some impulse. Very often she moved the upper part of her body rhythmically to and fro. In the ward she usually stood alone, leaning against the wall. Outbursts occurred from time to time, in which she got pale, started to shake, cried, and did not talk. Such outbursts lasted up to one hour. However, she did not lose consciousness. In the beginning it was difficult to make her eat. The alarming symptoms disappeared in the first part of her stay at the hospital, and after discharge from the hospital she continued her school-work successfully. In the ward the patient always showed a helpful attitude.

The analysis showed the following: She was deeply attached to her mother. She did not want to leave her. The fear of being left by the mother went back to her earliest remembrance. She had slept with her mother since earliest childhood until recently, when at the height of her illness she did not feel any love toward her mother and was afraid of being touched by her.

She showed great affection for one of her sisters, who was eleven years older than she. For a long time she had been sick with rheumatic heart disease. This sister used to tell the patient fairy stories over and over again. One of her earliest remembrances is that of having "fairy parties" with her favorite sister. There were acorn cups, bread, sugar, and water. A still earlier remembrance is that of being held and sung to by someone and rocked to sleep in a rocking chair.

Her hatred against her father was outspoken. There were many family quarrels in which the father became rather violent. She never liked her parents because they shouted at each other. When she was six, her father beat her sister with a strap; she ran to the roof, screaming, while he followed. The patient was terribly frightened.

Her brothers and sisters also used to fight. Knives and forks were thrown. At six, she wanted to stab her father. When she was five, the father used to kill chickens on a chopping block. She saw or imagined a chicken wriggling after its head was chopped off. She was terribly frightened and ran away. She also used to hear violent quarrels of the family in the next apartment.

The father seemed to represent to her a picture of wild and dangerous aggressiveness of which she was afraid. He killed chickens, beat her sister, and made loud noises. She protested against his violent aggressiveness by aggressiveness of her own. There was a masochistic attitude, with very early roots, which drove her to surrender. About her third year, she had the following dream: Big mattresses were moving toward her on tiny straight pins, threatening to crush her. When she awoke, the door was closed; she called, but the door seemed to be "far away and deep down."

Around her seventh year, she dreamed of a spinning wheel coming to chop her up. She was also afraid of a straight line moving slowly and continually in front of her eyes. At five, she was feeding chickens grass with a pair of scissors and "cut off a piece of her thumb." The blood spouted. She ran to her mother, crying, "I fed the chickens a piece of my finger." At seven, she hurt her nose which bled profusely. A little while later she fell while skating and broke her wrist.

She always had animal pets. A white rabbit died, when she was four. Her dog was run over on a railway line. It was cut open and bloody, and was a horrible sight. At six, she saw a woman in a coffin in a dark room. The patient started to laugh. When she was six and a half, an older sister died. (The sister had epilepsy, but it is possible that her death was suicide.) The patient saw the coffin.

Her attitude toward pain seemed to be closely connected with her early experiences. Pain gave her pleasure; the pleasure of masochistic surrender to the father. Everybody who came near her threatened her as her father did. Loud noises reminded her of the aggressive father. Her obsessional impulse to choke people expressed her repressed sadistic attitude. There was an early remembrance of her father putting his hands on her when she was sleeping between her father and mother, and she shuddered away from it.

Her insensibility to pain was partially the attempt to escape heterosexuality. She was completely ignorant in sex matters when she came to the clinic for treatment. The sex information she was given there increased her repulsion against sex. Death wishes and death fantasies were other methods of escape for her. When she imagined herself dead, she thought about immobility and a cataleptic state with preserved consciousness. With her sister she escaped into a fairy story world. She liked fairy tales, and it is characteristic that she mentioned "Sleeping Beauty" as a fairy tale which appealed to her more than others. She hated any kind of apparel, even shoes. At two or three years, she pulled her hat off. "I never liked hats." She hated it when other girls talked about dresses.

She overcompensated her sadistic attitude by an increased attitude of helpfulness. "I can't bear even to see flies killed." There was a strong desire to be loved, which has not been satisfied. She was afraid that others might not believe her, and might laugh at her. She thought that she was extremely ugly (which in reality was not true, although she did have acne which slightly disfigured her face). As a child she was too fat, and was laughed at while she was in school. Sometimes she felt that her head was bumpy and her nose disfigured. In one of her later dreams, her attitude toward her own body came out very clearly. "People look at me loathingly and hate me for what I am thinking."

There was another group of phenomena which deserve interest. "Last night, before falling asleep, I saw a man tumbling and falling in front of my eyes." At another time before falling asleep, she saw a chair with shoes piled on it. "They were putting piles of bread right before my face. The door looked far away; farther away than it should have been." At another time, before falling asleep, she saw cups and saucers tumbling over her face. "I was in the linen room, where I was folding linen. The shelves and the linen felt piled too high. They kept rising higher. I could not see straight. I had funny feelings. The lines were out of proportion. They grew."

At another time, she complained that she was sitting in class and the teacher looked far away. "I wondered what would happen if she should die . . . I felt very big today, high up . . . I always wanted to be tall . . . My forehead feels low." On another occasion, before falling asleep, she saw an exceptionally tall man falling from a diving board. As he fell, his face grew larger and came nearer to her. Later in the course of the treatment she felt as if her legs and arms did not belong to her and were separated from her. On another occasion she felt too tall, as if she were towering above everybody.

In the beginning, she had the following dream: "I dreamt of water again. It was a flowing river. Somebody was in a motorboat. Somebody had a cold and had to take medicine. There was something about a pumpkin pie." Her associations were: She loved to watch the water. It was beautiful. From her early childhood she went to Coney Island with her mother and enjoyed it. She would like to travel to distant countries. She would like to travel alone. She likes to read sea stories and about submarines. She likes motorboats because they rush so much. She likes rapidly moving things, but is sometimes afraid of them. She felt funny the day before. "I felt I would go mad if I didn't do something. I wanted to smash the dishes. I felt so wild. I felt like going crazy again. A crazy person does odd things, may kill people or may have suicidal mania. I often wanted to be buried under water. There are queer shapes and creatures under water. I like penknives, daggers and swords. I like stories about knights." Her mother had said something about pumpkin pies the night before. The patient did not like to eat;

25

but in her childhood she was very fond of sweets and she often had sudden cravings for sweets. She once dreamed that she was sent home because she ate cakes and meat at night in her sleep, but she denied this vigorously. Since her earliest childhood, her mother had to make her eat.

Her attitude toward speed was related to her sadistic attitudes. She wanted to do things quickly. She liked to walk quickly. She wrote very rapidly and her handwriting was difficult to read. She liked to rush. She often dreamed of walking fast, and of speeding trains. The fast movement also took her away from the present. In one dream she went up in a dirigible and in some way got out of this world. The slow-moving line in her childhood dream was extremely distasteful to her. In one dream she was in a fast-moving elevator that changed into a very fast train.

She often wanted to jump out of a window, and she felt herself doing so. When she saw someone on a roof, she felt afraid that he might fall off. She also often dreamed of wide expanses. In one dream she wandered with her brother to a huge garden. "I dreamed of babies. They played on a vast expanse of sand. Somebody poured out toys which were disproportionately large." Once while she was reading, the print appeared very small, no matter how near her eyes she brought it. One day she felt queer, as if she herself and the house were on stilts and crooked and leaning to one side.

In another characteristic dream, she was in school in the English class. She felt the beginning of a nervous attack. She was breathing fast and her heart palpitated. She waited in the corridor, leaning against the wall. Teachers and nurses passed her. The English teacher returned with a nurse, and had her taken home and put to bed. She knew that someone was outside looking through the keyhole and saying, "She will go to sleep soon." She felt rather dizzy and weak. They entered and did not find her asleep, so they grabbed her and pushed her down. The doctor said: "Do it quickly before the blood freezes in the brain." She struggled and lashed out with her legs, but her legs seemed to be quite loose and had a shorter span than usual. The doctor sprayed air or liquid into her face and she lost consciousness. The scene changed, she was on the street with someone who was leading her. She was much shorter and her head was hollowed out—just a bare, empty shell. The person leading her had his hand in the hollow of hers and was urging her along. "I don't know exactly whether it was I or another person, for I seemed to see the figure and yet be it." She felt happy, since she had no real head and could no longer think or worry. It seemed to her that an experiment was done on her in the room and made her this way. Then they passed by a railing where a short, ugly deformed girl was standing with a few other people. She asked for milk. This seemed to be the second stage of the experiment. Soon there passed a fairly tall girl whose head was in the shape of an octagonal plate glass. She seemed to be quite pretty. She was carrying what seemed to be a long, narrow bundle. A sign of recognition passed between them, that this was the first stage, and the experiment was progressing satisfactorily. The girl seemed to be her favorite sister. They said about her: "Every day, when passing, she can see Bobby (her sister's little son)."

The patient also had changes in the perception of time. Often, occurrences which had just taken place seemed to her to belong far back in the past. "I remember things—they are further back—it seems as if it had happened in a dream; even things which happened yesterday seem to be further back."

The important phenomenon of pleasure derived from painful stimuli is directly related to the scenes of violence between her parents, which she witnessed as a child. There were quarrels in which the father beat the mother. The patient wanted to be hurt by the hated father. She wanted to stab him. She felt the pleasure of painful stimuli for the first time when she was stuck by the needle when the physician took her Wassermann test.

She succumbed to the sadistic love object. This attitude was fully developed at the age of seven. At that time she dreamed that a spinning wheel came close to her in order to chop her up. This was an anxiety dream. There were other anxiety dreams. A mattress was coming on rolling pins to smother her. This nightmare again refers to her violent father.

Her hatred was not only provoked by the violence of her father. She slept with her mother and was deeply attached to her and to her older sister who was a substitute for the mother. At the height of her illness she was not able to maintain this homosexual relation. At that time, every relation to others provoked deep inner resistance, and she was afraid of being near anybody, and was obsessed by the desire to strangle people who were near her. Defending herself against masochistic subjection, she became sadistic. Disappointed in homosexual and heterosexual relations, she regressed to a sadistic attitude for which she tried to compensate by a particular kindness and readiness to help. The father chopping off the heads of chickens represented a castration threat. Her memory of cutting a part of a finger away with a pair of scissors points again to the castration fear and castration wishes. One may interpret her complaint that the chicken devoured a part of her finger as the fear that her penis may be bitten off and devoured. She also has very strong oral tendencies which she denied in the beginning of her illness. She tried to escape from these conflicts into the peace of death, which for her meant a cataleptic state. She would then have again been in a passive masochistic position, which she could enjoy without remorse.

Her moral problems are reflected in her attitudes toward space and time. When she awoke from her first anxiety dream, the door seemed to be "far away and deep down." After being crushed by her violent father, she reversed the situation. She was not below any more, but higher and farther away from the door through which a helping human could come in. At the height of her illness, other human beings were too close to her. Because of all these moral conflicts, space lost its stability. Things were falling from a cupboard. Laundry was piled too high and was in danger of falling over. Persons sometimes seemed to be too far away. Space widened to vast expansions. She and the house in which she lived appeared to her as if on stilts, crooked and leaning to one side. Her libidinal problems thus found an expression in the changing relations of space. Space relations are primarily determined by relations to other human beings. Space is for her an interhuman phenomenon; it reflects her relation to her mother and father; it expresses the various phases of her aggressiveness, and her struggle for a deeper relation to homosexual and heterosexual love objects. When she experiences the vastness of space as such, this is a secondary phenomenon.

It is difficult to separate problems of space from problems of time. The patient liked speed and motion. In her dreams there were fast-running trains and elevators. Momentum, which in physics increases the impact and the danger, expressed her aggressive and sadistic tendencies. Fighting against her aggressiveness and doubting every one of her actions, her life was not full of the present, and when the present had passed it seemed to recede; it was as if it had happened long ago. She tried, indeed, to go out of the everyday world into the timeless world of fairy stories in which beauty substitutes for aggressiveness.

Aggressiveness destroys and distorts the image of the body. Our patient experienced lengthening and shortening of her body, and distortions of her head. There exists an inner relation between outer space and the space of one's own body. When the dimensions of the outer space are changed, there is also a change in the dimensions of the body image.

The disruption and annihilation of space is similar in obsession neuroses and depression, except that neurotic disturbances are more easily shown to depend on attitudes toward specific love objects.

Our patient says: "When I felt so horrible today, the girls in school were separated from each other." One of her dreams goes as follows: "Sister was at home. Two firemen came in, tall as the ceiling and thin, in order to help her. She looked out of the window; the railroad stretched far. There was a music band and the sound retreated. They were playing a military march." One day she felt very small and things were remote. She felt anxiety; she wanted to have a Teddy-bear in bed so that she could touch something which was solid and real. In the auditorium at school, the girls looked small and the teacher far away. On a similar occasion she wondered what would happen if the teacher should die. "At six or seven, I was always afraid that Mother would leave me alone. I never wanted to leave her."

## FORM AS A PRINCIPLE IN PLAY[10]

When one watches children at play, one soon observes that there are certain principles that appear again and again. In a previous study by Bender (1932), it has been pointed out that motility is a factor in determining the form of children's drawings and games. Children often take toys, such as carts, trains, etc., and move them on the ground with outstretched arm in a curve or in a half-circle, the center of which is the shoulder joint. The plane on which the play takes place is seemingly one factor and the peculiarities of the motor apparatus are another factor. Klüver (1933) has observed drawings in monkeys which are determined by similar principles. In hopscotch, the figure in which the play takes place is determined by the range of jumping on one leg; the curved form is drawn with outstretched arms with the body as a pivot. Rotation around a longitudinal axis is one of the basic forms of movement. Köhler (1931) describes whirling as a form of play in apes. The principle of rotation is also demonstrated in the movements of the circular joints, such as the shoulder and hip, and, to some degree, also in the hand. In parietal lobe lesions with spontaneous turning around the longitudinal axis, Hoff and Schilder (1927) have also observed a tendency for rotation in movements in the circular joints.[11]

[10] From Bender and Schilder (1936).

[11] Subsequent to the writing of this paper, we developed the concept that whirling on the longitudinal axis was the characteristic motility of the schizophrenic child (already suggested by Schilder) and was, in part, the basis for the body image, ego boundary, and many other psychological problems (see Bender, 1947). Teicher (1941), working with Schilder, studied the motility of two hundred children, four to thirteen years of age, in order to determine the normal and atypical patterns of these postural responses.

Specific motor tendencies, therefore, find an expression in the play of children. Motility adapts itself to the plane on which the play takes place. The formation of foreground and background is basic for the play of children. When a child gets a number of lead soldiers or other toys for play, the form of his play is partially determined by the form of the field in which the play takes place. For example, three-and-a-half-year-old Joey puts soldiers near the border of the table and also on the bench. He also transfers them to the border of the wash basin. He puts a horse in the middle of a small desk calendar. He presses the head of the horse against the cork of a closed ink bottle as if trying to push it in and says, "I push him in this." He even attempts to put the soldiers parallel to the wall and is disappointed when they do not stay in this position. The geometrical and physical qualities of a given field are determining factors in the play of children. Joey's attempt to put the horse in the ink bottle shows that the form of objects is another determining factor. It becomes a symbol into which one can push something else. We will consider again the more primitive geometrical forms. Joey likes clusters of three men around a horse. He arranges soldiers in a row. He puts a soldier in each of three corners of the wash basin. He arranges soldiers and tongue depressors in forms of incomplete symmetry. The following primitive forms emerge: (1) a cluster; (2) a row; (3) an irregular star.

Observation of this child attempting to place his toys against the wall makes it clear that experiments with gravitational qualities are factors which have to be considered in the play of children. This child does not take gravity into consideration at first. In the play of Nora (four years old) and Rita (three years old), pushing objects over or allowing them to fall was a great source of pleasure. These are instances of active experimentation with gravity.

There is no question that the play of these children also has another meaning. Joey is continually commanding the toys which he puts in specific places. In the play of the two little girls, their delight in power and aggressiveness was obvious. The formal elements are, of course, not isolated parts in psychic life but are a part of the biological orientation of children. Knocking toys down satisfies the aggressive impulses of the children, but it also helps them to acquire a better working concept of the problems of physics connected with gravitation. To be upright or to lie down is partially a moral problem (aggression and submission), but it is also a problem in physics and a problem of the orientation of the organism to gravity and the physical world. Orientation means, for us, not only perception and knowledge, but also the motor side of the adaptation of the individual.

Larry (four years old) and Russell (five years old) showed a great interest in placing dolls, that had fallen down, into an upright position. Whenever the examiner pushed a doll down, Russell would stand it up again. Immediately after this play, Larry noticed a man cleaning the windows and said, "He will fall down."

In the child's later development, there is a tendency for clusters to develop into more symmetrical forms. The matching of objects plays a great part. Objects which are similar in shape and color are put into groups. For instance, Vivian's (nine years old) play with china toys consisted entirely in arranging them in different symmetrical forms on the table and moving them from one form to the next, sometimes transporting them by means of tiny carts.

We have mentioned the three-and-a-half-year-old boy who showed an interest in pushing a toy horse into an ink bottle. In older children, this tendency to put something into something else is still more obvious. The children put lead soldiers into carts, either lying or standing, and they try to pile in as many soldiers as possible, sometimes pushing the soldiers in rather roughly. It is a great satisfaction for them to have as many in the car as possible. If there are bigger and smaller cars, the smaller cars are put into the larger cars as well. Five-year-old Emmanuel, for instance, put one car into the other and said he would put them into the garage. The same principle prevails in even older children, as can be seen from the protocol of Charles, an eleven-year-old boy of average intelligence.

"They had a war. The Americans and the Indians. I am on the side of the Americans because that is my nationality." He is asked: What is the matter with the Indians? "They can't fight so good. I am only playing with them. Here is the battlefield." He puts all the soldiers in carts and puts them in another position. "Bang-Bang. That guy is dead." The Americans kill four Indians. One Indian knocks down an American. "They are having a war because they don't like Indians." He puts the small racer in the big truck. "That is the place where you carry things,

31

because they can't carry them in their hands; they are too big." He lines all the vehicles up and lines the soldiers up along the edge of the table. "I am going to line some over here too." In the course of later play, he places vehicles in a series, whereas they were parallel before. He likes to give orders to his lead soldiers. He always arranges the soldiers in groups.

This protocol shows an elaboration of the same form principle which we found in the younger children. The elaboration partially consists in adding meaning to the formal situation. This tendency is already present in the younger children. They put a soldier, for instance, in a car "because he is dead" or "tired" or "he has gone home." One gets the impression that the formal principle of putting something in something is more basic and is merely exemplified in the meaning added.

Children are never satisfied with any form which is reached. Form is merely a transition to a chaos, that is putting the toys in an unorganized heap. But new organization is immediately sought again. In older children, the groups have a more definite meaning; Indians, soldiers, pirates, etc. In younger children, however, grouping as such is the main purpose. Although the same principles return again into every new grouping, the new grouping is never completely identical with the previous one. Whereas, in the protocol of the three-and-a-half-year-old boy, tongue depressors and soldiers are brought into a symmetrical form without further comment, older children usually give some definite meaning to their groupings. It is as if they would have adapted the formal principles better to the total situation and its meaning. In this respect, it is particularly interesting to follow the development of a situation which we have called the automobile test. A toy man is put between three toy cars which are placed so that the front ends are all pointing toward the man. The younger children push the man and cars about without much regard for the inner quality and meaning of the objects. Older children start to move the car or, at any rate, to imagine a movement which corresponds to the structure and position of the car. In such an experiment, where James (seven years old) and Dorothy (nine years old) are present, the girl starts running the car and the boy runs the man down with the car and puts him into another car. He is asked, "What did you do?" "I

knocked him down, he was run over, the guy was carrying him."
"Why did you stand him up again?" "He will be run over again,"
said Dorothy. "The car will run over him and he will be dead."
In the midst of a discussion about death, Dorothy kisses the smaller
car and says, "Because it is little." She puts it in another car and
says, "I don't want it to get knocked over." The car, with its momentum, needs to be played with according to its structure. It carries
with it an immediate pattern for aggressiveness, but only older
children are able to grasp this situation. The younger ones express
aggression by merely knocking over. Of course, a complicated object
like a car does not merely carry the meaning of aggression, but it is
also, as mentioned before, a vessel and a container. The definite
meaning of an object depends, of course, on the total situation.

The following protocol exemplifies what we have said:

Five-year-old Emmanuel is shown a toy cowboy between two toy cars.
He says, "It bumps him. He better watch out—because—he is dead." He
knocks down the car. "Fall down car." Several other cars are now put at
his disposal and he piles up the cars. "I am making something. Put this
one on top because it fell down. Goes slow because it is broke." He lines
up the little cars against the wall. "It will crack." Knocks a big car against
a little one. "Now it cracks." Piles them up again. "Now I make a car."
He puts a little car in a big one. "It is broke . . . . I tell you so many times.
It broke itself I say. All the cars broke. Put it in the garage and get it
fixed. I bring it back." Gets men and puts them in the larger car. "They
are garage men to fix the car." The next day he gets a set of lead soldiers
with carts and wooden toys representing the various members of a circus.
He puts all the toys in the largest cart including smaller carts. He looks
all over the floor for more toys. "This is the march." He lines all the circus toys on one side and the lead soldiers on the other side and knocks
over the circus toys and then the lead toys. "They knock down, they go
to sleep. I fix them all over." He puts all the lead toys and the circus toys
in the cart again. He puts small autos, soldiers, elephants, etc., all in the
larger cart. Then he knocks them all out again. "They are dead, they got
run over."

In a little older age group, consideration for the actual meaning
of the toys is greater. Amad is nine years old and Leon is seven years
old. Following are some illustrative protocols of their play:

33

LEON: (with two cars and man) "The car is going to run the good guy over. He will die."

AMAD: "He don't die. He will get hurt and they bring him to the hospital and he will get better and when he sees that truck again he gets that man and kills him."

LEON: "The man is going to break the car up and burn the man in the car so it won't run over him no more."

ADULT: "How can he if he is dead?"

LEON: "The car got electric and burns him up. The car could fall. The feet must go on the electric and then the car could fall. This car was coming and he is strong, and he went back that way; then that car comes and he doesn't see it and he gets hurt and they bring him to the hospital. He gets better, sees the truck, burns it up, puts it on fire, and brings it in the river, makes the motor go."

AMAD: "He puts dynamite under it, then ran away."

LEON: "The car is coming and the man is going across and the car got the man run over, and the man got hurt. The car went right on the man's foot and the man got a broken foot. They bring him to the hospital. They gave him a stick and a foot to walk. When he sees the car he is going to take the wheels off and the motor off and put it on his car, and break that car and throw it in the river."

Irregular arrangement of several figures with small cars.

LEON: (immediately) "This is a good guy—this is a bad guy—this guy is going to kill this guy with a knife, so that he comes with all the guns and he is going to shoot that guy," etc.

The play becomes increasingly violent and many more of the lead soldiers are considered dead and piled into the car.

The purely formal elements are decidedly subordinated to and integrated with the mental content. Only when the play progresses do the more primitive form elements come more and more into the foreground. The play satisfies those instinctual tendencies of the children which correspond to the form of the play. In the preceding instances, the aggressiveness of the children is able to express itself in the play.

It is characteristic for children never to be satisfied with anything less than all of the available playthings. They want to get everything that is to be had, otherwise they feel restless and dissatisfied. The child is only temporarily satisfied when he has gotten everything that is in the room. They often ask where the toys came from and whether one could not buy all the toys in the store. The following protocol is very characteristic. Russell (five years old) is an aggressive, overactive child of inferior intelligence (IQ 71) and Larry (four years old) is usually shy and quiet on the wards, but has a history of temper tantrums at home.

The examiner knocks a doll over.

LARRY: "Take another one."

RUSSELL: "Me take another one."

LARRY: "Look at the two here."

RUSSELL: "Me throw it down. Stand it up. One doll, two dolls. Stand up one doll."

When the dolls fall down very easily, the chief interest of the children is to get them into an upright position. Whenever the examiner pushes the doll down, Russell stands it up again. Takes it into his hand. Russell is rather petulant. Larry takes the dolls in his hand in a protective way. He picks up the lead soldiers and looks at them very carefully. Russell wants everything immediately. He insists on it.

RUSSELL: "Give me all the mans."

When the toys are taken out of the drawer, he does not want to play with the toys which are given him but tries to take other toys out of the examiner's pocket. Larry does not show any constructive effort in play. He merely takes everything, in a rather protective manner, to himself and only lets a car run slowly over the desk. He does not let the cars collide.

Russell has seemingly forgotten that he wanted dolls from the examiner's pocket, but he is easily reminded of it. Puts his hand in the examiner's pocket and says, "No more, only matches." He appears to be disappointed.

Larry asks for the horse. "Let's see the horse." Russell immediately loses interest in what he has. Russell has a definite reaction pattern in that he wants everything and once he has it he is not interested in it any more.

RUSSELL: "The bad boy won't give me the cars."

Russell is somewhat dominated by the idea that something is withheld from him. In order to get the cars, he takes two pieces of paper and gives them to Larry. When Larry finally gives him the things, he has no interest in what he has asked for. Russell offers Larry the broken legs of a doll. Interest in getting something he shouldn't get makes any active play for him completely impossible.

It is interesting to notice that he wants to get the last thing that the other boy has. When something is given to Larry, Russell immediately becomes excited. Finally, he again gives Larry the broken legs of the doll, with a great gesture of generosity.

Larry could be induced to give the other boy everything.

In play, Larry seems to put the lead soldiers together without putting them in any action. He rather carefully avoids pushing any one of the figures down. He does not protest when one toy after another is taken away. He takes two trucks and, when given a doll which is named Doris (his sister's name), he makes a noise with his mouth, plays with the later car and tries to put the doll into the car.

The child is a little shy and does not even dare to take off the hat of the doll. When the examiner pushes the doll down, he heaps the two cars upon her abdomen and her face and he continues to play, covering the doll with the cars. Finally, he brings the car near the doll which is now standing, but he does not push her down. He brings it as near as he can. The examiner pushes the doll down with the car and he repeats it. He lets the doll fall down rather carefully. When he plays, he is very careful not to come too near the doll. He frequently covers the doll up with the cars.

He sees a man cleaning windows and says, "He will fall down." This is a child who restricts himself, in his movements, to small and rhythmic expressions. He is not very active in play. After he left the room, he had a severe temper tantrum and had to be placed in his room by the nurse. Later he became quiet and, on being sought out, it was found that he had defecated in the room and smeared the feces over himself and over the room.

One sees that emotional problems and formal problems cannot be completely separated. The experimentation of the child with form and configuration is an expression of his tendencies to come to a better handling of objects by action. By trial and error, he develops insight into the structure of objects. To the structure of the object belong the general spatial qualities, the laws of gravitation, push, and momentum. The child has to learn about lines, series, and groups. Furthermore, the child learns about the general form when something can be put into something else. It is remarkable that the same gestalt rules have been worked out concerning the general gestalt principles in visual motor patterns. These problems lead to emotional problems, problems of destruction, preservation, and protection. We are of the opinion that emotional problems and the so-called form problems are identical in their core. One could, for instance, consider the problems of impact and putting one thing into another as specifically sexual problems (as, for instance, Klein has done, who sees in every collision in the play of children a symbolic hint of parental intercourse). If one merely puts the emphasis on a sexual interpretation, one neglects biological connections which are at least as important as the sexual. One could, with some right, consider the interest of the child concerning parental intercourse as an application of his general interest in impact and putting one thing inside the other. In the children of our group in which the play method of approach could be used (under ten years) there was no difference between boys and girls. The individual fate of the single child very often determines the formal principles specifically used. In one of our children, the motive of attacking from behind was outstanding. In some children, the impact problem plays a greater part and, in others, the tendency to put things into other things is predominant. In other words, there is a general trend of psychophysiological organization which is not rigid, but is, more or less, a mode of procedure adaptable to the biological situation. Form principles reflect merely the general plan of psychophysiological organization.

The form of the organism and its motor possibilities determine the play of children. Rotation of the total body around its longitudinal axis and circular movements of outstretched limbs are of special importance. Motility adapts itself to the plane on which the play takes place. Play starts with the formation of foreground and background. The child undertakes continuous experimentation concerning the geometrical qualities of lines, angles, and clusters. In three-dimensional games, the child is particularly interested in whether something can be put into something else. Further experimentation concerns gravitation, push, pull, and momentum. The experimentation with space and mass (geometry and physics) is based on the instinctive drives of children and, therefore, is dependent on their individual emotional problems. The definite form of the play is adaptable to the biological situation. Form principles merely reflect the general plan of psychophysiological organization.

37

## SUMMARY

Every tonic and phasic activity, in any part of the body, may gain importance from the formation of perception. Disintegration of the imagination suggests that optic imagination develops from indistinct vortical movement with vague color impressions, to loops, ellipses, and circles, and finally, to distinct crossings, angles, and definite shapes of all varieties.

This preliminary impression is supported by Bender's studies of visual motor patterns. These visual motor patterns develop in stages that can be observed by following the development of the drawings of children in the first few years of life. Observation of these stages proves the development which has been suggested by the observations quoted previously.

Tachistoscopic experiments demonstrate that the stages of the ontogenetic development of the visual motor pattern of the child are recapitulated in the individual development of every sensation, imagination, and perception.[12]

Development from the primitive stages of experience to complete experience is connected with the process of active reality testing, which participates in the creation of gestalten. The testing process is a motor process; tonic and phasic motility lead to repeated contacts with the outer world. In connection with this process, a better differentiation takes place between what belongs to one's own body and what belongs to the outer world. I do not think that sensations are projected into the outer world and so become perceptions. The division between the outside world and the body is always present. The decision as to what belongs to the body and what belongs to the world is based on testing and constructive efforts. The primitive object is, at first, variable in its orientation in space. The early investigations of W. Stern (1924) and the newer work of Bender (1938) show that children are insensitive to changes in the orientation of objects, especially in regard to right and left, and below and above. In copying, they very often change direction without being aware of it. In the imaginations of adults, similar transpositions in space may be observed. Definite forms, other than loops, are finally

[12] See Ross and Schilder (1934). This report on tachistoscopic experiments includes two protocols on children.

conceived, in their correct spatial relations. Primitive form principles are often exaggerated (Bender). Primitive gestalten develop into more complicated ones. A whole may be created by piecemeal gathering of single pieces, as observed by Klüver (1934) and myself in eidetic images, by Freud in dreams (1900), and by Poetzl (1917, 1928) in experimental dream studies and in optic agnosias. I think that collecting and adding pieces, putting pieces together as in a jigsaw puzzle, plays an important part in the psychology of the senses. A continuous testing, changing, and rechanging process occurs until the final shape is reached. The same process can cut the whole into pieces, without any regard for form and configurations which may mature from configuration. Optic experience, then, has two principles: piecemeal construction and destruction, and organization in definite configurations which may mature from primitive to higher stages of development.

We do not live only in an optic world. We are directed toward a world which appeals to all the senses. When we see an object, we anticipate that it can be grasped, smelled, and tasted. Every object has an appeal to all the senses. This principle expresses itself in the phenomena of synesthesia. Primitive experiences are very often rhythmic; they repeat the same object, and instead of one object, several pictures may appear. We may say primitive experiences have a tendency to multiplicity. In primitive experiences, the size of objects is variable; the localization of the experience is uncertain. Changes often occur in a rhythmic way. Variability—in size, number, direction, space, distance, and rhythmicity—is probably the most important characteristic of experiences in the primitive visual field. These primitive experiences remain in the background of fully developed experiences. Primitive shapes in motion can be prematurely stabilized. Hallucinations show many characteristics which we find in primitive experiences. Investigations of this type establish a basis for a better understanding of hallucinations.

Similar principles, with characteristic changes, are valid for other senses. Sound travels in space. It has a tendency to repeat itself, which comes out clearly in hallucinations. We turn toward the sound and we begin to repeat the sound, if it is language. Jacobson (1932) has shown that action currents are present when we imagine verbally. Construction of the object, with continual interchange, until a comparative stabilization (gestalt) is reached, seems to be the basic principle for the organization of the senses. It seems that the vestibular apparatus is also necessary for the maintenance of this construction. This is understandable, since the vestibular apparatus has such a close relation to the tonic apparatuses.

In smell and taste, another motility becomes paramount. In smell, the "object" smell must be taken in, either through the process of breathing or through sniffing. The turning of the head in the direction from which the smell comes plays a less important part. It is a "taking in" from the outer world, in order to sample. The tonic principles of the optic and acoustic spheres are replaced by the rhythmic principles of breathing and sniffing.

The movements of the mouth, which makes tasting possible, are of a much more complex nature. Sucking occurs when the nipple is put in the mouth of the newborn. However, there are continual movements of the mouth as if the infant were trying to get an object. Later on, the mouth movements, combined with movements of the head, follow the object. After a source of nourishment has touched the mouth, the mouth closes tightly and the sucking starts, which accounts for the possibility of taste. In adults, movements of the tongue bring the object of taste, which has to be chewed by the action of the jaws, to receptive surfaces. It is remarkable that even in the imagination of taste, the movement of the jaw and tongue occur, and swallowing is initiated. Secretion of saliva occurs even in the course of imagination, and we have every reason to believe that secretory changes are occurring along the whole gastrointestinal tract. In other words, in the whole field of taste, phasic motility is necessary in order for perception to occur, and a reaction occurs in the motility and secretion of the gastrointestinal tract. Secretion and peristalsis are primitive responses to situations. Although they are not voluntary or conscious, they serve the whole attitude of the individual.

It is essential to study basic motor attitudes of the individual in connection with perception. We can turn either toward an object or away from it. We have reason to believe that turning toward an object is more primitive than turning away from it. An object appeals to all senses at once. It is initially perceived as in motion or movable. Only in late development is it perceived at rest. Orientation toward the object and away from the object is represented in voluntary action. Tonic reactions, which are not as fully conscious and voluntary as the majority of phasic actions, are necessarily always present. Every action is based on a background of posture in which the individual is oriented to the outside world. As Koffka expresses it, posture is in direct relation to the spatial framework. A posture must necessarily be a reaction to the force of gravitation. Action can only be understood as emerging from the continuous tonic adaptation to one's environment or pulls. When an individual turns toward an object he may either want to touch it or incorporate it. Incorporation has been considered as the final aim. However, every step is, in itself, a final end, even if it does not lead to touch or incorporation. We do not want a world which can be completely subdued and incorporated. We expect the object to offer resistance to the final incorporation. We need a world we can cling to and lean upon—a world which offers us protection and security. Grasping takes the object partially into the body, a process which is completed when the object is taken into the mouth. But, primarily, grasping does not serve to incorporate an object into the mouth; rather it serves as a help in the fight against gravitation.

The whole path—from visual perception, or hearing, or smelling an object, through tonic and phasic action to final solutions—is, from the beginning, connected with the reactions of secretions, the smooth muscle of the gastrointestinal tract, and the whole vasovegetative system. The entire system gets is final shape by the continuous interaction between the tendencies toward and away from objects.

The construction of an object is essential in itself, and not merely because the object might sooner or later be of immediate use. We need and want an independent world. Even the relation of grasping and bringing to the mouth is not a primary one. The child primarily uses grasp in order to get the support of an independent object.

# II

# The Body Image

According to Preyer's observations (1882) the child has, in the beginning, the same attitude toward the parts of his body as he has toward strange objects. The child watches his arms and legs in motion as he would watch the flame of a candle. He looks at his grasping hand as attentively as at any foreign object. He observes himself and touches himself in the bath, especially the feet (39th week). He bites his finger, arms, and toes so that he screams with pain (409th day). He bangs his own head with violence (41st week). He presses one of his hands, with the other, firmly on a table, like a toy. This interest in observing one's self diminishes in the second year. It is as if the child now knows his body and has no further interest in it. Preyer (1882) and Bernfeld (1925) conclude that a child has practically no knowledge of his body at first and has to distinguish it from other objects by kinesthetic, motor, and visceral data. Bernfeld correctly says that it is a question of coordination of optic, tactile, and other experiences with the motor body ego. Preyer, and Dix (1911-1923) have emphasized the importance of the pain experience in this development. But, on the other hand, Dix reports that even in the 10th month the child's actions against his own body do not provoke the pain reaction one would expect. Thus, a ten-month-old child bangs his head against the wall as if it were a foreign object; with others, in the earliest months, a bleeding wound provokes no pain reaction. It seems that pain reactions toward the

---

[1] From Schilder (1935).

42

internal organs are stronger at this age. Preyer and Bernfeld also emphasize the importance of internal organs for the creation of the body image. It seems that some parts of the body can be dissociated from the body, even late in development. Bernfeld correctly says that the body ego is present from the beginning, because some organs obey the needs of the body from the beginning.

A nucleus of the body image is present in the oral zone from the beginning; head, arms, hands, trunk, legs, and feet, grow in single relays to this nucleus. Bernfeld comes to the conclusion that there is a primary development starting with the oral zone, and that a secondary refinement differentiates the body image from the outside world. This process can act in two directions: if the child finds the body ego too big, the mother has to be eliminated; in other cases it is too small and the toes have to be added. According to Bernfeld, compliance of the body or disorder in the organ functions are the main factors in this development. Bernfeld's formulations are based on analytic material and are very similar to my views. It is true that actual empirical material about the child is very limited; Bernfeld's summary is based on his study of adults.

In any case, the problem of the development of the body image arises. We do not know in detail how this development takes place. We have reason to believe that there is an inner development, a maturation in all phases of psychic life, and that there are inner factors, which are given in the organisms and are comparatively independent of experiences, which determine this development. But we see that the process of maturation always gets its final shape through individual experiences, and we should not neglect this influence of individual experience.

The general principle may be explained by Gesell's experiment (1929). In a pair of identical twins, Twin T., beginning at 46 weeks, was trained twenty minutes daily, for six weeks, in stair climbing. Twin C. was not. At 48 weeks, T. scaled the stairs for the first time without assistance. At 52 weeks, he was an expert, while C. could not climb, even with assistance. But at 53 weeks, C., without training or assistance, climbed the stairs. Similar experiments have been made by Breed and Shepard (1913) concerning the pecking of young chicks. It is obvious that even in functions in which maturation of the central nervous system is undoubtedly of great importance, training plays a part, at least in some phases of development. At any rate, T. was superior to C. between the 48th and 52nd weeks. We see that even the way that maturation develops is dependent upon the factors of experience, but we do not know the later development of the twins trained in this way. According to the experience of psychoanalysis, we have to at least reckon with the possibility that their psychic attitude in walking and climbing stairs will be different throughout their whole life.

Concerning the image of the body, we have to suppose that there is a factor of maturation which is responsible for the primary outlines of the postural model of the body. But the way in which these outlines develop, the tempo of development, will be largely dependent upon experience and activity, and we may suppose that the finer trends of the body image will be still more dependent upon life experiences, training, and emotional attitudes. There is no reason why one should join either of the extremist groups: those who believe experience, learning, and conditioning are in the foreground (Watson, 1930) or those who believe experience means little or nothing (Köhler, 1929; Koffka, 1928; Wertheimer, 1923; and Wheeler, 1929). Freud himself has always emphasized that, besides the factor of anatomy and structuralized function, there is the factor of experience and attitude. There will be functions which are determined merely by anatomy and physiology, but even in those, the psychic influence and the influence of experience will, according to our best observations, play some part. In other experiences, especially those concerning the libidinal structure of the postural model, experience will play an outstanding part; but, even so, experience will be connected with anatomy and physiology. I have often emphasized that the central factor of the organism and the personality very often determines which part of the anatomy will be used.

One has to suppose that the body image not only has ontogenetic development but that there is also phylogenetic development. It will, of course, be difficult to determine this phylogenetic development.

Preyer and Bernfeld emphasize the important part that pain plays in the development of the body image. We know very little about pain sensation in animals. Hempelmann (1926) has collected material on this subject. The pain reactions of the lower vertebrates are rather limited. This is so even with birds. Human beings reach the highest level of pain sensitivity. Can we consider pain sensitivity to be one of the important factors in the building up of the body image? Von Uexkuell (1927) considers pain as a biological necessity. It is a sign of one's own body and serves to prevent self-mutilation. This is especially necessary in carnivorous animals. Rats devour their own legs when the sensory nerves are cut. It seems, at any rate, that pain is one of the important factors in the organization of the otherwise labile structure of the body image.

We are still more uncertain about invertebrates. We can never know whether the violent defense reactions of earthworms are really an expression of strong irritation of the nervous system. When an earthworm is cut in two, the part of the body which does not contain the higher centers makes more violent movements. In the arthropods, especially insects, lesions and mutilations, which according to our experience would be apt to provoke pain, do not have any particular external effect. If the antennae and the whole abdomen of an ant are cut off, it may quietly continue sucking honey. A caterpillar, the rear end of which is injured, may gnaw itself when the anterior end is turned toward the wound. A cross spider devours its legs when they are broken off. A male spider, gnawed at by the female during copulation, may continue the act. According to von Uexkuell, a dragon fly starts to eat up its own body when its rear end is pushed between its jaws.

We are justified in believing that we are dealing, in all these instances, with an incomplete organization of the postural model of the body, and we may come to the general conclusion that the psychological integration of the postural model of the body is characteristic of the higher levels of phylogenetic development. It is remarkable that in the instance of the rat, the cutting of the sensory nerve disintegrates the postural model of the body, so that actions occur which, in their structure, are similar to the actions of the invertebrates. Apparently, the rat which devours its own legs has a body image in which the optic part plays a less important role. One is also reminded of the human cases of nonperception of one side of the body because of lesions of the tactile sphere, in which the optic impression is not sufficient to preserve the unity of the body image. Experiences of this kind are warnings against the over-evaluation of optic factors in the building of the postural model of the body.

It is necessary to mention here another remarkable phenomenon, the so-called autotomy. This defense reaction is to be found not only in some invertebrates but also in lizards. By a special reflex, which has its center in the lumbar region of the spinal cord, the lizard is able to throw off its tail when caught by it. The vertebra breaks at the preformed weak point in its middle. Decapitated lizards also show this reflex.

It is clear that we also have a mechanism which changes the body image at a very deep organic level. It is a diminution of the body image which goes into the body as such. But we see, on the other hand, that there may be organic differences in the coherence of the structure of the body so that a psychological and organic dissociation of parts of the body may become simpler. The mechanism of expansion and contraction has, therefore, a deep organic level, but we find the same mechanism again, in the psychological structure, as emphasized before.

Ferenczi (1919) regards autotomy as a tendency to throw away an overloaded organ. He considers it a basic reaction of life and compares it with the withdrawing of psychic energy from an unpleasurable experience. He considers ejaculation from this point of view. He finds a similar tendency to push out the genitals, which are loaded with displeasure. He mentions worms which are likely to push out their whole intestines. Others burst, as a whole, into single parts. Although I doubt the validity of Ferenczi's explanation in detail, I do consider that the general principle of trying to find analogies to psychological processes in the organization of animals is absolutely justified.

When dealing with genetic psychology, we should not forget that objects in primitive thought and objects in fully developed thought are not the same thing. Just as the body is a construction which takes place according to the total situation, objects have their meaning only in the specific set of circumstances. We are too much inclined to believe that the circumstances in our thought are the only ones that matter. In my *Medical Psychology* (1924), I mentioned Volkelt's (1914) experiments on spiders. When a fly is put directly into the mouth of a spider, it is not accepted. It is only accepted when it flies into the web and the spider has the opportunity to seize the fly actively. The spider's object is not actually the fly, but the concussion of the fly with the web and its subsequent activity, leading to the fly and the connected series of impressions. Similar instances can be found all over the field of animal behavior. The following well-known instance, taken from Köhler, belongs to the same category. Regarding cleanliness, Köhler (1931) tells us he has observed only one chimpanzee in captivity that was not coprophagous (feces-eating). Yet, whenever an animal stepped into feces and lost its footing, it would hobble away until an opportunity was found to clean the foot, just as a human being would in a similar predicament. The hand was never used in the process of cleaning, although but a moment before the same substance was being conveyed by hand to the mouth, the animal refusing to let it go even with severe punishment. In cleaning his foot, however, the ape would make use of a stick, a piece of paper, or a rag, and his gestures showed unmistakably that the task was a disagreeable one. This was also the case whenever any part of the body was dirty; the filth was removed as quickly as possible—and never by the naked hand. Feces are viewed differently according to the total situation. I have chosen this particular example because it pertains, at least indirectly, to the body image. We may suppose that the lack of coherence in the body image of animals will vary according to the situation.

When a child draws a hand with an enormous number of fingers, it does not follow that he has the same perception of this part of the body in any other situation. When he disregards spatial relations in drawings, it does not mean that he would disregard them in other circumstances.

The same problem is met in the whole realm of primitive thought. To us, the number "2" has a pretty well-defined connotation, but in primitive thought, the "2" in "2 apples" and the "2" in "2 men" are very different things. According to Levy-Bruhl (1923), the numerals (in the Kuki Chin group of the Tebeto-Burman family) are restricted in their sphere so as to apply to some special kinds of objects. We may come to the general conclusions that connotations and objects are constructions which fit in with particular situations. It seems that primitive thought and primitive levels of development are more prone to create objects and connotations according to the actual situation, and that they do not feel the necessity to coordinate the various situations. When objects are seen and connotations are created which satisfy the needs of a multiplicity of situations, it is a sign of a higher level of psychic development.

In primitive thought, there is a greater esteem for the enormous variety of situations and no attempt, or only an insufficient attempt, is made to find a method which is fitted to all those situations. I do not believe that the thought of an adult person ever gets completely away from creating new connotations and new object perceptions according to the urgent need of a single situation. Our body image is certainly not always the same. The body image is different according to the use we make of it. The logical thought of clear consciousness tries, of course, to construct the body image so that it fits at least the majority of situations. Development of the body image in some way runs parallel to the development of perceptions, thought, and object relations. The undeveloped body image therefore shows deep characteristics. It shows a greater tendency to transformations; it is easier to expel parts and take other parts in. But even this incomplete and incoherent body image is used differently according to the various aspects of the situation.

## THE EMOTIONAL PROBLEM IN BODY IMAGE[2]

In the course of our life, knowledge about our body increases; but it is a slow process, going on throughout our whole life. At first, the child knows very little about his body. According to Preyer (1882), the infant has the same attitude toward his body as toward other objects. He follows, with his eyes, the movements of his arms and legs in the same way he would follow a candlelight. He touches himself, especially his feet; he bites his fingers, arms, and toes until he cries with pain. Even pain sensations are not well organized. The body image is constructed in the course of our individual life. When the state of consciousness changes, the body schema becomes more and more distorted.

But the image and appearance of our body are also dependent on

[2] From Schilder (1934b).

48

our emotional life, and change along with the emotional attitude toward the body. The openings of the body have a greater physiological and psychological importance than most of the other parts of the body. We feel the mouth, the anus, the nose, and the genital opening in a particular way. The openings of the body are not only emphasized by the particular sensations which they furnish, but they are also invested with particular libidinal interest. The structure of the body image also depends on libidinal tendencies. The genitals play a particular part in the body image. There are always sensations coming from them. In many persons, the anus and its surroundings assume a similar importance. The eye, with its great importance for libidinal life, is always felt in some way. The body image, in any human being, does not have the same clearness in all its parts. The important parts give more sensations and provoke different emotional attitudes. The body images of different persons show characteristic differences.

Every disturbance in the emotional life will, therefore, immediately react on the body image, and libidinal disturbances will provoke changes in the image of the body. From this point of view, let us discuss a case of neurasthenia in a boy of twenty, who considered himself gifted.

He was studying law, but he felt that he could not concentrate any more. He complained about itching in his hands and feet, and in his anal and genital region. He also complained about constipation. Erections disturbed him. His attention was distracted from his studies and he had to interrupt them for a year. This is rather a common picture of neurasthenia. Neurasthenics are people who give too much attention to their bodies. How did this patient come to the idea that the parts of the body which he mentioned deserved special attention? When he was four years old, his mother gave birth to his sister. He was in the next room and heard his mother moaning. He got the idea that the physician was torturing her. In the analysis, which lasted several months, he brought forward that he imagined that the physician who was assisting at the birth was brushing the toes of the mother, causing her intense suffering. The boy had this idea from observing his father wiping his feet with his hands when he came home in the evening. The boy had suffered from an itching skin disease early in his life. Itching is a painful sensation that has to be relieved by one's hands. We do not know very much about our body before we touch it. The boy's research on his body, in this case, was intensified by the itching skin. The development of his body image must have been affected. We know from many observations that children are particularly curious about the openings of their bodies. They put their finger into every body opening they can reach. Such intensified investigation must lead to an early consciousness concerning the openings of the body.

The anal and genital regions are subjected to more sweating and eczemas than other parts of the body, especially in childhood. The anal region of this boy was irritated not only by his own hands, but also by his mother. She was always interested in bowel movements and often gave him enemas. She was also interested in a swelling of his genitals, probably a hydrocele. She often examined them, which he resented very much. The parts of his body to which his attention was drawn by his own actions, by the actions of his mother, and by the observations he made of others, were the parts which later on were associated with neurasthenic preoccupations. Between his fourth and fifth year, his intensive anal interest culminated in a fear that animals, like rats or dead chickens, would crawl into his anus when he was defecating. The patient was not manifestly sick at this time and did not show abnormal trends in the latency period. Between his twelfth and thirteenth year, a diarrhea, which seemed extraordinary to him, disturbed him very much. He had sadomasochistic fantasies at the same time. He imagined himself being cruelly tortured. He became more and more conscious of his body. Erections and ejaculations were a new source of worry. Itching sensations and the neurasthenic disturbance mentioned above developed. The unity of the body image is disrupted when libido is too unevenly distributed over the body, since some parts are invested with too great an amount of libido. If the patient had enjoyed the parts of the body overloaded with libido, he would have presented a picture of perversions, with anal-sadistic, and perhaps homosexual, trends. But since his superego protested against perversions, a neurosis appeared, in association with the same organs from which he derived pleasure in early childhood.

An understanding of the body image cannot be arrived at from the point of view of psychoanalysis alone. We have to study the data of brain pathology, which shows that the function of the parietal lobe is indispensable for self-perception of one's own body, the body image. This concept of the body image goes beyond psychoanalysis —and psychoanalysis has not considered the subject sufficiently. So far, it has neglected experiences concerning the body as a whole. How does the child experience his body? When you find that the neurasthenic patient has developed a characteristic attitude concerning his own body in early childhood, which corresponds to the later symptoms, there is at least a great possibility that the two sets of facts have something to do with each other. When we hear, for instance, that a child of four has a fantasy that his mother was tortured by a physician who brushed her toes, we must believe that his adult neurasthenic sensations in the feet have something to do with the childhood situation and that this situation expressed tendencies which later on play a part in the genesis of the neurosis. These early tendencies are not due to innate patterns alone. They depend a great deal on the attitude of the person who brings up the child. One can make a child self-conscious concerning his own body and parents will do so concerning those parts of the body which are important to themselves; or there is a transition of the body image of the parents to the body image of the child. We cannot overrate early childhood experiences; they necessarily have a formative effect on later life. The experience of one's own body is the basis for all other life experiences. It is astonishing to see how little interest psychologists and psychiatrists have given to this problem. The whole field of somato-psyche has been neglected. The life of a human being is a unit and anything that has happened in one's life can never be completely lost. Early life is of greater importance than later life. But the early occurrences are not more than the basis of our later life. We do go into the future, but present and future are based upon the past.

These problems are problems of organic neurology. The concept of the somato-psyche comes from Wernicke (1906), a psychiatrist who was primarily interested in brain pathology. But the concept of the somato-psyche is a psychological concept. The psychological and the physiological approaches must lead to the same conclusions. The body image is based on the structural organization of the human organism. It is based on physiological data, but these get their final synthesis from the personality.

All life experiences, the inner life history, take part in the elaboration of the body image. Our inner life history is also the history of our relations to our fellow human beings and to the community in the broadest sense.

Levy (1932) has shown, in an interesting study, that children who became conscious of a part of their own body, also became conscious of the same parts of the bodies of others. A boy with an inverted nipple was extremely interested in the breasts of other persons. When a child has difficulties in walking, he develops an interest in the feet of other persons.

The body image belongs to the community. Whatever we may do, the images are never isolated. There is a continual interchange between our own body image and the body image of others. We want to know about them. We want to project parts of our own bodies into others. We are never completely contented with our own body image. It is in a continual state of flux, it is always changing. For example, we change by dancing. Limbs change their gravity, the circular movements make parts of the body fly away. Clothes change our body image. They make us appear larger. They help us to expand beyond ourselves. We put on masks. We walk on stilts. We may even become a part of a horse we ride. In carnival festivities, we may grow immense noses and immense heads. Sometimes we want to contract. Sometimes we tie the bodice tight and wear tight clothes. We do not respect our physical boundaries.

Infants have very little reaction to pain. The same holds true of animals. Are there states of ontogenetic development in which the body image is undeveloped? And is the incomplete pain reaction a sign of insufficient integration of the body image? We must study the libidinal structure of the body schema before we can try to give an answer to these questions.

Two factors apparently play a special role in the creation of the body image: one is pain, the other is our motor control over our limbs.

Preyer (1882) has especially emphasized the role of pain. We have to acknowledge that pain belongs to us in a special way. Bernfeld (1925) stresses the importance of the fact that our intention acts on our bodies in a more immediate way, but every sensation contributes to the building up of the body image. There is no fundamental difference between the various sensations in this respect. Sensations are always the sensations of a person. There is the central factor of the ego with its intentions, strivings, and desires. This central factor uses sensations and perceptions.

Attempts have often been made to attribute to the sensations which come from the inside of the body a decisive importance in the building up of the body image. French authors have talked of a coenesthesia, but there is no question that the sensations coming from the inside of the body have no inner meaning before they are brought into connection with the body image. None of the numerous French writers has taken pains to study the actual experiences we have regarding the inside of our body. I do not think that coenesthesia, the so-called "Gemeinempfindungen," has any decisive part in the construction of our bodily self. Our bodily self is built up according to the needs of the personality. It is true that pain is an important factor here. It helps us to decide what we want to have nearer to our personality, to the center of our ego, and what we want to have further away from it. This decision and choice must be closely related to the motor activities; but what is true of pain is also true of any other sensation. Every sensation has its own motility. Sensation has, itself, a motor answer. Continued activity is therefore at the basis of our bodily self. We choose and reject through action. Bernfeld's contention thus finds its proper place.

We may say that the body image is the creation of the dominating will (Nietzsche's *Herrschaftsgebilde*). Since optic experience plays such an enormous part in our relation to the world, it also plays a dominating role in the creation of the body image. The optic experience is also experience by action. By action and determination, we give the final shape to our bodily self. It is a process of continual active development. Under the influence of the inner drive we can only separate artificial sensory experience from inner activities and libidinal strivings, which emanate from a central personality.

The development of the body schema probably runs, to a great extent, parallel with sensory motor development. Luquet (1913), who has studied children's drawings, talks of the synthetic incapacity of the child: "The thing is not there as a whole. The details only are given and, owing to the lack of synthetic relations, they are simply juxtaposed. Thus an eye will be placed next to the head, an arm next to a leg, etc." Of course, drawing is a rather complicated psychic activity and it may be difficult to determine whether this synthetic incapacity is at all based on sensory difficulties or whether it is merely due to motor incapacities. But the child is completely satisfied with his drawings, and therefore I believe that the way in which children draw human figures really does reflect their knowledge and sensory experience of the body image. They express at least the mental picture they have of the human body, and the body image is a mental picture as well as perception.

Goodenough's study (1926) contains material which is of the greatest importance regarding the problem of the child's body image. The way in which children draw fingers deserves special interest in this respect. They may multiply the fingers; they may draw them in a straight line. It seems that there is a close parallel between the optic development and the understanding of special relations in the body image.

Piaget (1928) has studied the development of the connotations of left and right in children. Between the ages of five and eight, the concepts only have a meaning in relation to their own bodies. Between eight and eleven, they can also apply them to others. Only after that time can they use left and right connotations freely for others, for objects in space, and for themselves. Piaget distinguishes three stages: egocentrism, socialization, and complete objectivity. He believes that this has to do merely with judgment and reasoning, but I discern, in the development of the left and right connotation, a development in the body image. According to Koffka (1928), the picture of an ear, mouth or finger may not be recognized by a child, although he is able to recognize these parts on a complete body. At any rate, we gain the impression that, from the point of view of sensory motor development, the child brings more-or-less isolated and unrelated experience into a complete form by continual effort. Even then, the parts are not in such a close relation to the whole as they are for the adult.

## THE CHILD'S CONCEPT OF THE INSIDE OF HIS BODY[3]

It has been pointed out by Hartmann and myself (1927) that as far as direct experience goes, we know nothing of the organs inside our bodies; all that we are actually aware of is a heavy mass. The sensations which become part of our subjective experience relate only to the surface of the body or to a fraction of an inch beneath the surface. The body openings too, from the point of view of

[3] From Schilder and Wechsler (1935).

psychology, are experienced only a small way under the surface. Bodily sensations, except that of weight, are concentrated on the surface and what we know of our organs is acquired intellectual knowledge or something that we have learned. Normally, our sensation would never disclose to us the existence of heart, lungs, and intestines. Our direct experience of our own body is based on visual and tactile impressions, on perceptions of the weight of the body and its various parts, and on the happenings on the sensitive surface. These conscious data are of psychological significance not only for the individual, but in every sort of libidinal relationship.

The psychological problems involved in the castration complex are not only concerned with the surface, and with certain secretions of the body, but also with the insides of the body as well. It is reasonable to assume that the castration complex is operative in the pregenital stage of development and comprises the wish to preserve the whole body intact, including the inside of it, and also includes the fear of any sort of bodily injury. The fear of parting with partially digested food, the contents of the intestines, the feces and the intestines themselves (anal-intestinal castration complex) was the moving factor in an adult with schizophrenia, with profound regression, described by myself and Sugar (1926). The fear of dismemberment is one of the most powerful factors in psychosis. Bromberg and myself (1933a) have drawn attention to the part played by this fear in alcoholic hallucinations. According to Klein (1932), the desire to tear out and destroy the interior of the parents' bodies is conspicuous in the psychology of little children. The child is also afraid of being robbed of his own viscera.

An inquiry into children's knowledge about the interior of their bodies may, therefore, throw light on a number of psychological problems.

A systematic inquiry was conducted with forty children, four to thirteen years of age. Younger children were not selected because of the nature of the problem, which relates to conscious material and, therefore, makes it essential that the children questioned should be capable of expressing themselves in words.

The children were asked, "What is the inside of your body made of?" or "What have you got inside your body?" It was not easy to formulate this first question, since, generally, not much interest is evoked about the inside of the body, as all our attention is directed to its outer surface. Next, the examiner pointed to the child's head and to his own and asked what was inside; the same kind of question was asked, in the same way, with reference to the chest and abdomen. Sometimes these parts of the body were tapped or a fold of skin on the child's arm was taken up and he was asked what was under the skin. Sometimes the muscles of the upper arm were pressed and he was asked, "What is that?" In a few cases, some further questions were asked, as will be indicated.

A boy, aged four and a half years, who was a badly behaved child, said that there were "bones and potatoes" in his body. A four-year-old child of a physician said, "Body, face, heart, and stomach."

Other answers were as follows: Kathie, age six (M.A. 5-0). "What is inside of you?" "Blood." "Under your skin?" "Blood." "What else?" "What I eat."

Patrick, age six, average intelligence. "What have you got under your skin?" "Food." "How does it get there?" "I eat it." "What is inside of your head?" "My brain." "How did it get there?" "God made it." "What is inside of our body?" "Food." "And in your chest?" "My soul." "What is under your skin?" "Blood and bones."

Harry, age nine (M.A. 6-10). "What have you got inside you?" "Flesh like a skeleton." "In your head?" "My brain."

Anthony, age eight (M.A. 7-0). "What is inside you?" "Blood." "In your chest?" "A lot of bread." "In your stomach?" "Fish." "What is inside my stomach?" "Chicken." "In my head?" "Your brains." "Under my skin?" "Muscles." "What have we got in our chests?" "A lot of water."

Alfred, age ten (M.A. 7-0). "What is there under your skin?" "Me." "In your chest?" "Tubes." "In your belly?" "Bowels."

Joan, age seven (M.A. 7-0). "What have you in your chest?" "Milk." "In your stomach?" "Food." "In your head?" "Brains." "Under your skin?" "Flesh."

David, age seven (M.A. 7-2). "What is inside your head?" "Me." "Under your skin—here?" "Me." "In your chest?" "Bones." "In your stomach?" "Bones."

Two sisters came into the hospital because of precocious sexual activities. Frances, age eight (M.A. 6-8). "What is inside your chest?" "My heart." "In your head?" "My brain." "In your belly?" "Food, my stomach, sweets, and ices." "Under your skin?" "Muscles." Anna, age eleven (M.A. 6-8). "What have you got in your head?" "My brain." "In your chest?" "My heart, my lungs, and my bones." "In your stomach?" "Food."

Marion, age eight (M.A. 8-8). "What is inside you?" "What we eat." "In your chest?" "I don't know." "In our heads?" "Our brains." "Under our skin?" "Bones."

Raminos, age nine (M.A. 10-1). "What is inside you?" "Flesh." "In your stomach?" "Blood." "How does it get there?" "When I eat." "In your head?" "My brain." "In your chest?" "Flesh." "What is the heart?" "Flesh and blood." "What is your belly made of?" "My stomach and vegetables as well." "What is under your skin?" "Muscles and bones, when you eat you get like that."

Thomas, age ten (M.A. 11-2), gave a full description and drew a diagram as well.

Joseph, age twelve (M.A. 10-6). "What have you got inside you?" "I don't know." "In your chest?" "My heart." "In your stomach?" "Bones." "What have I got inside me?" "Flesh and fat." "What kind of flesh?" "What you have eaten." He knew however that what we eat and drink is in our stomachs.

Helen, age thirteen (M.A. 11-1), gave the following primitive type of answers: "What is there inside you?" "Bones." "In your chest?" "Food." "Under your skin?" "Flesh." "How does it get there?" "God made it of dust." "What is in your belly?" "My stomach."

The average eleven-year-old child gave the correct answers. Therefore, the majority of the children selected were ten years old or younger. Only six children were older. Two children were four years old and three were six years old. These children could not be questioned very satisfactorily. One eight-year-old had an M.A. of 4-8. One young child said that under his skin and inside himself was "me." Six of the younger children did not know that the brain was inside the head.

The head, we suppose, of all parts of the body is the least "private" or "improper." It is one of the exposed parts and counts as part of the face. In this regard, the child's knowledge is, of course, a reflection of the attitude of his elders. However, generally speaking, neither the heart nor the lungs are regarded as improper to speak about and, yet, the only children who knew anything of these internal organs were those whose attention had been called to them by their immediate surroundings. Normal adults do not pay attention even to those internal organs which are entirely inoffensive.

When the younger children were asked what was inside the body, the typical answer was that it contained the food recently eaten. Although this may, at first, seem surprising, it is nevertheless self-evident. It is the child's *direct* experience. Otherwise, he knows little or nothing about the interior of his body, but he does know what it is to put food into it, an important libidinal act in the child's experience. He pictures even his chest as being filled with bread, milk, or meat. Later on, he thinks of the food as being simply the contents of the abdomen. Even if he has heard of the stomach, it is unimportant in comparison with its contents. If he knows anything at all about the muscles and flesh, he believes that they make their appearance under the skin as the direct result of the food he eats. The statement that there are bones and blood inside the body ranks second in the children's typical answers.

Answers to direct questions may not seem entirely satisfactory. In every language, the terms used for the bowels have a rather vulgar flavor. Perhaps children know more than they say and do not say it simply because it seems unsuitable to them. That sort of thing is familiar in child psychology. We often noticed that if these children, who were under observation because of behavior problems, were questioned about the differences between the sexes, they either would not or could not say anything about the sex organs. They would say that boys wear pants and girls wear dresses, or they would say that girls have long hair and boys have short hair. If we showed them an undressed doll (without genitals) they would say, "It is a girl." If we made a penis out of modeling clay and put it on the doll, the majority of children exhibited a delighted expression and said, "Now it is a boy." In this instance, by modeling the penis, the adult made it clear that the child had nothing to be afraid of if he showed that he understood. Many of the prohibitions imposed by society have reference to words, and children will speak only if they can do so without using forbidden words.

So we must bear in mind the possibility that the younger children's typical answer, "There is food inside the body," does not represent the complete expression of what they believe or know, but is partly their response to the particular question in a given situation. Even so, the answers are noteworthy; they indicate the concrete nature of childish thinking. The body has inside it what we put into it; the food we eat enters directly into the structure. When adults shut their eyes, they perceive the body merely as a heavy mass (an experience suggesting the morula stage of embryonic development), whereas the child's picture of the interior of the body corresponds, rather, to the gastrula stage. Perhaps there is more in this comparison than a mere play of words. When we think of the form of the organism, we can really imagine only a few possibilities. It is either solid or hollow, and the purpose of the cavities in it is to receive something. There is also a similarity between children's ideas about their bodies and the experience of some melancholics. They describe themselves as a kind of tubular bag which simply receives everything put into it. Schilder and Sugar (1926) quote a patient who said that people took away his food, his bowels, and his feces, a complaint which becomes more comprehensible when we compare it with what children say.

Children also conceive of alligators, reptiles, etc., in the same way, as has been shown by the work of Bender and Woltmann (1936) through the analysis of children's reactions to puppet shows, their own art work, their dreams, etc. The anxious small child is afraid of these objects as devouring bad parent figures. When Klein ascribes, to children, a tendency to tear out the insides of their parents' bodies, it becomes more intelligible if we bear in mind the fact that food and bowels may be very much the same thing in the child's mind.

In conclusion, there is yet another inference which may be drawn from these records of ours. Two of the children said that they themselves were under their skin and inside their bodies. Now, it is one of the paradoxes of our bodily experience that our sensations relate to the surface of the body and yet we do not regard this as our body proper. The skin can be removed from the deeper tissues. We are inside our skins and know nothing directly of the interior of our bodies. Thus, it would seem that our bodily experience, apparently so constant a phenomenon, melts away. There are phrases which psychologically indicate that we can strip off our skin, such as "Jump out of our skins." I have observed a case which was instructive in this connection. A girl of fifteen suffered from a severe form of chorea, which proved fatal. She complained that her hands and feet were paralyzed and said that if only her skin would peel off she would be all right again. Her hair and teeth were not part of her. She maintained that an artificial rubber skin had been put over her real skin. She said that other people also wore masks, were "made up," and looked unnatural. Everything, including her skin, was dirty. Abnormal sensations evidently due to organic causes led her to deny the reality of her skin; this gave her the sense that both she herself and other people were unreal.

It seems, then, that sometimes we think of our skin as our most intimate possession, for example, think of the phrase, "to save one's skin," which means to save one's life; while sometimes we think of the skin merely as the envelope of our true selves and of what is inside us. But, in the deep infantile strata of our minds, we are not perfectly certain whether there is anything inside us except what is crammed there from the outside.

# III

# Personality Development

### INFANTILE EGO DEVELOPMENT[1]

Ferenczi (1913), in discussing the developmental stages of the sense of reality, considered the primitive stage to be that in which the individual, resting in the mother's womb and free from all desire, considers himself omnipotent. A further stage appeared to be that in which the child, by crying, compels the people in his environment to gratify his wishes. Later, he aims to change the course of external events according to his wishes, until, finally, he does justice to life by his own activity. In current psychoanalytic theory, all of these manifestations of a magical view of life are considered to be narcissistic trends. The ego invested with narcissism ascribes exaggerated abilities to itself. Thus, we do not deal here with ego instincts which bring us into the closest relation with the perception of objects, made possible through vision and hearing, and the senses of smell, taste, and touch. We must especially adhere to the point of view that every image, whether it be a perception or a representation, and every thought, indeed everything that deals with objects, contains within itself a call to action.

Evidently, we are here dealing with a very deep-seated characteristic of the organism. One might say that every sensation also has an efferent component. The motor response, in connection with the primitive organic manifestations, serves precisely as proof that something receptive has transpired. Receptivity and motor respon-

[1] From Schilder (1928a).

siveness might be regarded as the basic pattern of physiological events, even when the physiological event transpires without consciousness. When the knee is struck, the pull of the tendon produces the patellar reflex as a motor response. We may assume that the body is protecting itself against an external aggression by means of this reflex. The grasping movements stand at a much higher level. It is conceivable that, at a primitive stage of development, every object is seized the moment it is perceived. We are able to observe this directly at a certain stage in the development of the suckling. Schuster (1923) has noted the reappearance of such primitive grasping reflexes following brain lesions. This grasping may manifest itself in various psychic situations. We differentiate, from compulsive grasping, grasping behavior which much more closely approximates the volitional. The grasping is an incorporation of something, a making something one's own. It is not very different when the nursling opens his mouth with the desire to incorporate objects which approach him (feeding reflex). This is a tendency which likewise becomes manifest in the adult after brain injuries (Wagner-Jauregg, Bettelheim, 1924). We therefore assume the existence of a primitive tendency to master the environment.

There also exists, alongside this way of controlling the external world, another way, which can best be studied in connection with hallucinations. A number of hallucinations bring with them the tendency to grasp for the hallucinated objects. The so-called occupational delirium is to be understood in this way. I was able to observe, most clearly, something of this sort in a patient who could always be made to hallucinate under suggestion, and then would immediately begin to grasp for the hallucinated objects. Equally significant, in connection with hallucinations, is behavior which is determined through identification. One patient, for instance, hallucinated a cow and began to carry out the chewing movements. She therefore identified herself with her hallucination, and her chewing movements arose out of her identification. Something similar occurs in connection with cases of so-called muscle sense hallucinations, when the patients express in speech that which is hallucinated.

We might, therefore, in a general way, maintain that every image carries within it a tendency to action. This activity may merely take cognizance of the object as such or it may issue from identification with the object. We may consider the former type as the more differentiated and as manifesting a series of developmental stages. The muscle sense hallucination as we have described it above, undoubtedly constitutes a more differentiated psychic phenomenon than the compulsive grasping of the suckling or that which follows brain injury.

To reach for, to grasp, and to carry to the mouth are, therefore, attitudes which belong to every image. All these attitudes have no regard for the object—they not only appropriate it as their own and overpower it, but they also break it up and destroy it. (Compare Abraham's [1927] stressing of the libidinal sadistic component in this connection.) The impulse to gain mastery over things, the prototype of this impulse, appears to be primarily associated with the ego instincts, but it is also a precondition to sexual behavior. Here too, the object must somehow be grasped, held, and overpowered. Thus, there appears to exist a common ground to both ego and sexual instincts. The destruction of the object is, as has been mentioned, often associated with grasping, holding, and incorporation. The ego instincts, therefore, bear the closest relation to those aspects of the sexual instinct which we designate as sadistic. Freud (1920) goes even further and designates sadism as a death instinct, which becomes detached from the ego under the influence of narcissistic libido, so that it asserts itself by preference in connection with an object. "This death instinct then appears in the service of the sexual function. In the oral stage of the organization of the libido the conquest of the love object is still bound up with its destruction, later on the sadistic trend becomes separated off, and finally, at the stage of genital primacy, it takes on the function of overpowering the sexual object only to the extent required for the purpose of the sexual act." For Freud, the death instinct coincides with the ego instinct, since every individual strives for a natural living out of his life function, toward death, which is part of this. Hence, for Freud, the self-preservative instinct and the death instinct are the same thing. The death instinct would, therefore, have self-destruction as its object; only later is it thrust aside by the ego. Sadism thus directs itself, first of all, against one's own person, and only secondarily against the outer world.

63

It seems to me that the existence of a death impulse is questionable. The impulse toward death may be only the wish for a rebirth in the disguise of erotic strivings. The striving toward the external world, toward grasping and mastery, seems to us so elemental that we cannot look upon it as a derivative of the impulses to self-annihilation. Finally, it must be considered as questionable whether the sadistic aspects of sexual life are to be looked upon as ego components of sexuality or whether this sadistic component is not common to both sexual and ego impulses, along with the grasping, holding, and mastering, which points to a common instinctive basis from which both originate. According to Freud, the dominant task of psychic life, perhaps of nerve function generally, is to keep the organism free from stimuli, to maintain the inner tension at a constant level, and he sees in this the strongest reason for belief in the evidence of a death instinct. But is this not a property of every instinct, even the sexual, and does it not belong to the very nature of instinctive behavior, that as soon as inner tension is relaxed it creates for itself new aims, new tensions?

Freud attributes to all instincts the general characteristic that they seek to re-establish a former state. He designates this characteristic the repetition compulsion. This phenomenon takes place independently of the pleasure principle. But is not this re-establishment of a former situation, this repetition compulsion, insofar as it is at all a psychic experience, already part and parcel of the general laws governing psychic function (namely, that instinct strives after release of its tension)? It would be more correct to state that instinct strives after the object which brings release with it. Is not this former state sought, therefore, because it contained both pleasure and interest for the individual? Freud stresses the fact that in the dreams of those suffering from a traumatic neurosis, the traumatic experience repeatedly recurs. But is not this recurrence, insofar as it is not conducive to pleasure, a general characteristic of psychic function, unrelated to instinct, to conserve impressions, especially when they have reached a certain degree of intensity? It is conceivable that continuous recurrence of the same situation tends to minimize the effect of the original experience, but is one justified, on this account, in looking for this at the bottom of every instinct? Even if we follow the current basic principles of psychoanalysis, and look upon everything psychic as instinctive, it is the mastery of the present which takes precedence over the past, in instinct activity.

Thus, I find myself in disagreement with Freud's theory of the death instinct and the repetition compulsion, and consider to be ego instincts only the tendencies to seize, to hold, and to master, tendencies which are fully in accord with the general laws of instinct, namely, to strive after an object and to turn to new objects with a renewed ardor.

Of the remainder of psychoanalytic literature, reference to the ego instincts is found only in Staercke's paper, "Psychoanalysis and Psychiatry" (1921). He differentiates a tonic stage (a stage of rhythmic repetition), a stage of lying and dissimulation, and an idealistic stage. He derives his cue for the setting up of the first mentioned stages from the observation of the movements and behavior of primitive organisms. But is this difference in motor reaction sufficient proof of a difference of instinct? There can be no doubt, of course, that attention to the environment tends to defer a momentary motor reaction. Therefore, Staercke justly maintains that the ego instinct heightens the threshold of discharge. In this sense one can also, to a certain extent, subscribe to the further stages of the ego instinct established by him. Naturally, the question arises of whether this division is not after all a superficial one. Lying and dissimulation are very complicated attitudes, which hardly give us an insight into the structure of the ego instincts and cannot be taken as definite stages in the development of these instincts.

It is the outer world, then, which causes the emergence of instinct. Without attacking the general question of the reality of the outer world, we will hardly be able to gain deeper insight. Psychoanalysis is generally disinclined to see, in the outer world, anything but projection phenomena. It views the primitive organism as something which does not differentiate between individual and environment. This differentiation is undertaken only on the basis of instinctive attitudes. But instinctive attitudes are only possible in connection with objects and we have no ground for the assumption that objects can ever be created solely from within, unless traces of them are already present in former evolutionary stages. At any rate, in the domain of psychology we are ever obliged to assume the existence of an outer world.

The body itself is, in a certain sense, environment; only sensation cannot be said to be so. But is it possible to assume the existence of developmental stages in which sensation takes the place of perception? Such a state would, at any rate, know neither object nor subject, and the possibility of displacement from subject to object would be eliminated. It is much more likely that environment somehow impinges upon the primitive organism and makes itself known as environment. Subject-object adjustments can only follow experience with the outer world. In addition to the phenomenologically irreducible object experience, the experiencing of the environment contains a number of psychological characteristics. It is the environment which contains the real sources of satisfaction, since, even if we were to assume that the suckling hallucinates the milk, the continuous absence of nourishment will prevent the arousal of the feeling of pleasure. In my opinion, reality possesses a certain irreducible character, which can also be recognized through definite psychological forms of experience belonging to it. There exists, within us, a permanent striving to master reality, and it is only in connection with the objects of reality that we experience that transitory state of peace which we know as satisfaction.

We have now arrived at the point where we can inquire into the more subtle structure of the ego in Freud's sense. Its core consists of ego instincts with their tendency to master the environment. These ego instincts do not direct themselves toward the environment in an uncoordinated and chaotic manner, but become organized, by means of identification, into orderly entities, and these must now be more carefully considered.

As a result of identification, an outside person becomes incorporated into the self. At the same time, the quantum of libido which was bestowed upon that person is withdrawn into the self. As long as the object with whom identification takes place still remains partially outside, it naturally also retains part of the object cathexis. Identifications take place with a great many people. Each of these identifications organizes, or binds together, instinctive attitudes. The identifications with the father and mother are most important. But every love relationship depends upon an identification and the breaking up of a love relationship very likely does not mean an entire giving up of the identification; there is retained within the ego a remnant of the identification with its cathexis. Indeed, it is decidedly plausible that this residual cathexis may be greater than that which was originally accorded the object of identification.

We will see later on how this conception gains support from the fact that, very likely in connection with every difficulty, libido is not transferred directly from one object to another, but is first of all withdrawn from the object into the sphere of the ego. Freud also thinks that every object cathexis leaves a trace within the ego. One notices this in women who appear to be changed after every erotic relationship. One may therefore reach the general conclusion that every object-libidinal relationship, in fact every relation to an object, leaves behind it an alteration in the ego, which is, at the same time, preserved by any one of the many part configurations of the ego ideal. We have every reason to assume that the identifications of the ego ideal, the images of the various persons, are always retained, to a certain extent, in the ego. In other words, the structure of the ego ideal is not a homogenous one. It is built up of coordinated identifications.

One cannot be satisfied, however, with this statement of the organization of the ego ideal. Along with this organization, which one might designate as a horizontal one, there also exists a vertical structure. We have absolutely no reason to assume, for instance, that the mother identification, which takes place in the course of one's life, always takes place in the same manner.

New characteristics in the beings who surround us constantly come to light. A given person's characteristics are perceived differently by the newborn, the one-year-old, and the three-year-old, than they are by the five- and ten-year-old, and by the adult. The ego ideal, which develops out of the identifications with a given person, continually reconstructs itself anew in various ways, although all the ego ideal constructions, which spring from the mother identification, for instance, are held together by a common bond. But one must, at the same time, maintain that the identifications of a given age period should in some way show common features and accordingly we would defend the general point of view that the ego ideal constructions show a vertical stratification in accordance with the stage of developmental organization attained. It may now be of interest to see what constitutes the psychological structure of such

67

a primitive ego ideal. We have, in accordance with Freud, looked upon the ego ideal constructions as compromise formations between the repressive forces originating from identifications and strengthened by the ego instincts and the libidinal impulses.

The ego ideal, therefore, does not merely reflect the identifications of the moment, but also carries within itself a representation of the instinctive or real self. When we speak of a primitive instinctiveness, we must also assume a corresponding primitive ego ideal. The ego ideal, for instance, which represents the rule of cleanliness and those primitive self-evident adaptations to society, must not be viewed in the same way as one views the ego ideal constructions of the adult. The early identification with the mother does not take into account at all the riper fullness of her personality, but only certain, very definite, traits of hers. Indeed, even these traits can be seen by the child only in the light of his stage of comprehension. When, for instance, the child ascribes magical attributes to his parents, his identifications and, by the same token, his ego ideal must be permeated with magic. One might say, in a general way, that the height of organization of a given stage of instinct development has its counterpart in the ego ideal of that developmental period. These vertically superimposed ego ideal constructions will, in accordance with this, not be of equal significance as regards their repressive tendencies, and one might ask whether the different repressions issuing from the different ego ideal constructions do not in reality differ in their quality, so that a repressive tendency of a deeper level remains active, while one of a more superficial level is abolished, and vice versa. Later, I will show that something of this sort actually does take place in schizophrenia.

The conception of the organization of the ego ideal thus far given, still does not suffice. We must make it clear that a number of identifications possess common characteristics. For instance, both the father and mother identifications will contribute to the idea in the child's ego ideal construction that he must not soil himself with feces, must not play with feces, and the like. In other words, every identification will possess certain features in common with others. It is especially the more general requirements of society that become, in this manner, deeply engraved in the individual.

That which is done by the majority of people in one's environment will acquire an especially significant representation in the ego ideal. The finer characteristics, in the personal make-up of those with whom an individual identifies himself, undoubtedly become part of the ego ideal in quite a different manner. We are, therefore, approaching a new arrangement in the construction of the ego ideal and would make a distinction between those parts of it which are, so to speak, the impersonal precipitate of a host of identifications and those which still retain, in their identifications, personal characteristics of the love object. It is probable that those manifoldly rooted traces of manifold identifications bear a more intimate relation to the primitive ego ideal constructions than they do to the more highly differentiated ones.

This also carries the possibility of a bridge to an understanding of group psychology, since it is probable that the individual member of a group identifies himself not only with the leader, but also with the other members of the group (Freud), so that the identifications with all of these individuals leave traces in the ego ideal. In this connection, we will refer briefly, at least, to a new constellation of problems. Does there exist any relation between the degree of fixity of the individual features of the ego ideal constructions which are derived from a multitude of identifications, and the dynamic significance of the instincts as modifiers of the identifications? Does the ego ideal, in these cases, contain less of the instinctive, or real self, than in other cases? Is this, perhaps, the reason why it is so difficult for us to withdraw from the group? Is the deeply engraved multiplicity of identifications within the ego ideal responsible for our difficulty in going against the commands of the group? Is that part of the ego ideal which has been constructed out of the multiplicity of identifications the most firmly knitted part? Is it more difficult to shatter this aspect of the ego ideal than that which is constructed out of more individual identifications? The problem of communal life comes to light in this connection, and we shall see that this problem is also of great importance in the psychology of paresis. Are not all of these personal attitudes, which directly reflect the structure of the environment, general requirements of a society which demands adaptation to reality? Is it justifiable, then, to assume that the testing of reality, and for that matter, questions of reality and truth in general, stand in the closest relation to these

69

precipitates of manifold identifications, or otherwise stated, to that which every community requires of us? One sees, however, at the same time, that all the demands which the environment makes upon the individual are taken up by him, at first directly by way of the ego instincts, but that they receive their fixity through contacts with social life. One sees, at the same time, that this portion of the ego ideal stands in close relation to the perceptive self.

There is no doubt that the self can very readily become dissociated into its component parts. Freud has pointed out that the scolding voices of alcoholic hallucinosis are nothing but the voices of conscience. It is society, which in this way dissolves itself again into its individual identifications—and each of these identifications again assumes its own note; it is altered by the instinctive background.

We will now have to ask ourselves what we are to understand by the term "narcissistic stage"; what is the psychology of narcissism? What about the ego instincts at this narcissistic stage? According to psychoanalytic theory, the intra-uterine existence of the embryo is one of blissful contentment. Every need is satisfied. In criticism of this assumption, it might be naturally stated that the embryo not only moves within the mother's womb, but it also grows, and if the psychological viewpoint were to be brought seriously into accord with the biological one, we could hardly look upon a rapidly growing organism as blissfully happy. At times, the condition of peaceful sleep is akin to that of the embryonic state, even as regards the position of the sleeper, and certainly a state of profound sleep must be designated as one of bliss. Otherwise, how would we be able to renounce our daily interest so completely? (Freud.) Is it possible to even conceive of such a state of bliss with no unsatisfied desires? Do we perhaps enjoy sleep only because we awake in the interims of sleep? This sort of psychologizing has many a snare. The notion of a state of blissfulness must always be brought into relation with an object, even though it may be only the happiness that comes from the renunciation of an object. However, we know too little about the psychology of the embryo to say anything definite about it.

When we observe how matters stand with the newborn, we see that he directs activities toward certain elements of the outer world. He responds to auditory, tactile, and gustatory stimuli (Canestrini,

1913). Analytically speaking, it might be said that a partial cathexis of objects in the outside world has already taken place. In part, we must attribute these cathexes to the ego instincts since the presence of the impulse to seize, to hold fast, and to incorporate objects must be taken for granted even in such primitive organisms. How does the infant experience objects? We have every reason to assume that his cognizance of the structure and nature of the environment is in no way as complete as that of the adult. Even in the adult, feeling about an object becomes intensified when the perception of it is inadequate. This leads to the important question of how the infant recognizes his own body during this primitive stage, since the body presents two plans of attack. It appears on the one hand as an object, in the same way as the objects in the environment, while, on the other hand, it mediates the sensations by which one is aware of one's own body. The body is thus both perceived and felt. What is of prime interest here is sensation, which renders the body bodily. Whether the cognizance of one's body is gained by means of sensation only or whether it is also perceived, is a problem which we cannot consider in detail now. In my opinion, both elements enter into the situation.

Concepts, and very likely ideas also, arise out of sensations and perceptions. And there can be no doubt, when the question of a dividing line between personality and environment is raised, that concepts and ideas are attributes of the personality and not of the external world. Naturally, however, the things referred to by a given concept or idea belong to the outside world. But does not every instinct presuppose that sort of externality, which is to be differentiated from the subjective reaction? Even one's own body becomes the goal of a particular instinct (that part of the body which is identical with its perceptive mechanism).

In other respects, personality and environment are only relative concepts. It is impossible to conceive of a perception without at the same time thinking of some process going on in the body. Sensation is the subjective reflection of a perception. If we did not place the term "sensation" in opposition to the term "perception," they would lose all their meaning. Of course, a transitional stage between sensations and perceptions is entirely possible. Afterimages must certainly be looked upon as sensations, although, not infrequently, the spot on the wall which corresponds to a projection of the sensation, at first strikes us as a perception. It is doubtful whether a condition can even exist which does not permit of a differentiation between personality and environment, between sensation and perception. It might be possible to assume an undifferentiated zone between personality and environment which reflects both, since it is probable that even in the most primitive subjective states there is already some environmental participation, some indication of the total structure, even though the decision is as yet impossible, with reference to its individual elements, as to whether they belong to the personality or to the environment. I am certain that, in these primitive developmental stages, personality and environment approximate each other more closely. The external is much less differentiated. However, a close relation already exists between the infant's seizing and holding movements and that which we describe as the environment. The ego instincts, therefore, have a closer relation to the environment, and we have already described the intimate association between ego instincts and the perceptual phenomena. In accordance with this, we must also assume that an organism which is without movement and activity, experiences the environment only in a rudimentary form. No organism, however, can be thought of as entirely without movement and, in the last analysis, it can only be a question of quantitative differences in the motility of organisms. The undifferentiated zone between sensation and perception is more closely related to the organism than to the environment. Nevertheless, the existence of an outside world and of subjective reactions must be attributed, even to the consciousness of the amoeba.

In the newborn, ego instinctive stirrings are already present; the outer world is there, but in an incomplete state. We have every reason to assume that the newborn's consciousness of his body lacks completeness. It is clear that during the state of inadequacy of the organism's experiences, the possibilities are better for ascribing a given element now to the organism, now to the environment. The resultant zone of indefiniteness makes the phenomenon of hallucination (projection) possible, as well as the phenomenon of personification. But the psychological fact of externality is a pre-existing form of experience and is not explicable on the basis of projection.

This pre-existing notion of an outside world and its form embraces only that much of it which relates to behavior tendencies associated with the newborn's perceptions. But perceptions and behavior tendencies must be related to a world of reality. The final evaluation of both organism and environment is derived from the side of instinct by way of projections, identifications, and personifications.

Accurate estimates of the environment are constantly gained through identifications. We are, therefore, justified in assuming an environmental reality which furnishes points of attachment for the ego instincts, although this ego instinct reality contact appears from the start to be associated with a libidinal form of contact. This is true even of the organism's primitive conception of the outer world. For instance, this is the case with respect to the sucking activity of the nursling. The less developed the image of the outer world is, the fewer are the opportunities for object cathexis. I have already stressed the point that the cathexis of the outer world is very incomplete, when one takes into consideration the isolated objects of the environment as such. The recognition of these objects is facilitated through an identification with persons of the environment. The first identifications must therefore constitute an important step in the forming of a conception of the outer world. It is through these identifications that the environment acquires its final form. The less certain the guiding lines for the estimation of the environment through these identifications, the more extensive is the region of indefiniteness and the greater is the amount of libido directed toward the self and toward this zone of indefiniteness, which is more related to the self than to the environment.

As long as the ego instincts remain unorganized into differentiated groups through identifications, the image or concept of the outer world must remain less differentiated and more indistinct. This is more or less the condition of the primitive organism. Organism and environment are nearer one another at this time; the activity of the organism is capable of affecting only a minor portion of the environment, and, because of this, its value to the organism as a source of satisfaction is less than are those satisfactions which come to it without any special exertion on its part, perhaps only in consequence of a mere wishing and hardly perceptible, purposeless

73

activity. Since, during this state, the organism requires but little libido for the outside world it will have so much the more at its disposal for its own body and its own sensations. Further development of the ego instincts, even though rendered possible through the identifications, is guided by the environment. Along with this, phylogeny, which gradually becomes activated in the course of the individual's development, also plays an important role.

In the case of illness, this clustering of the ego instincts around ego ideal constructions is interrupted and the perception of reality becomes distorted or undifferentiated. The ego instincts lose their goals. In the place of a highly developed ego, there is a more primitive one, and new identifications may set in which no longer respond to the reality of the outer world, but, rather, to the child's primitive ego ideal constructions and regressive instinctive attitudes. Projections will now follow in a much freer fashion.

I believe, therefore, that one should speak of a narcissistic developmental stage only when the outer world is perceived merely in its outline, when the organism itself is not sharply differentiated, and in the presence of a wide zone of indistinctness, which naturally is more closely related to the organism. During this state, the individual does not as yet busy himself with ego ideal constructions. The primitive environment attracts little libido to itself; the main portion of the libido remains with the body and with the zones of indefiniteness. We should speak of a narcissistic regression, on the other hand, in case the ego ideal constructions become largely destroyed, so that only the more primitive of these constructions retain their cathexes. Interest in and the libidinal significance of the environment suffers, in this condition, as does the conception of the outer world. Along with this, the grossly organic structures remain intact, as do the psychic constructions related to them, which in a general way assure perception of the organismal structure. These, as we will see later, become disordered in amentia; the zone of indefiniteness again becomes widened and the relation between organism and environment again becomes uncertain.

By narcissistic libido, we mean libido which is not attached to some part of the outer world, but remains attached to the body as well as to the ego ideal constructions. Delusions of grandeur presuppose the existence of an ego ideal construction. A wish to be

God precedes the delusion that one is God. A profound narcissistic regression with an extensive destruction of ego ideal constructions cannot go hand in hand with grandiose delusions. Neither can one designate as a grandiose delusion a primitive sense of omnipotence in the sense of a primary narcissism caused by repression. We should not confuse narcissistic cathexis with the narcissistic stage. The central manifestations of a narcissistic regression are, above all, hallucinations and the rearrangement and distortion of identifications so that they become more primitive and are no longer in accord with reality.

Ego ideals are connected with every stage of development, except the narcissistic stage. These are the prohibitive tendencies concerning pleasure in urinary and fecal function, belonging to early education and early primitive identification with the parents. The ego ideals develop in close correspondence with the various libidinal levels and find their final development by identifications connected with the Oedipus complex. Every one of these various identifications will add to the repressing tendencies and will have an influence on the direction of the repressions. Thus, there is a vertical structure of ego ideals which will vary in every individual and will be basic for the final direction of repressions. The ego ideals not only have this vertical organization, according to the age and stage of libidinal development, but they also have a horizontal organization. The child does not identify himself with only one person; there are the father, mother, nurse, brothers, and sisters, etc. Their attitudes toward life and toward the libidinal needs of the child necessarily differ. They will tend to agree in many ways, for instance, concerning elementary cleanliness or concerning a general tendency toward the outer world. But they will be different in the intensity with which they themselves act and with which they educate the child. In many ways, they may be totally different. Accordingly, in the child's ego formation, there will be parts which will be strong and coherent and other parts which will be unhomogeneous in their structure. Vertical and horizontal organization in the superego are of equal importance for the final organization of the personality, whether libidinal tendencies are freely acknowledged, merely repressed, replaced by their opposite, or replaced in a symbolic way. Even the type of symbolic substitution will be dependent upon the temporal organization of ego ideals and simultaneous identifications. It does not matter whether the superego formation is ascribed to the early stages, as it is by Klein, or to the oedipal stage, as it is by most analysts.

## INFANTILE SEXUALITY[2]

Infantile sexuality was first explored by Freud (1905). His observations center around the Oedipus complex. He observed that children between the ages of three and five show apparent sexual interest in the parent of the opposite sex. At the same time, death wishes are directed against the parent of the same sex. He observed that a child has sexual feelings which are not so very different from the sexual feelings of the adult. Although more primitive sexuality also plays a part, the sexuality of a child of this age centers around his genitals. This formulation was developed in the years around 1900, but has undergone considerable transformation since that time. Freud speaks, later, of the phallic organization, meaning that at this stage of development girls and boys alike are chiefly interested in the phallus. The other parts of the male sex organs do not have any specific interest for the child. The girl feels handicapped by the fact that she does not possess this valuable organ.

According to Freud, infantile sexuality also has a preoedipal stage. In this preoedipal stage, children show a general love of their own bodies (narcissism), i.e., oral tendencies, anal interests, and urethral interests. As I have previously indicated, Freud's own formulations concerning narcissism are not very definite. Sometimes it is considered as a very primitive stage preceding all other sexual manifestations and sometimes it is considered as a stage following other autoerotic tendencies. Most analysts differentiate two types of narcissism; a primary type occurring at birth, and a secondary type, which reunites the other autoerotic pleasures with the unit of the primary narcissism into a new entity. According to most of the current psychoanalytic formulations, narcissism merely has one's own body as the object. One loves one's self and nothing else. According to Freud, a real relation to love objects occurs only in the stage of the phallic organization. But toward whom and toward

[2] From Schilder (1942a).

what objects are the oral, anal, and urethral interests directed? Is there no object at all? Is there, at this stage, no definite relation to the father and mother? Such a theory can scarcely be considered satisfactory when one recognizes that a knowledge of one's own body is acquired in no way prior to a knowledge of the bodies of others (compare *Image and Appearance of the Human Body,* Schilder, 1935).

A further difficulty for psychoanalytic theory arises from the fact that the later attitude of Freud concerning sadism and masochism was rather indefinite. In earlier psychoanalytic theory, sadism and masochism were considered as partial desires of sexuality, which were directed chiefly against love objects of the same sex and chiefly in connection with anal tendencies. At the present time, sadism and masochism are considered as fusions between the death instincts and erotic tendencies. According to Freud the death instinct is never experienced directly, which is a rather difficult conception. But if, in the preoedipal stage, homosexual anal and sadistic tendencies prevail in relation to the love object, some conception of the love object must be present. Klein (1932), whom most of the English analysts follow, has indeed come to the idea that the Oedipus complex, and the object relations involved in it, originate not between three and five years, but much earlier, probably at the end of the first year.

Freud had always acknowledged the great importance of oral tendencies in sexual development. Abraham (1927) has taken up this idea and placed great emphasis on it. The first stage of sexual development was considered not only as oral but also as cannibalistic. A subsequent anal phase has also been strongly emphasized by him and an anal phase of special destructiveness was postulated. Klein has taken up the train of thought of Abraham and now comes to the formulation that the child is extremely aggressive around the first year and tries to attack the parents with all the methods at his disposal. According to her, the child wants to steal the penis of the father, which is supposed to be a part of the mother's body. For the child, the images of the parents are combined. Furthermore, he wants to scoop out the contents of the mother: her breasts, her food, and her intestines. In this attack, the child not only uses mouth and hands but also feces and urine, which he considers as poisonous weapons. Naturally, the child fears the counterattack of the parents, who may use the same tools. The child also introjects the violent parents into himself and, if not threatened by the outside, feels threatened by a terrifying superego, which is no less destructive than the outward forces.

Freud himself had protested against this conception and most analysts refuse to date the Oedipus complex at such an early age and also reject the assumption of the predominance of oral sadistic trends (compare, for example, the paper by Reich, 1936). At any rate, the age the Oedipus complex starts has become an open question. There can be no doubt that object relations of great strength can be observed in very early childhood. In the analysis of patients who have lost a parent at a very early age, vestiges of very strong object relations can be found fairly often. I share the doubts of many analysts concerning the correctness of other statements of Klein, which are based upon a method of rather arbitrary interpretation of the play of children. However, it is correct when she states that children are much more aggressive than we have thus far suspected—but she has completely neglected the fact that the child is also constructive and does not have only destruction at heart.

A further difficulty arises, in the modern development of psychoanalytic theory, from the problem of female sexuality in childhood. From the very beginning of his studies, Freud was very much impressed by the idea that children are interested only in the male sex organ. He found that the little girl considers her body to be incomplete and feels that she has been castrated, and that she envies the boy for his penis. He believed that boys have the same opinion about the inferiority of the female body without a penis. Freud based a good part of his opinions of female psychology on the castration complex. According to his opinion, half of mankind (or even a little more than half) must needs believe in its physical inferiority. More independent female psychoanalysts, like Horney (1924), stress the fact that a little girl soon gains the insight to realize that she has a valuable organ in which she can receive something. I myself have spoken about the female pride in "caves" of the body, which is no less original than the pride the boy displays in his penis. Freud had never accepted the fact that the little girl can be proud of her receptive organs, the possession of which she dimly perceives.

A rather queer defense for the basic tenets of Freud, concerning the female castration complex and female sexuality, came from Rado (1933). He stated that the girl, being aware of her defect, fantasies the possession of an illusory penis and creates a whole system in order to fortify herself in this illusion. Observation of children, and the careful analysis of adults, for me confirms Horney's (1924) point of view. The little girl is not merely concerned with the absence of a penis, but finds satisfaction in her own sex organs. She does not want a penis any more than the boy wants the female sex organs. Of course, the girl and the woman sometimes wish to be masculine and to be endowed with the corresponding organs, but the reverse is also true of the boy and the man. They also badly want the organs, the sexual experiences, and the possibility of the other sex.

It was one of the great discoveries of Freud that human beings suffer great anxiety concerning their sex organs. This is the castration complex. These fears are manifested at a very early age. Since the penis is a protruding organ the boy is afraid that it might be cut off, and since the girl is in possession of an opening she is afraid that it might either be occluded or forcibly enlarged. Since she has a vague conception that she has a receptacle of value in her body, she is afraid that this organ might be taken out of her body. The fact of the castration complex was first seen by Freud only from the point of view of the male and he never changed his opinion in this respect. However, it soon became evident to him that his original conception was too narrow, since human beings are not only afraid that something might happen to their sexual organs, but they are generally concerned with the integrity of the total body. It is true that the protrusions and holes physiologically and psychologically play the most important part in the body. This was hinted at in his original formulations and put on a broader basis in my studies on the body image. Protrusions and holes were then considered as symbolic of male and female sex parts.

The concept of the castration complex had to be enlarged; now we even speak about gastrointestinal and oral castration. In the current pcychoanalytic literature, it is suggested that the separation

79

of the child from the breast of the mother after the feeding act, and especially weaning, plays a part in the castration complex. The act of birth has even been considered as an experience of castration to the child, from whom the mother's body is taken away. The general tendency in present psychoanalytic literature is to consider every separation from the mother's body as castration. It is perfectly true that there is something in common in all infringements on the integrity of the body, but the body is more than just an annex to the sex parts. It has a definite value in itself, and it is arbitrary to view the integrity of the body merely as an aspect of the integrity of the sex parts. Some analysts emphasize the point that one can talk about a castration complex only in connection with the phallic phase, but what the phallic phase is and when it starts has become rather controversial. Personally, I prefer to speak about the wish for the integrity of the body and the fear of being dismembered. I am inclined to believe that this dismembering motive is of fundamental importance and the castration complex is merely a partial expression of it. The extension of the castration idea to separation from the mother is more or less arbitrary and does not take into consideration the complicated processes which are the basis for the constructive acts which lead to a well-developed body image of ourselves and others.

One cannot discuss the castration complex without studying the relation of the child to his mother and father. In the earliest stage of development of psychoanalytic theory, the father played a much greater role than he does today. This is a natural consequence of the fact that psychoanalysis, in its earliest years, was proud to drive the psychoanalysis of the adult back to the age between three and five. Around 1920, it was considered rather radical when Freud postulated that no analysis was complete which did not elucidate this period. Before the advent of Klein, it was not considered possible to analyze children younger than three or four years of age. It is true that, in 1918, Freud came, through analysis, to an infantile scene (observation of the parental intercourse) which had taken place when the patient was one-and-a-half-years old. Naturally, psychoanalysis, from its beginning, always had a tendency to go farther and farther back into early childhood. After all, Freud started with the study of adult sexuality and its traumatic sequences. The most important phase in psychoanalytic theory put the critical age between three and five. At the present time, psychoanalysts are concerned with still earlier experiences. For the child around the age of one year and younger the mother becomes more and more important. Nursing and weaning become the paramount problems. The penis of the father seems to be less important than the nipple of the mother, and the mother becomes the fundamental love object for both boys and girls. It is she who provides food.

In analysis today, the intake of food is considered only from the point of view of a sexual function. This is the easier way since, in the course of development of psychoanalytic theory, the function of the ego instincts has become less and less clearly defined. In the beginning of psychoanalytic theory, when the ego instincts were defined as serving the preservation of the self, the meaning was clear. It is not clear to say that the ego instincts are death instincts and, as far as can be observed, have only destructive functions. When, further, the ego instincts are considered as silent whereas the tumult of life comes merely from the libido, it becomes useless to speak any longer of the duality of instincts, which was previously one of the cornerstones of the Freudian theory. I am not interested in whether this theory of instincts is dualistic or not, but it seems to neglect the specific differences which exist between the human attitudes toward sex and toward self-preservation. Furthermore, if the ego instincts are silent, we are indeed faced with a pansexual theory otherwise justly decried by Freud. To consider food intake merely from the point of view of libido is arbitrary, to say the least.

In addition, psychoanalytic teachings concerning infantile sexuality all too frequently neglect the motor functions of the child. Beside motor functions serving the intake of food and aimed at the destruction of animate and inanimate objects, there are constructive motor activities, which appear in the play of children and in their actions toward persons and objects in real life.

Freud himself must have been aware of theoretical difficulties, since greater emphasis was subsequently put on the ego, which, in its psychoanalytic sense, was supposed to have a synthetic function: coordinating the diverse drives and demands which come from the libido (the id) and the demands of the superego (conscience). This synthetic function of the ego is in no way restricted to a particular

81

part of the personality, but is a general function of the psyche, which we have called constructive.

In spite of the objections of some analysts, I believe in the Freudian conception of the three parts of psychic apparatus. The connotations of the superego, ego, and id are valuable, since they point to important differences in various aspects of human personality. But one should be careful not to consider superego, ego, and id as definite entities to be treated as if they were three different persons.

One should never forget that the individual has a powerful motor apparatus directing him toward the world. The need of the child to get impressions from this world and the need to do something in it is really enormous. The child wants to do something in this world, wants the world to exist, and, especially, wants his love objects to be in it. Only against this background do the findings of psychoanalysts concerning infantile sexuality gain their full meaning. Infantile sexuality exists and every careful observation of the child clearly confirms this. Freud's assumption concerning the Oedipus complex is based on sound observation of the child as well as of the adult. Again and again the attempt has been made to prove that the genital sensations of the child are fundamentally different from the genital sensations of the adult and are devoid of true sexual character. Observation of children decidedly speaks against this attempt at evasion, which is repeated in the literature again and again (e.g., Harms, 1936).

The hostility of children against any rival in sex and love is also obvious. The statements of Freud concerning the Oedipus complex are therefore valid. Discussions among psychoanalysts show that they are no longer able to see the Oedipus complex as the distinct entity it appeared to be when Freud first discovered it. It is difficult to say when the Oedipus complex starts and it is also difficult to say that it ever declines, that the early attitude toward the parents ever loses its importance. Von Markuszewicz (1936) justly points to the many contradictions originating from any attempt to systematize our knowledge about the phallic organization of sexuality.

There cannot be any doubt that so-called "partial desires" exist. Mouth, urethra, and anus mediate sexual sensations, apparently of great strength and great importance. The descriptive statements of analysis which come chiefly from Freud himself are unquestionably true. It must be further emphasized that adult remembrances, in analysis, of feelings concerning the Oedipus complex and the "partial desires" confirm the interpretation we have derived from the observation of children. Erotic tendencies, connected with the skin, sensations, seeing, and being seen, cannot be doubted either. In observing children and analyzing adults, one comes to the conclusion that every function of the body and every part of the body does not serve erotic gratification only, and I am even inclined to extend this statement to the genitals proper, although I am conscious that this may be an overstatement. The older psychoanalytic formulation, which speaks of the narcissistic, oral, anal, sadomasochistic, homosexual, and genital levels, has the great advantage of being clear. I still think it is basically correct.

The theory of the oral stage of sexual development and oral libido is assuming greater importance in the newer development of psychoanalysis. It is, nevertheless, unsatisfactory. No attempt has been made to differentiate oral libido from the merely nutritional function of the mouth. On the whole, I think present-day psychoanalysis has neglected the fact that we have to eat in order to live and that does not prove the all-importance of oral libido. Balint (1935) has justly pointed to the great difficulties we incur when we view the scheme of sexual development too rigidly. It is also very difficult to finalize a clear insight into the nature of the object relations in the different stages of sexual development. Personally, I have very serious doubts concerning the strength of the aggressive tendencies in childhood and have indicated, in the course of these discussions, that there is a much stronger undercurrent of positive and constructive tendencies in the relation between the child and its surroundings than most psychoanalysts currently suspect.

Psychoanalysis has justly stressed that the relation to love objects changes during development. There is progress in the relation between the child and his love objects insofar as he learns more and more to appreciate them, and in the child as well as in the adult the development of genitality parallels the depth of relations to other human beings. In recognizing the place of infantile sexuality, psychoanalysts have put greater and greater emphasis on the earliest stages and have been more and more inclined to underrate the developments which take place later. The plasticity of infantile experience does not end after the first, second, or third year of life. Every new event and every new person, every new sexual contact, may become of paramount importance. Life is not merely a mechanical consequence of earlier experiences, although the patterns formed in early childhood may have a very great importance since it is difficult to dissolve them by new experiences. In studying infantile situations and infantile experiences, we should not forget that it is difficult to come to clear conclusions transcending the mere observational, since language—the most reliable sign system—is either absent or not developed in the young child. The play method used by Melanie Klein can easily mislead and one should never forget that the reaction of the child is deeply influenced by our own attitudes, by the experimental setup, and by the situation. One can address one's self to very different sides of a child's personality. In the analysis of adults, the difficulties in tracing back the steps to the experiences of the very first years of life are considerable. It is often impossible to attain direct remembrances, and one cannot always safeguard against errors in reconstruction. However, when used with sufficient care, the method is valid. It has enriched our knowledge of infantile sexuality, and its usefulness is far from being exhausted.

This, of course, is not a complete report on the present status of psychoanalytic knowledge of infantile sexuality. A mere repetition of the prevalent psychoanalytic theory was not intended. I have tried to show the historical development of the problems and the fundamental results obtained by the psychoanalytic methods.

## DANGER SITUATIONS—FEAR, GUILT AND ANXIETY[3]

The newborn child is helpless. He is completely dependent on the mother who puts him to the breast and supports him, feeds the child, and gives him protection. The child takes hold of the mother by grasping and sucking, and thereby also gets its nourishment. There is, in addition, babbling and crying, and a rather diffuse motility which undergoes a gradual process of adaptation. It is doubtful whether the child is aware of his complete dependence as

[3] From Schilder (1942a).

such. He may have a feeling that he has greater power and that his crying is an action which leads to the immediate satisfaction of being fed. Ferenczi (1913) speaks of levels in the development of the reality principle. We have reason to doubt whether the child feels as helpless as he actually is. He likes to sleep, but he also likes to be awake. He enjoys nursing, babbling, motility, and, indeed, urination and defecation. Furthermore, he also enjoys stroking and being stroked. He does something himself; he develops great activity in sucking, grasping, and all the efforts to maintain his equilibrium, and he does not seem satisfied without activities. He particularly enjoys being threatened in his equilibrium, unless the maintenance of equilibrium becomes too difficult.

From a merely descriptive point of view, we should say, therefore, that there are enjoyments and satisfactions, threats and deprivations; and there is experimentation with dangerous situations and an attempt to overcome them. The child does not merely want satisfactions—he has interests and strives for a better adaptation to his situation.

The preceding material may be expressed in tabular form as follows:

| Danger and Discomfort | The Positive Side | Experimentation |
|---|---|---|
| Pain, hunger, nausea, tension, itching, cold. | Well-being, food, enjoyment, absence of tensions. | Pleasure in small pain, and experimenting with a variety of sensations. |
| Loss of equilibrium. | Support. | Pleasure in rocking. |
| Restriction of movement. | Pleasure in moving. | Play in motility and babbling. |
| Fear of being deprived. | Security in food supply. | Play with deprivation. |
| Fear of dismembering. | Security of body integrity, aggression. | Play in aggressiveness. |

Psychoanalytic theory stresses the dangers in the life of the child and the life of human beings in general. It holds that individuals merely want to escape from dangerous situations and be in the state of the greatest amount of positive feelings and rest. The latter is especially emphasized. The basic psychoanalytic attitude, although not formulated in this way, largely coincides with the point of view of Schopenhauer, who believed that there are no genuine satisfactions and that pleasure originates only when we have escaped displeasure. An active interest in experimentation and a turning to the outer world in a spirit of trial and error investigation, guided by an inherent interest in the world, are generally neglected factors. It is my opinion that, in human existence, danger, enjoyment, and experimentation have the same importance, and although linked with each other, no one of the three can be eliminated as an important, distinct dynamic. In relation to the danger situations, we meet three fundamental attitudes: fear; anxiety (and dizziness); and guilt.

We shall first consider fear. Fear arises when a definite situation in the outer world threatens definite damage. Contrary to many current opinions, the child is directed toward the outer world from the earliest stages of his development. There are threatening persons, threatening animals, and threatening inanimate objects, especially loud noises, such as thunder. Later on, the same fear may be related to something inside the body. Isaacs (1933) reports on childhood hypochondriac fears in which the organs were experienced as wild beasts; but these fears were based on a frightening incident which had occurred previously. The threatened damage is loss of support, loss of love (love, according to Watson, is correlated to stroking; we would rather define it as a series of skin sensations due to the motor activity of another person), loss of food and clothing, or loss of the integrity of the body. According to Klein (1932), the child feels threatened not only by the muscular aggression of the adult but also by his urine and feces. To a child, the mother is a continuous source of food. This is not only because the child is nursed—the mother also gives other types of food. Love experiences do not consist solely in getting food, but also in being stroked, kissed, bathed, and protected against the cold, either by the warmth of the mother's body or by clothes. One might say that the three fears—loss of support, loss of love, loss of food—are very closely connected with each other. The loss of integrity of the body is related with fear of attack by another person. But children also consider deprivations as attacks, so that all the fears of childhood can be summarized in the fear of attack, since the fear of deprivation is merely a subgroup of this general fear.

We speak of anxiety when the individual feels threatened, but not by a definite object—he is not quite clear what is threatening him. The analysis of both children and adults has shown that the contents of anxiety and fear are basically identical. If we study cases with anxiety neuroses, we find two definite types. In the more common type, the anxiety centers around the fear of a threatened separation from the love object, especially by sudden death. In the second type, there is a fear of dismembering and annihilation. The case of anxiety neurosis previously discussed combines features of these two types.

Any kind of danger provokes aggressive tendencies and any type of aggression is connected with the fear of a counterattack. If restriction of motility provokes rage, one may suspect that a counterattack is expected. Fear of punishment may occur when a child has learned that other children's parents punish forbidden acts by deprivation. The child may either realize that there is retaliation for his own aggressiveness or he may feel that he is caught in an intricate system of orders and warnings, which he does not understand, but which he must obey to escape punishment.

The feeling of guilt originates when the individual feels that he deserves punishment. When there is a clear feeling of guilt in connection with the fear of punishment, the right to punish and the justification for the punishment is fully acknowledged. Often the punishment is not only expected but is wished for, since the expectation of punishment is still worse than the punishment itself. Also the performance of the punishment may soothe the parent and so renew the love relation between the parent and the child. We owe our knowledge of this process to Freud (1919) and Rado (1928). Finally, one may identify himself completely with the punishing agent outside the self and erect a superego inside, and then administer punishment to himself either in thoughts only or in action. This feeling of guilt may be either conscious or unconscious. Feelings of guilt may originate from every action which may lead to the disapproval of the parents or the parent substitutes, outside or inside of ourselves. Freud has stated that feelings of guilt originate only from aggressive tendencies for which one wants to be punished, but I think that this formulation is too narrow. Since the feeling of guilt is connected with a danger which is not fully perceived, feelings of guilt and anxiety are often met at the same time.

I have discussed the problem of dizziness in detail in a previous communication, so that only a few remarks will be sufficient here. Dizziness seems to occur chiefly when the dangerous situation is connected with the loss of support and the fear of losing one's equilibrium. These terms should be accepted in their broadest sense, since dizziness may result from every difficulty in orienting oneself in relation to the outer world, as well as the difficulties of moral orientation in general. Our patient, a severe case of depersonalization, complained of dizziness—as do all depersonalization cases—expressing her great inner difficulty in getting into proper relations with others and with herself.

Until now, we have followed rather closely the descriptions and formulations of Freud and his pupils, who have indeed shown the great insecurity under which human beings labor. The question remains, how do human beings in general and children in particular, protect themselves against this danger? According to Freud, they must either renounce relations with the outer world to some degree and regress, or they must create a different world by projecting into the outer world problems which are within themselves, and changing the outer world to suit their own desires. By these methods, they desperately struggle for security.

According to our whole formulation, there is no reason to believe that the primary state of individuals is one of insecurity and danger. Individuals seek self-protection after they have been threatened, and they approach the world primarily in a spirit of interest and experimentation. It is true that, at the beginning of life, the child is often threatened and hindered in this state of experimentation. He is not only threatened by the dangers described, but he is particularly threatened by aggressive love and smothering by the adult. Adults have the tendency, mentioned above, to not respect the child as an entity, but to use him merely to fulfill their own desires, as a neurotic toy. We know that children desperately strive to protect themselves against this approach; and that which we may call the aggressiveness of the child is merely his attempt at self-defense in the erotic and social spheres. In the relations between children and adults, we may ask, what function does the relationship serve for the child and for the adult? In the relation between adult and child, there must be a way of giving love and helping each other which does not merely push the child into a neurotic and dependent position. Genuine tendencies to help one another are present in the child as well as in the adult. Naturally, the adult has the greater possibilities and responsibilities in this respect.

When the child and the adult experiment in the world, they have a genuine pleasure in this world and in its existence. They want to have a world outside, and this world consists of individuals who are acknowledged as social and sexual human beings. It is true that such a development occurs only during constructive efforts and experimentation. The genuine tendency to help these entities belongs to this process. It cannot be denied that a continuous process of identification and projection takes place, by which the individual builds up the outer world and persons therein, but the line of these reconstructions is drawn by their reality. Real satisfaction can be gained only when we have succeeded in building, in this way, a personality outside of ourselves not as we want it, but as it actually is. Of course, we approach this by a process of gradual approximation. Quite in the same way as perception functions in the deepest trends of this process, the outside person is at work too. Klein has made the interesting and correct observation that children make a differentiation between the good mother and the bad mother. They are not the same to children. In neurosis and psychosis, one may find the same mechanism. One of my patients with a severe obsessional neurosis felt that an actress, in whom she was homosexually interested, changed her appearance continually. She was sometimes taller, sometimes shorter, sometimes slim, and sometimes broad; even the color of her eyes changed. An eleven-year-old Negro girl said, when her mother called for her at the children's society, "This is not my mother; my mother is taller and has bigger eyes." She persisted in this reply.

Now every human being has different aspects. When we return from a voyage, those persons whom we especially love are not at all

identical with our expectations. We are astonished and it is sometimes very difficult to bring the two pictures together. At the moment we are separated from a person, our fantasy starts working
and rearranging the data, or a reconstruction takes place. This reconstruction does not lead to a picture which is identical with
reality. Other human beings can hardly be perceived "as they actually are" and their appearance changes with changes in our attitudes. Naturally, they too actually change. They wear different
clothes. For example, it is sometimes difficult for a man to unite the
picture of a woman he has slept with with his view of the same
woman under different circumstances. One is different in the morning, at noon, and in the evening. One is different if shaved or un-
shaved. If individuals are followed over a long span of their lives,
these changes merely become more obvious. The mental pictures
of parents are liable to change more than any other picture. The
mother of a suckling, the mother of a two- or three-year-old, and
the mother of a five-year-old are not only very different from each
other, but are also different from the mother of an adult. In every
phase of the development of the child, the mother changes. Or, to
put it paradoxically, the mother is a series of different pictures.
The difference between the single pictures may be enormous. In a
sense, we deal with a strip of pictures. Even the single picture has
several phases for the child. In every moment, the mother fulfills
different functions. She is the mother who gives food, clothes, and
caresses, which are three facets of the good mother, but she also
denies food, support, and caresses, and these are facets of the bad
mother. Punishment is merely another form of deprivation. One
strip is of the good mother and another is of the bad mother. It is
probable that these strips are always in relation to each other.
However, in the course of development, the constructive process
integrates these strips more and more, and after puberty they are
fairly well constructed into a unified picture of a fellow human
being.

Severe emotional problems beset patients who disrupt the picture
of a beloved person into a multiplicity of pictures: the obsessional
patient was torn between love and hate in every one of her human
relations; the Negro girl had severe emotional conflicts with her
mother. Often, life is seen as a series of threats directed against the

individual in every phase of existence. This is a distorted view and is closely connected with the concept that the individual wants merely satisfaction and rest. World and experience are indeed disturbing if one merely wants to withdraw and rest.

However, human beings have a genuine interest in the world, in action, and in experimentation. They derive a deep satisfaction when they venture into the world. They do not experience reality as a threat to existence. Organisms, and especially human organisms, have a genuine feeling of safety and security in this world. Threats come merely from specific situations and deprivations. Even then, discomfort and danger are experienced as passing points, which finally lead to a new security and safety in touch with the world. Human beings, furthermore, are not merely interested in other human beings from the point of view of getting satisfaction from them. Just as they want independence, socially and erotically, for themselves, so they also want social and sexual independence for other human beings. It is true that contradictory tendencies to bring this other being into a subservient relation do exist. Even the picture of another human being may be split in two. But the tendency to help the other person and to give gifts is the final recognition of the other human being as a personality.

A case which has been rather thoroughly analyzed may serve as an illustration:

The patient suffered from such severe anxiety that she could not stay alone in her apartment; she felt that only certain persons, such as her husband and some of her friends, could protect her. With the approach of anxiety, she felt she might go completely to pieces, scream, and become violent or insane. She had had an early insecurity in walking. Her mother did not give her sufficient supportive help. She was particularly afraid of walking on an inclined terrain. Previously, she had experienced dizziness and vomiting in the subway. Although these experiences were partially directed against the mother, there was probably, in this respect, an organic basis for her insecurity that could not be ignored. The insecurity in walking and equilibrium were reinforced by erotic insecurity. Her mother was possessive but not demonstrative, and the erotic advances of the patient to her parents were rejected, especially by the father.

From stories by a Polish maid, concerning burglars and violence, and from cruel behavior by this maid and her mother, further insecurity originated. This actual threat became the more dangerous since it was not counterbalanced by erotic satisfaction. Early sexual play with the brother had merely increased her feelings of guilt. There was a definite fear of being dismembered, but she also felt exposed to another threat— that she might be exploded from inside by too big a penis, by a child, by a drug, or by an enema. There was also an enormous hunger reaction; she wished to ingest huge quantities of food and to be stuffed up. It was of paramount importance for her whether or not she was empty or hollow inside. She had the wish to have the male sex organ in her vagina. Her orgasms were wonderful feelings that her insides were turned out. She had the feeling that an orgasm was something definite inside her, like a substance which merely came out. Thus she felt threatened from inside and out.

In our previous discussion we have, in some degree, neglected the threats which come from the inside of the body of the child and which manifest themselves by tensions. It is characteristic, in the thinking of the child, that the inside of the body is generally regarded as something which has been stuffed into the body. The studies of D. Wechsler and myself (1935) have shown that the young child believes the inside of his body to consist of the food which has been taken in.

Only the presence of the love object can protect this patient against the inside and outside dangers. We would not be justified in saying, as does Klein, that the presence of the love object assures her merely that a love object is not destroyed, although this point has some justification. It is incorrect to assert that the love object allows the projection of the destructive inner self and so diminishes the danger of being destroyed by terrible forces inside. The patient's anxiety consists of being alone and going to pieces. There is no fear of dying. This latter point, seemingly, belongs to an anxiety neurosis type in which the object relation is less burdened with destructive elements. The patient occasionally experienced the analyst as thirty feet or miles away. This is less an expression of fear of being separated from the analyst than the expression of destructive tendencies against him. The patient was proud of her strength by which she might destroy. She felt she had enough weapons of destruction so that the penis was not necessary for her. However, she sometimes used her toes to make figures and to express her feelings. From an early age, there was masturbation connected with enormous anxieties and feelings of guilt. For her, masturbation meant destruction of her sex parts and an inability to conceive. For a while she felt that her breasts were hardened. In early childhood, she thought children were born from them. This is an expression of the wish for a child. After she was married, she developed an exophthalmic goiter. Interestingly, one of her first remembrances consisted of her brother biting her neck. (This was partially a family tradition.) In the period before puberty, there was mutual masturbation with another girl. Masturbation was connected with storytelling and ended with a strong desire to urinate. There was also mutual explorations of their bodies, centering around the breasts and urine. The feelings of guilt connected with these activities were as outspoken as the fear of being caught by the mother. She could not recall the content of the stories.

Her aggressiveness made it difficult for her to let a man take the initiative. She also felt that, taken all-in-all, there were no real men (in her dreams, the famous he-men of the screen appeared as feminine). She did not want to give much food to her guests and there was also a lack of sexual generosity. She did not want to give in to a man unless the man gave himself completely. As in all cases with anxiety neurosis, there was also a fear of being trapped. She did not want to be restricted in her motility; in addition, being trapped also meant for her to be deprived of power, to be included in something like the mother's womb. Her neurosis started shortly after the death of her father, when a story of infection with gonorrhea was told, which reminded her of the dangers of sex and masturbation.

Any attempt to give a halfway complete interpretation of such a complicated case would fill a volume. The case at least offers clear insight into danger situations. She was afraid of being cut to pieces, being deprived of her genitals, especially being emptied, exploded from the inside, and hardened in the body. Furthermore, she feared being crushed, incarcerated, and deprived of her motility. She also feared not getting food or enough love. Threats came chiefly from the parents, from the brother (partially also from an older sister), and from a Polish maid. Each one might also put something danger-

93

ous into her. Furthermore, she was afraid of her aggressive tendencies, which might increase the aggressiveness of others. She wished to take the part of the aggressor, which was chiefly experienced as masculine. The love objects outside reassured her of their existence. They were less dangerous in reality than in fantasy. She had not destroyed them as yet. She also wished for their existence since she wanted to have objects independent of herself. She really needed love objects who, in spite of everything, and especially in spite of her strength, had remained independent.

Human problems are primarily problems in the world, and by identification with the dangerous object an inside danger may follow, but this is merely a reflection of the outside danger. It is true that the individual wants to go back to outside objects. It is also true that all threatening dangerous situations are in close relation with primitive wishes. The patient may have felt that an attack from her mother was at least some form of close contact with her, and to take a part of her mother or father into herself might have been a deep satisfaction, although connected with untold dangers. Still she suffered severely. Unconscious satisfaction involved some cruelty toward the patient. She had tried hard to get her satisfaction in the way of a child undaunted by the dangers and pain connected with it. This attempt survived in her neurotic symptoms. Her final attempt to get satisfaction, as a person, had failed. When she was able to get some gratification by ruling over the persons around her and by making them tributaries, she merely tried to adapt herself to a defect in her relations to the world and in her satisfactions. The statement that a neurosis is a symbolic satisfaction of infantile desires has to be qualified.

## SOCIAL AND PERSONAL DISORGANIZATION[4]

In the first few months, or even years, the child finds himself in a distressing situation. He is completely dependent upon forces unknown to him. Food is given him at intervals, which he cannot understand. He experiences hunger without being in possession of definite methods of getting relief. Furthermore, he is exposed to uncanny gravitational influences which sooner or later lead to

[4] From Schilder (1937a).

94

painful experiences. In the process of continuous experimentation, the child has to discover what he can do in this dangerous world, which threatens him continuously with deprivation of food and love and an encroachment upon the integrity of his body. He needs the continuous guidance and help of those around him. The child needs sensual gratification through being stroked, kissed, cleaned; that is, he needs tender care or, in one word, love. He also has to find out by what methods he can gain these gratifications.

The child is continually experimenting. He has to learn about the quality of objects, as well as the quality of his own body and the bodies of others. Lauretta Bender and I have observed that children of three and four years put objects against the wall and expect that they will stick there. They experiment further with configurations and symmetry: putting toy soldiers in series and groups, reorganizing the groups and pushing the soldiers down, having one group fight the other, etc. They experiment with holes and openings. How much can one put into a box? How can one take it out? How many soldiers, how many little cars and animals, can one crowd into a bigger car? What is the significance of the edge of a table or background? Experimentation of this kind takes place continuously. Such experimentation is also necessary when the child wants to build up the experience of his own body or his body image (Schilder, 1935).

By trial and error and continuous experimentation, the child comes to an appreciation of the forms of the outer world. He learns about the consistency, weight, and size of objects. In the same way, he has to learn about the consistency, size, weight, and texture of his own body and the bodies of others. Children are not theoretical scientists. For the child, experimentation means gaining security concerning dangers and, furthermore, the gratification of power concerning objects. He tries to reach gratification of his needs concerning food and love. It is evident that he has to experiment in a social way in order to get this gratification. Gratification and security come to the child chiefly through adults who take care of him. His direct contact with objects is comparatively limited at the beginning of his life, and, even in these contacts, the social factor is paramount.

In Pavlov's work with conditioned reflexes, salivation at first occurs with almost any sound; individual and social experimentation is in the process of formation. When a conditioned stimulus is elaborated by any specific agent then all related stimuli have somewhat the same effect. When, however, the chosen stimulus is repeated many times, these extraneous stimuli become gradually ineffective. In the process of so-called "differential inhibition," very specific and very fine differentiations take place.

Differential inhibition is best obtained when a sound of a chosen wave length is followed by food, whereas other sounds of different wave lengths are not followed by the unconditioned stimulus. Differential inhibition is a process of trial and error which leads to a better insight into the quality of the object (in this instance, the wave length of the sound). The differential process also leads to a more appropriate answer, by the organism, to the situation at hand, in both the motility and the vegetative spheres. Differentiation takes place under the guidance of experience. Experience is construction and reconstruction under the guidance of biological needs or through the guidance of the goals and aims of the individual. One might say that, at first, the child forms general attitudes, but it is better to say that he transfers attitudes which have been successful in one case and learns, merely by trial and error, whether such a transfer of attitudes is successful or not. The dog has no reason to differentiate between the sounds of different wave lengths until it finds out that only specific sounds are followed by food. Children primarily use connotations and words in the same way. One child said, "People die of pneumonia." He had apparently heard, from adults, of a specific case where this had happened, and he had no reason to think anything else about death before having new experiences with the subject. This is probably the structure of every general connotation, which only gets its final meaning by continuous contact with reality.

Our psychological approach therefore stresses the gradual shaping of experiences under the influence of action and trial and error. Configuration is the result of a continual interplay between action and impression; experienced constructions are often given up for new constructions. This whole process is directed by the vital drives, which get their final meaning only through continuous interchange with other human beings. Socialization is, therefore, the fundamental form of human experience. The attitude of the adult will be decisive for the child, either in increasing fear and insecurity or in giving the child a higher degree of security. Only the child who receives encouragement will dare to continue with the experimentation which makes a relation with the external world necessary. Only this continuous experimentation will help the child to find his way to lasting gratifications. Every discouragement will provoke a paralysis of the trial-and-error probing mechanism. Attitude and connotation will be the chance result of one situation and the child will be badly adapted. One might almost say that, in such a case, connotations and words will not convey a clear meaning. Discouragements therefore lead to wrong attitudes. There is an inclination, at the present time, to underrate the intellectual life. However, connotations and words, ideas and ideologies, are merely one aspect of the total attitudes, which are, naturally, also emotional attitudes. Fears, inhibitions, and complexes also express themselves in the wrong way of thinking, which may be either conscious or unconscious in the psychoanalytic sense.

Psychoanalysis has shown that, in the sexual field, early deprivation, intimidation, and punishments lead to severe distortions in personal development. One might say that this early complication in the child's life interrupts his process of testing the world and so leads to attitudes which are fundamentally wrong. As Freud has shown, such an event, in an individual's development, may remain without visible consequence until an actual situation, implying deprivation or punishment, reveals the aberration in the individual's approach to the world. And so, a neurosis may be defined as a wrong attitude resulting from the interruption of the process of testing and probing. I have emphasized that, from earliest childhood, this process is guided by relations to other people. The attitudes of the mother are of fundamental importance for the whole development of the child. We have characterized deprivation of food and love and encroachment upon bodily integrity (by tying down, castration, mutilation, and pain) as the two fundamental dangers to the child. Both might provoke wrong attitudes in the child; either an attitude of withdrawing and giving up with an incomplete mastery of the situation or an attitude of blind aggression. Therefore, the attitudes of the parents lay the groundwork for the child's social

97

adaptation. The child who is badly adapted, from a social point of view, will be a continuous element of disorganization in society (which after all consists of individuals).

Why has the erotic aggressiveness of parents (such as spoiling, and the stressing of partial tendencies in their children) not been mentioned as a source of social maladaptation of the child? Such attitudes of the parents bring the child into a passive position, force him to premature and one-sided attitudes, and hinder the free process of trial and error which the child would undertake if not under specific erotic pressure.

It has been mentioned that a free process of differentiation of testing can be interrupted, checked, and hindered in every phase of a human being's life in which deprivation and threat become paramount. Deprivation and threat to the single individual are the characteristics of a dissociated and disorganized society. If we study the development of the child, we often see that deprivation and threat are formidable only because insight into the true nature of the danger has not been gained. The modern psychotherapeutic procedures instigated by Janet, Breuer, and Freud, force the individual to acquire insight into the structure of a danger situation, make it less terrifying, and so remove its paralyzing influence. Individuals threatened too much by real or imaginary danger may develop a complicated and dangerous defense system as a counter-reaction. This defense system may lead to an attitude of cruelty in relation to other human beings, to acts of dismembering and physical violence, or to acts which deprive others of food or love. Even the neglect of other human beings' justified claims to obtain satisfaction in food and economic values in general, and in love or social values, may make such an individual dangerous to society.

A disorganized society is a society which neglects the justified claims of the individual to a free development of his attitudes and potential. Then he will not be able to attain gratification in the sphere of food, love, and security, economic as well as emotional. Such a disorganized society will provoke personality distortions in the single individual, who either does not understand the threat and answers with increased counteraggression or is hindered in his development, by the threat. These wrong attitudes in adults will be transmitted to children and will be detrimental to their erotic and social development. The distorted children will, in turn, add to the disorganization of future society.

On the basis of such a psychological approach it is logical to attempt to deal with the disorganization by individual and social therapy. The individual has to be led back to the point where—threatened by insecurity, deprivation, and destruction—he has given up free emotional development and testing. Very often this point is marked by wrong ideologies concerning sex, morals, and other attitudes. This point is, furthermore, marked by incomplete understanding of the meaning of work and by substitutions of vague general connotations and phrases for observation of situations and facts. This is the deepest meaning of psychoanalytic procedure itself, and similar procedures which have originated from psychoanalysis.

I am in deep sympathy with the opinions of Ogden (1934) and Korzybski (1933) when they state the importance of the correct understanding and meaning of words. The individual has to understand his ideology, his mode of living, and his aims and goals, with their historical development and relation to the problems of society. This process of understanding is not merely intellectual, but has an emotional basis. It is, after all, based on the human being as a totality. In the individual case, psychoanalytic technique or a technique similar to psychoanalysis will be indispensable in the searching process, which will help the individual to give up attitudes developed under threat and deprivation. From a social point of view, there is the task of making individuals understand their words and ideologies and making them recognize where they encroach on the security of others, thus adding to the general disorganization of society. Analysis of the destructive and depriving social ideology, on the basis of what we know through analysis of the individual, is one of the paramount tasks of sociological psychology. Insight, the psychological attitude of one individual, has immediate repercussions on other individuals and should not remain merely a theoretical insight. Those who fail in this respect should be relentlessly forced to gain insight into the genesis of their ideologies. This procedure, according to the optimistic belief of psychoanalysis, should involve the cure of the individual who has contributed to the disorganization of society.

Some instances may illustrate these principles. There is a type of juvenile criminal who has been pushed into a passive and dependent position by weakness of body, severity of education or the aggressive tenderness of his parents. In the mind of the child, passivity is linked with the danger of being attacked. This is reflected in the whole body. The openings of the body, especially the anus, react with sensations, since the superior force of the attacker merges with something in the body or may even disrupt the unity of the body. Another line of response consists of fears concerning the individual's own reason for aggression—the penis. Passivity, weakness, and homosexuality become, in this way, connected with one another. The formation of such a complex is favored by the general tendency of our society to coordinate strength with masculinity and weakness with femininity. Such attitudes pervade family life. A reaction sets in against this enforced passivity. The defense measures will become stronger as the individual is increasingly deprived of reasonable satisfaction in the erotic and economic spheres, and as the economic system increasingly corroborates the pressures exerted by the family on the individual during childhood. The restricted action may appear in the child as more-or-less severe behavior problems, and in the adolescent and adult as an action of alleged strength and courage (assault or holdup), in which the aggressive weapon (knife or gun) symbolizes not only increase in strength, but also increase in virility (penis).

Asocial acts of this kind are based on an individual history of the type described, but they take place only in a specific setting, where the individual finds ideologies of a similar type and is assured of social approval of the asocial act, at least by a small group. It is even sufficient that an *imaginary* group of this type should exist. In such a series of events, the following social and individual events are of importance: (1) a wrong appreciation of physical strength; (2) a wrong ideology concerning masculinity; (3) a faulty judgment concerning social forces and the importance of the individual's own social group; (4) a lack of insight into the factors that provoke the individual's revolt against his parents, which is transmitted to society; (5) attitudes of the individual which are the result of aggressive and erotic tendencies of the parents in relation to the child; (6) the family pressures which enforced passivity; (7)

economic deprivation imposed upon the family and transmitted to the child; and (8) the ideologies of the parents and their group, and the ideologies of the group in which the individual lives. This is not and cannot be a systematic discussion of all the factors involved, but it may open the way to a theory which takes social factors more into consideration.

# IV

# Language, Thought, and Symbol Formation

## THE DEVELOPMENT OF LANGUAGE[1]

Observing language development in the child, we note that first he expresses his sensations and feelings by crying, then follows a period of babbling, then one of voice imitating, then the beginning of language comprehension, and finally, the use of language for communicating and naming. In this language development, there is a period in which the child utters speech sounds taken over by imitation, but their meaning, as such, does not come into his consciousness. In this period, the child produces concept signs simply as memories and does not conceive of them as signs. C. and W. Stern (1922) refer to these as sham concepts and write: "The child applies his words not only to individual objects exclusively, as for instance to the mother, but also to a series of similar objects, as for instance the word 'uncle' to all men, or 'pip-pip' to all flying creatures." Furthermore, the early phases of the child's language development show a progressive change in use and meaning of one and the same word. Meaning is mostly extended to other instances (occasionally it is limited to fewer) or it is transferred to a new instance and the previous meaning is given up.

According to C. and W. Stern, at this stage the child is not aware that each word has the function of continuously representing one definite meaning; to him, naming is a momentary reaction and previous experiences have only a subliminal aftereffect. First word

[1] From Schilder (1924).

meanings are only symbols of familiarity based on associations. The child's behavior in extending to insects the "pip-pip" learned in seeing flying birds, for example, may be described as follows: The child directs himself toward a category of things, but has no interest in differentiating within it, and produces for the entire category a concept sign not familiar to us—but to him it means, more or less, "flying." However, he does not equate nor confuse birds and insects. This is an example of how concept signs change; the problem of changes in meaning in the psychology of language is mostly one of changing concept signs, rather than of actual changes of meaning. Aphasic disorders also affect the concept signs primarily, though the disorder of these, in turn, does not affect thinking itself. Thus, the view that thinking and speaking are identical must be emphatically rejected. Rather, there is a path from thinking to speaking which is to be apprehended only by studying the relation of the word to its meaning.

All languages have speech sounds which imitate the sound qualities of things, but in more advanced languages there are fewer of these sounds. The speech sound, in general, does not map the qualities of the object it refers to. Other speech sounds do, with certain affects and moods, as suggested by their physiological organization; these are called "vocal gestures." Gestures are closely related to language; there is a natural language of gestures. It is probable that sounds which coincide with gestures of the mouth region play a role in the genesis of speech.

Naturally, these two factors can explain only the joint appearance of certain psychological content and certain sounds, but not the meaning relationships between the sounds and what they designate. To explain this relationship, we must assume a specific act, the meaning function, or as it has been less fortunately called, the symbolic function of the spoken word. The language training of the deaf-mute Helen Keller was sharply divided into two phases by her startling experience of suddenly becoming aware of meaning. Yet, the process by which the child acquires speech must not be equated with the evolution of speech. It has been proven that the child does not form words independently, but builds his language by what adults relay to him. Stumpf's (1900) son had an idiosyncratic language, but the basic material was derived from the language of

103

the environment. The ontogenetic development of the child's language is thus by no means a reproduction of phylogenetic development, since the child finds himself given a particular linguistic milieu. Or, in the language of biology, a cenogenetic change has taken place in the evolutionary series.

The function of the child's language apparatus is more transparent than the adult's, and, therefore, in it we obtain a glimpse of how he adopts the language of his environment, and also of the modes of functioning which play a significant role in language development in general. Romanes' well-known example, in which the word "quack" is transferred from a duck to a coin with an eagle on it, and then to all coins, represents in striking form the process of change in meaning, which plays such a great role in language. The child's adopting the language of his environment presupposes his inherent capacity to do so. The growing child's predilection for imitating a particular language, replete with sound imitations, interjections, and vocal gestures, which adults convey to him, must rest on peculiarities of infantile language which bear on phylogenesis.

## PSYCHOLOGY OF LANGUAGE[2]

It seems worthwhile to consider language from the viewpoint of constructive psychology. A newborn child is rarely completely quiet. When awake, he is always making some noise, either crying or screaming. Soon the child starts babbling, which is apparently a more-or-less playful action. Even deaf children start to babble, but do not continue. Imitation of what the child hears from others comes comparatively late. The child understands language before he can use it. An awareness of emotion as expressed in words and an appreciation of the melody of speech precedes the understanding of the content of words. The connection between words and objects is formed gradually, as the name of the object and the object itself are brought simultaneously to the attention of the child. This is the mechanism of the so-called conditioned reflex[3] and the child reacts,

---

[2] From Schilder (1936).

[3] Schilder has shown (1929a) that Pavlov's term is not appropriate. Conditioned reflexes are not reflexes in the common sense; however, he here uses Pavlov's phraseology in order to facilitate understanding.

in many respects, to the presence of words as if the object, as such, were also present; the word has become a sign of the object. The object is not merely a sensory and intellectual impression but a summons to a set of actions. These actions may be voluntary movements of striated muscles, but they may also consist of involuntary innervation of smooth muscles and glands, as in Pavlov's experiments, where, when a conditioned reflex is formed, there occurs not only the secretion of saliva but also a change in the total motor reaction of the dog. When the food stimulus has been connected with a light signal, the light becomes a stimulus for food. When the signal comes, the organism prepares itself for food. This same relation exists between the word and the object which it means. The word functions as a signal for an attitude of the organism, which may express itself either in an action or in a change in the innervation of visceral organs, in the broadest sense. The solution to the problem of the meaning of a sentence, which has been so puzzling to investigators, will be found in the preparedness of the organism toward the object promised by the signal. This preparedness is not merely a physiological state, but is perceived by the individual.

Logicians have always declined further analysis of the signal function of words, by saying that the variety of sensations, representations, and feelings, and their changing character, indicated an occurrence in psychological experience which was completely different from meaning in the logical sense. Attempts to relate meaning with functions of the psyche which are better understood from an empirical point of view have been decried as psychologistic. If we take action based on experience and attitude toward objects as the unit, objections of this kind are not possible, and the highly artificial distinction between impression and expression must be given up. The irregular sequence of disconnected shreds of representations and images, and the irregular fluctuations of feeling and feeling tones, have significance only in being a part of a total situation, which culminates either in action or in preparedness for action. Actions are indeed definite, even more definite than the preparedness for action; this, in our opinion, constitutes meaning.

This discussion of the signal function of the word takes for granted that language exists and is merely transmitted by the adult to the child. Watson (1930) and Russell (1927) have emphasized that words act as signals in the process of conditioning. Russell is of the opinion that the structure of sentences must be considered differently. He thinks it cannot be explained in a behavioristic way. He believes that the correct use of relational words—that is, of sentences—involves what may be correctly termed perception of form (this involves a definite reaction to a stimulus which is a form). The first words of children usually have the significance of sentences. The child expresses pleasure by the word which names the object. The word "sugar" says: "Look how nice it is; I would like to have it." Sugar and spinach are not simple data of experience which wander into the child's head; both objects have been built up by a series of constructive processes, not only in the child's mind, but also in the child's actions. We speak of an object merely when some kind of stability in action has been reached. A word which designates an object of relative stability becomes a reliable basis for action and a definite entity or concept. If you forget that objects are products of construction in which trial and error play such an important part, and you forget about the motor part in every perception, you will misunderstand the sign function of language and the meaning of meaning (see Ogden and Richards, 1925).

One may ask how words have acquired such signal functions for man and why man has decided to take words, and not movements of the fingers or of the toes, as signals for objects. To get an answer to this age-old question it is necessary to go to observations on children who have not, as yet, acquired the signal function of words, through education. This is the period of spontaneous crying and babbling. The crying of the child is an expression of biological needs. It very often ceases when the biological needs are satisfied. Bernfeld (1925) justly calls it an instinctive action for a definite aim. The crying stops when the child starts sucking. From the beginning, the oral apparatus is the center of important biological functions. Taking food is connected with noises; the smacking of lips, for example. When sucking is replaced by chewing and biting, other specific noises occur. To make these remarks more graphic, consider a dog devouring its food. Delboeuf (1901) relates the "Ma" sound, which plays such an important part in the early utterances of children, to the sucking movement of the child. Wundt (1904) emphasizes the fact that the organs of the mouth which serve eating are named by sounds produced by the same function. It is possible to hypothesize that speech is the expression of an oral tendency to get hold of objects, and thus expresses the wish to devour the object. Darwin emphasized the importance of speech and singing in the sexual activities of animals. The mouth and vocal organs serve manifold biological needs, and this, their primary function, enables them to produce signals for objects.

In babbling, the child experiments with sounds. According to Esper (1933), author of an excellent paper on language, the stimuli which lead to babbling are chiefly internal. So-called stimuli are probably never only internal or only external. We react to the world according to our internal state. There is no purely internal state because we are always directed toward the world. Internal and external are correlated with each other. Once he realizes that his efforts can produce sounds, the child tries to reproduce the sounds he hears. In experiments on acoustic imagination, Parker and I (Parker and Schilder, 1935) found subjects who could imagine the sound of a tuning fork only if they imagined themselves hitting the tuning fork.

The child babbles because diffuse motor activity is as characteristic of motility as continuous sensation (as in idioretinal light) is characteristic of the perceptual side of psychic life. Not only the vocal organs, but also the motility of the total body of the suckling, are continuously in action. The organism is in a continuous state of fluxion from a sensory, as well as from a motor, point of view. These primitive sensory and motor activities are, in many respects, rhythmical in character. They probably represent a primitive tendency toward adaptation. The babbling corresponds to the vortices and currents in the visual field. It is a field of action. Rhythmical function also goes on in the electrical field, as is shown by the Berger rhythm obtained from the cortical region, especially from the occipital region of the cortex. It is characteristically modified by incoming sound, as Weaver and Bray (1930) especially have shown.

Continuous activity is necessary for the child to gain understanding of sounds. He has to reconstruct them. There is no mere coincidence of motility and the sound of babbling. Modern psychology is not inclined to put emphasis on imitation. Allport (1924) tends to reduce imitation to conditioning. Still, imitation undoubtedly does exist in language, as the investigations of C. and W. Stern have shown. It is a genuine tendency. When one observes the behavior and utterances of children, one continually finds instances of imitation. Children often answer a question, which has previously been directed to another child, with words almost identical with those the other child used. Analysis of the meaning of imitation is necessary. In this example, it merely may be simpler for the child to repeat. The repetition may express admiration for an intelligent answer by the other child, or may even be based on a wish to be completely like the other child.

In Pavlov's experiments, conditioning means preparedness and does not mean a mechanical sequence of events. When a child babbles continually, after he has heard himself babbling, he may do so only because the sound has given him full control of a particular set of muscles and he wants this whole situation repeated. Motility of the entire body brings the organism into continuous touch with reality, and so creates new sensory impressions. There is no fundamental difference between the vocal organs, the mouth, and the other organs of motility.

Our relations to objects are twofold. First, we try to get hold of the object—motility serves this purpose. We grasp with hands and mouth and we are directed toward the object or away from it. The second relation is that of identification. We may identify ourselves with the object, may try to become like the object. We act in the same way as the object acts. As a matter of course, we must have some inner relation to the object in order to desire identification. The identification mechanism cannot occur prior to and be more primitive than the object mechanism, as Freud himself and many other analysts are inclined to believe. Although the object relation is a necessary prerequisite to identification, identification is an independent biological attitude, indicating the social character of living beings and their experiences. (This problem is very fully elucidated in Schilder, 1935.) Whatever the relation between imitation and identification may be, they belong close together. In psychoanalytic terminology, identification is a specific psychological mechanism explaining conscious imitations as well as actions which we may class as "unconscious" imitations.

Direct imitation of sounds which do not have the character of speech (onomatopoeia) does not play a very important part in the development of language. Whenever it does occur, the explanation is simple: sound emitted by an object may easily become a signal for the object (e.g., sounds produced by the mouth during eating are natural signals for the presence of food; noises emitted by the sexually excited person show the particular state of mind present; and noises concomitant to vital functions are signals to others, indicating the biological state of the individual). All noises emitted by the mouth have an immediate social character and social consequences, which, in the course of events, may be sought by the individual, who will then feel inclined to give the signal again. Signals, by their very nature, have a social function. It is possible that signals may acquire their final meaning only by the effect they have on the social group. According to the investigations of Frisch (1915), the homecoming bee starts dancing, touching, and pushing other bees, which thus receive its contact and smell. The other bees then leave the beehive for the feeding ground. One could call this dance a signal. The dance probably has a decided individual function for the bee; it acquires the signal function since it expresses itself in motion which makes itself felt. This is a signal, irrespective of whether the bee wants to signalize or not. It has a social function and leads to social actions. It is hard to believe that this social function is merely a side effect.

Noises provoked by eating are a signal to others, whether or not one wishes them to be so. Generally speaking, signals have a social significance. Pavlov's dogs relied on some unknown force (if the experimenter were not in the room) to supply the food after the light signal. The signal was a promise. We might speak of signals and promises in terms of "promising thunder." We cannot provoke the lightning ourselves. Of greater importance are signals produced by ourselves, or by other living beings, to express a definite announcement that something else will come, as lightning is a sign that thunder will come. When regular sequences occur, the beginning of the sequence signalizes its continuance. Words are self-produced signals. At first, signal systems are always comparatively crude and have to be worked out in a process of gradual adaptation by trial and error. But signs and signals are never as reliable as the object itself. The development of the modern rules of contract bridge is an amusing instance of this kind. To look directly into the hands of the other players would certainly be a simpler and more reliable procedure than to indicate the strength of a hand of cards by one's bidding.

The drops of saliva in Pavlov's experiments indicate that the dog expects food, or in objective terminology, that he is prepared for it. The light or sound which provokes the conditioned reflex is a signal of the food to come. The dog cannot produce these signals himself. By the drops of saliva the dog expresses its appetite; the meaning of the drops is that the dog wants food. The meaning of the light or sound signal is that food is promised. The saliva indicates that the promise was understood, that the meaning of the signal was clear.

In Pavlov's, and Bechtereff's (1926) experiments, the signals were chosen arbitrarily by the experimenter. In language, the adult chooses the word for the child. That language signs were chosen as a by-product of the vital function of devouring is merely a historical derivation. It is remarkable that Pavlov's progress in experimentation is closely connected with the substitution of "artificial" signals—such as a bell, metronome, light, or skin irritation—for the natural ones of sight and smell of the food.

If sound or light acquire a signal function it is at first inexact and only later becomes precisely differentiated. In the words of Pavlov (1928, p. 298), differential inhibition "must occur when from any definite agent a conditioned stimulus is elaborated, then all similar and related stimuli also have somewhat the same effect. But when the chosen stimulus is repeated many times these extraneous stimuli gradually become ineffective."

Pavlov further writes:

We have made a conditioned stimulus from the mechanical irritation of a certain place on the skin. At first after this conditioned reflex is established other points of the skin also show the same effect when they are stimulated, and the closer they lie to the first point, the stronger their effect. This spontaneous generalization of the stimulus has a special biological significance, and is the expression of the irradiation of the excitation in the mass of the cortex. By repeating the stimulation of our chosen point in the skin and accompanying it with feeding, and not accompanying the stimulation of other points by feeding, these latter become inactive; now they are differentiated, negative, conditioned stimuli. This kind of inhibition we call differential inhibition.

Differential inhibition fulfills a still more complicated task; it forms the foundation of the differentiation, delimitation or separation of the compound stimuli which have been previously extended in the cortex of the cerebrum by means of the coupling activity [Pavlov, 1928, p. 298].

Similar results may be obtained with sounds of different frequency. In the process of differential inhibition, very specific and fine differentiations take place. Differential inhibition is a process of trial and error which leads to a better understanding of the quality of an object (in this case, the signal character of the excitation of the skin and of sound). Differentiation takes place under the guidance of experience. Experience is not mechanical repetition, but is, rather, construction and reconstruction, under the guidance of biological needs or the goals and aims of the individual. We may say that the stimulation of the skin and the sound are at first general concepts and only later become specific connotations, in the process of differentiation.

The term "general concept" is perhaps not quite correct. Before a specific connection, the dog merely has no interest in or reason for differentiation. Children use concepts and words in the same way. For example, one child said, "People die of pneumonia." He had heard from adults that this had happened in one specific case and, until he acquired new relevant experiences, he had no reason to think that pneumonia was not the cause of all death. Probably every general concept gets its final meaning only by continuous contact with reality.

The child believes that the single case fits everything. Schilder and Wechsler (1934) call this "the principle of undue generalization." One may say that thinking starts with general concepts, although this is incorrect if we use the term "general concept" in the formal logical sense. The general concept of the child is a single experience, taken without analysis as representative of many other experiences. In the experiments of Pavlov, a differential inhibition takes place. With sound, this differential inhibition may occur when the sound is repeated often enough, but the differentiation takes place more quickly and more correctly when the unconditioned stimulus follows only the one specific sound, whereas the other sounds are not followed by the unconditioned stimulus. We obtain a specific insight into the nature of a signal only by trial and error, or by way of fulfilled and disappointed expectations.

Dogs do not talk, of course, but we may expect that if we form a so-called trace reaction, the dog may think in the meantime, "Now after awhile I shall get food," and it is probable that the image of food will come into its mind. The behaviorist will say that we have no proof of this; but if one experiments on human beings, one can easily prove that an electric shock, repeatedly given to an individual five seconds after a signal, is soon psychologically anticipated. It may even be reproduced with hallucinatory vividness. It may be that we deal with the simplest case of a memory image and, furthermore, with a hallucination. In such a case, the memory image is a part of the inner preparedness for the unconditioned stimulus and belongs to the total reaction. The past situation returns in the service of the present. The memory image and the representation are a part of the conditioned reflex, in Pavlov's sense. If the word is really a signal for the object, the picture of the object and the memory of the object must be closely related to the word. We should not forget that the object or its memory image also provokes a set of reactions or actions. In Pavlov's dog, the conditioned reflex is not only the secretion of saliva, but is also motor reactions which lead to the grasping of the food. This side is not fully apparent only because of the artificiality of Pavlov's experimental setup.

The meaning of the word comprises, therefore, the object (its representation or memory image) and the motor reactions and physiological reactions connected with it. The object is the foundation for the concept and the word is the sign for the concept. To have an intention or direction toward an object in thinking is related to a reaction of the total organism. The meaning of a word may become founded in organic reactions rather than in the memory image. We then deal with thinking which is to a great extent independent of imagination. The object is supposed to have some kind of stability. A word that designates an object forms a concept purporting to be a definite entity, which is unchangeable, and which therefore offers a reliable basis for actions. One may, of course, say that the word "horse" means a specific horse, or it also may mean all horses. In the latter case, we deal with a general concept, although it is easy to prove that, in everyday life, these general concepts are actually far from being general. They merely claim to be a possible basis for action in an unlimited number of cases. If one tries to use general concepts as a practical basis for action, one soon finds out that they are approximately as reliable as the sound which conditions drops of saliva, before differentiation has taken place.

What we call a word, or what we call a sentence, is always more or less arbitrary. For instance, when I say the word "horse," and nothing else, I imply that I do not intend to be explicit and do not want to commit myself. The *concept,* in the logistic sense, is a mere abstraction which does not exist. In other words, everything we say —be it letter, syllable, word, or sentence—yields sound patterns which we use as signals for the total situation that should be the basis for our actions. Sentences offer problems of their own, although language becomes flexible only through them. Characteristically, in a sentence, an object or a fact is considered as having different aspects or parts standing in different relations to each other. One can say that the different grammatical forms of a word, and the different prefixes and suffixes, are subdivisions of the word. However, the different grammatical forms have meaning only in a sentence and not in relation to the single word. The prefixed or suffixed word is merely a word which can be divided into part sounds but not into part meanings. In our attitude toward objects, we do not want objects that are completely stabilized. We tolerate a motionless, changeless object only for a very short time, and then divide it into parts and consider its different aspects.

The history of the "indivisible" atom is interesting from this point of view. What are the qualities of the atom? Does it move? Does it stand still? What is its form? Even the "indivisible" had to be divided and subdivided until there finally remained a mysterious energy quantum, which has either no definite velocity or no definite place. The atom has become divisible, has lost its constancy and stability and is now much more inconstant than an object of the senses. The development of physics is dependent upon basic psy-

113

chological principles of psychic experience (as pointed out in Schilder, 1928). The development of the theory of the atom shows that psychologically we cannot tolerate constant and static entities. The stabilized object is a psychological borderline concept. We see sides of the object, parts of the object, and also like to see the object in pieces. We put the pieces together and try to make a new unit out of them, which we again destroy.

If language consisted only of words, it would not have sufficient flexibility, and could not picture the breaking of the objects into parts and pieces. Grammar leads to a rather complete breakup of words and so reflects the breakup of situations and objects which, as emphasized above, play such an important part in perception. On the basis of the same qualities, the constructive process becomes possible. Since grammar chiefly reflects the breaking up of the object or the construction of the object, the relation of the whole to the parts and pieces becomes the most important content of sentences and grammar. The expression of attributive relations is, therefore, one of the most important functions of the sentence. Grammar develops language into a scientific system for breaking up and composing total situations.

Psychic life is active and constructive. We always intend to do something, and we build up. We have emotions and we are continually acting. It is probable that different types of action are necessary for different psychic acts. When we construct an object and when we construct relations between objects, the psychic activities involved must be different. We are much more conscious of our activities when the construction is complicated. In judgment, this may appear like a definite agreement or disagreement, but it should be understood only from the general point of view of construction of object relations, which are necessarily connected with a higher degree of organization.

I have already pointed to the fact that the import of a judgment merely means that the individual is emotionally directed toward the object. Sounds, in language, contain, in themselves, the fact that they mean more than mere sounds. One may easily call this the expression of the import. It is also true that the sound which, for the dog, has become a promise that feeding will occur, is no longer like any other sound. It has gone through many more constructive

114

processes. For the dog, the sound has the import of feeding. The previous feeding experiences are the foundations to which the sound relates. We also understand why import is the interpretation of the foundation. I would state, however, that it is no longer so important to go into every detail of the relation between signal and fact; the general insight that we deal with constructive processes is what is of outstanding importance.

One sees that it is not so difficult to reach a biological and physiological theory of language, if one considers the principles of the constructive psychic energies. Words and sentences have signal functions. They are signals for objects. Objects are not merely given to the individual by passive reception, but involve a continuous process of construction and reconstruction. The individual takes parts of the objects, puts them together, rejects other parts, and molds and remolds the object. This remolding, reconstructing, and rebuilding process is based upon a continuous interplay between sensory and motor functions. With the construction of the object, the first steps have already been taken toward using the object for the biological purposes and aims of the individual, since the whole process of construction is guided by the biological needs of the individual and, later, by the situation. When an object is signalized, the sensory motor attitudes connected with the construction and utilization of objects come into play. The meaning of a word and of a sentence is the sum total of the sensory motor attitudes concerning the expected objects. This sum total is unified in preparedness for action, or in action itself. Words get their signal function by being by-products of the process of getting hold of food and sexual objects. They were psychological phenomena of excess energy not immediately used for hunger and sex, and have primary directness toward leading to the satisfaction of urges from which they originated. Signal functions have an immense social significance. They are signal functions not only for one individual, but for the whole community. Signal functions are, at first, inexact indicators of biologically important objects. By continuous testing, they are reconstructed so that they become more reliable guides to action. The material for the signal function is taken from the vague background of continuous motor activity and unrest of the small child with his undifferentiated needs. The constructive process also

115

gives motor perfection to language. The further elaboration of language takes place by trial and error, biological satisfaction and disappointment, which leads from the use of single experiences as patterns for action to individualized action fitting specific situations.

## THE CHILD AND THE SYMBOL[4]

The child draws at the age of three or four years, scribbling, making loops and crisscross lines. An incomplete oval and a circle soon emerge. Later on, the circle is combined with a straight line, and primitive drawings of the human figure appear. The child attaches one or two lines to the circumference of the circle, which, for him, serves as a satisfactory picture of a man. Arms may be added next, and it may be a long time before a definite body is drawn. The development of drawings of the human figure has been carefully studied by Goodenough and she was able to show that the drawing of the human figure can be used as a measurement of intelligence in children (Goodenough, 1926).

The child is even satisfied with a very incomplete product. The circle with the appended straight lines is indeed a picture of the human figure, but can such a picture be called a symbol of the human figure? Such terminology will obviously not help us to a deeper understanding. We have to assume that the visual motor organization of the child is different from that of the adult. The perceptual motor organization in children can be studied particularly well with configurational drawings, such as those used in the gestalt psychology studies of Wertheimer. Bender (1932, 1938; Bender and Schilder, 1936) has studied the development of the visual motor gestalt patterns in children. The child's world, in the visual motor field, obviously has primitive organization patterns. The drawings of the human figure, however, do not merely reflect visual motor organization from the point of view of uninterested perception. From the earliest stages, children show an overwhelming interest in the human face. The whole psychophysiological organization, and the emotional interest, of the child are represented in the way in which he draws. This is particularly true con-

[4] From Schilder (1938).

cerning his drawings of the human figure, but it also applies to his every attempt to make the pictures of objects.

One might ask whether these primitive lines symbolize the human figure for the child and whether we are entitled to use the term *symbol* in this connection. This has to be answered in the negative—the child experiences primitive units of gestalt and draws accordingly.

A human figure is such a primitive gestalt unit. When an adult draws a perfect picture of a human figure he says by means of it, "I am interested in the human figure, I enjoy reproducing it. I want others to see what I can do and participate in my activity." The basic psychological trends in the child and in the adult are not different in this respect. It is obvious that any drawing is a sign of interest in the object which the drawing depicts. However, a picture pointing to an object in a more or less complicated way, should not be called a symbol. We only have the right to speak about a symbol when the sign does not give, to the person who uses it, a clear idea of the object which is meant, but merely points in the direction in which the meaning is sought. A symbol is, therefore, a sign, the referent of which is not clearly known to the person who uses it. However, the sign should contain within itself the hint that it stands for something else. If the experience that the sign means something else is not sufficiently represented in the consciousness, one should not use the term "symbol."

Psychoanalysis often speaks of symbols when the meaning of the sign is, according to the terminology of psychoanalysis, unconscious to the person who uses the sign (picture), i.e., is not known to him. Psychoanalysis calls, for instance, a stick which appears in the dream of a girl, a symbol for the penis. However, the dreamer does not consciously know this meaning of the stick. Only by a process of interpretation is the fact, that the stick might mean more than a stick, brought into consciousness. I have proposed to call such pictures (signs) not symbols but symbol-like. The child, in his drawings, is obviously not interested in symbolism, but strives for a mastery of the world, which he reaches step by step.

D. Wechsler and I have studied the attitude of children toward death.[5] We were struck with the realistic way in which children

---

[5] Reported in full at the end of this chapter, p. 132 ff.

dealt with the rather difficult question of death. Bright, six-year-old Edward C., for instance, when asked how one knows that someone had died, answered with, "One listens to the heart. I saw my father and my mother dead. They were good people. I think they are still under the dirt." Edward also distinguished clearly between his own observations and what he had been told. He said, "A kid told me about devils. I don't know whether it is true. How should I know if they are in heaven, I am not a fortuneteller. I heard somebody say that the angels take the soul but I am not sure about it. They read it out of the Bible; I did not see it myself. But I am sure they are lying under the ground." Why? "I saw it."

However, children do not always have such a critical attitude, they may accept convention. Children do not always make an attempt to solve the contradiction between convention and observation. For instance, six-year-old George says, "Dead people go down in a big hole and they put a lot of sand on them. Then they don't feel anything. When we are good we go to heaven. We don't feel nothing up there. The hole that they put people in is near to heaven, right next to it. If you are bad you go to hell and burn up. Nobody can help you. It hurts but you don't know if you are burnt or not."

Of course, the child does not use words and connotations in a correct way. He is prone to generalize unduly and use insights which fit a specific situation as if they would fit other situations having only a superficial similarity to the first. He is not sensitive to contradictions and is not capable of bringing the different parts of a situation into definite connections. However, he struggles hard to come to a grasp of the world which consists of single objects related to each other. There is a continuous process of testing and trial and error going on, which appears in the language as well as in the action of the child. We came to similar results in our study of aggressiveness in children.[6] The child also demands simple orientation. Five-year-old Milton answered the question, "Do you like to hit kids?" with "Then you are bad." Why are you bad? "Because they hit you back." What is a coward? "A cowboy." This obviously shows that Milton had difficulties in getting an orientation in the world of words.

In the instances studied, it is obvious that symbols, in the sense

[6] See Chapter V, p. 161 ff.

formulated supra, do not play any part. Children have an incomplete sign system and incomplete connotations at their command, and they try to work them out in a continuous process of experimentation, in which the aims and drives of the total personality play the leading part. Many of the situations which are interesting for the child are not accessible for direct experimentation. The higher degrees of aggressiveness, for instance, cannot be performed in reality but are performed in fantasy and play. The fantasy and play appear as a continuation of experimentation in a more plastic situation. Charles, for instance, lets Indians and cowboys kill each other in elaborate play. In his aggressiveness in real life, he has to be much more modest. He uses primitive gestalt principles in the arrangement of his miniature soldiers. In the same way as many other children, he likes to put soldiers into cars and even to put one little car into a big car. This principle of enclosure is obviously a formal principle, but does it not point to something else? From a psychoanalytic point of view, we know that the interest in boxes and their contents may point to an interest in the womb. Of course, such an interest is forbidden to the child. The free process of experimentation is hindered either by the difficulty of the subject matter or by threats which originate from the situation or from the attitudes of adults. We are entitled to call a picture, which originates under such a particular situation, symbolic, when it clearly points to the underlying situation and symbol-like when the relation between the picture and the underlying situation can be detected by a more complicated technical process of interpretation. For instance, Griffith (1935) tells of a boy who used boats to symbolize the place of origin, the birthplace of the child. Griffith thinks that fantasies such as hiding in rabbit holes, crawling inside the hose, and living in a coconut are also symbolizations of the birth problem as conceptions, as a little house inside a big house, hundreds of eggs inside of a big egg, and a little box inside of a big box. However, it would be wrong to forget that the child has, besides interest in the womb, an interest in security and protection and also a definite interest in the general biological problem of being enclosed, sheltered inside and outside. Symbols and symbol-like pictures will only occur when the process of experimentation has been prematurely interrupted and the child is afraid to live out his

119

interrupted or forbidden drives. In the single case, it may be diffi-cult to differentiate where the direct experimentation, the approach to reality, has stopped and where, instead of it, incompletely de-veloped images, symbols, appear. However, we have reason to be-lieve that the manifold sexual problems of childhood express them-selves very often in symbols and symbol-like pictures.

One of the most important tasks in the orientation of the child to the world is the acquisition of a clear perception of his own body —the body image. The child solves this task with great difficulty and it is a long time before he can decide which part of the world belongs to his own body and which part belongs to the outer world. Very closely connected with this fundamental problem are the problems of the integrity of the inside and outside of the body, orientation about the sex organs, and the fear of being robbed of the insides of the body or the fear of being cut to pieces or dis-membered. Many of these problems appear in the psychoanalytic literature; the writings of Melanie Klein, for instance, emphasize the problems of introjection and projection as an aspect of identi-fication.

The relation of these important problems to the problem of symbolism, in the narrower sense, is not a very close one. The attempt to gain an image of one's own body and preserve this body for the satisfaction of one's needs is a problem of adaptation in the emotional and perceptional sphere. However, whenever the ex-ploration of the body meets difficulties, pictures of symbolic char-acter are liable to appear—interest in the sex parts and the excretory functions will have substituted for them an interest in the other parts of the body or an interest in objects in the outside world, which may serve as symbolic substitutes for the organs. We might, in this connection, define symbolism as experimentation which is retarded in comparison with the general state of development, in the perceptive and emotional spheres. Since such specific adaptation difficulties play an important part, we should not neglect the role symbolism plays in the life of the child. However, we should also remember that the child has an enormous urge to live in reality and do things in reality, and that he comes to reality by a process of maturation and a process of constructive experimentation. It would be wrong to consider the development of the child merely from the aspect of the symbol. It is much more correct to see the development of the child chiefly as an aspect of constructive adaptation. Symbols appear where the trial and error process is interrupted. They are, therefore, danger signals on dangerous points of the developmental process.

Primarily, we are entitled to offer the child guidance to reality. In particularly difficult problems, it may be of help to point to them, at first, in the veiled form of the symbol, in order to relieve anxieties of the child which might be provoked by an immediate hint to the dangerous problem. We should consider fairy stories which we offer to children from a similar point of view. So far, we have overrated the need of children for fairy tales, myths, and fantastic stories which distort reality. If such symbolic material should be necessary for the guidance of the child, one should not forget that the purpose is not to have the child remain in the symbolic sphere; rather, he should have the opportunity of approaching the reality of his level of maturation and experimentation, untrammeled by fears that may have necessitated the preliminary use of symbols or symbol-like pictures.

The puppet shows used by Bender and Woltmann (1936) as a psychotherapeutic method are especially adapted to allow for a free expression of infantile aggression, and permit an unusually facile projection of the child's problems into the puppet characters. These puppet shows contain realistic characters like Casper, a policeman, a father, a mother, and cannibals, and there are also animals like crocodiles and monkeys. Occasionally, there is a fantastic character like a witch, along with the magic elements belonging to such characters. In the figures of the plays, the child sees his own problems and expresses himself freely, at first concerning the characters of the play, and learns in this way to understand his own problems. It may be easier for the child to understand his fear of aggression from the mother when he is shown a witch and he may understand his counteraggression better when it is, at first, experienced toward the symbol of the mother. However, sooner or later he will have to understand his attitudes toward his mother in order to use his faculties in free play.

The child approaches the world in a continuous process of constructive experimentation, which is determined by the maturation level and by the individual factors of psychological development. One does not have the right to call these products of experimentations "symbols," even when the approach to reality remains incomplete. These processes of experimentation come out in children's drawings, in the formation of concepts, and in the language products of children. Symbols and symbol-like pictures are signs which point to an unclearly seen referent. The incompleteness of the symbol-like picture has to be revealed by specific methods. Symbols and symbol-like pictures appear where the experimentation process belonging to a specific maturation level is prevented by danger and threat. Symbols are, therefore, danger signals concerning the adaptation of the child to the world. Their primary aim, however, is to go to reality as such, and, in the literature of children and in puppet shows, the use of symbolic material is only justified when the immediate approach to reality would be too difficult. The symbol should not be a purpose in itself but a step toward the final mastery of reality according to the maturation level.

### Psychoanalytic Remarks on *Alice in Wonderland* and Lewis Carroll[7]

Lewis Carroll's *Alice in Wonderland* and *Through the Looking Glass* are classic stories for children. As far as I know, nobody has tried to find out what is really offered to children through these stories.

One would expect that authors writing for children should have had a rich life and that this richness of experience might transmit something valuable to the child. Charles Lutwidge Dodgson (the real name of Lewis Carroll) lived a rather narrow and distorted life.[8] He came from a religious family. His father was interested in mathematics. His mother is described as gentle and kind. None of the biographies contained anything about the deeper relations between Charles and his parents. In none of the books can anything be found about his relations to his brothers and sisters. He was the oldest of eleven children, eight of them being girls. We merely hear that he gave theatrical performances for them and that he died in

---

[7] From Schilder (1938b).

[8] The following sources were used for this article: Reed (1932), de la Mare (1932), Herrick (1932), McDermott (1935), Moses (1910), and Collingswood (1929).

1898, at the age of sixty-five, at his sister's house, where for twenty years it had been his custom to spend Christmas and other holidays. In his childhood, he amused himself with snails and toads as pets. Furthermore, he endowed earthworms with pieces of pipes so that they could make better warfare. He also built something like a railroad. He matriculated at Christ's Church, in Oxford, his father's college, when he was eighteen. He was always a brilliant pupil. He spent the greater part of his life in Oxford, where he lectured in mathematics. He was ordained deacon in 1861, but never proceeded to priest's orders and very rarely preached. This may have been partially due to his stammering, a symptom shared with others of his siblings (one of his biographers sees in this a hereditary taint, due to the consanguinity between his mother and his father).

*Alice in Wonderland* appeared in 1865. In 1867, Carroll made a trip to Russia with Dr. Liddon. The diary of this trip is meager and dull (McDermott, 1935). He showed a great interest in churches. In 1871, *Through the Looking Glass* appeared.

Carroll had no adult friends. He liked little girls and only girls. He had very little interest in boys, but he occasionally showed interest in juvenile male actors. However, Bert Coote, one of the child actors in whom he was interested, had a little sister who may have been the real cause of Carroll's interest. When a friend once offered to bring his boy to him, he declined and said, "He thought I doted on all children but I am not omnivorous like a pig. I pick and choose."

*Alice in Wonderland* originated from stories told to Lorina, Alice, and Edith Liddel, the three daughters of the college dean. He was particularly attracted to Alice, who was then about seven years old. He had photographed her in a pose which, in its sensual innocence, reminds one of pictures of Greuze. His interest in his child friends usually ceased when they were about fourteen and he exchanged correspondence with them when they grew older. In his numerous diaries, there is not the slightest suggestion of neurotic interests. His friends, interviewed by Reed (1932), testified in the same direction. He was a prolific writer of letters to little girls, in which he tried to amuse them. Some of his poems addressed to little girls are not very different from love poems. The dedication of *Through the Looking Glass* reads:

123

Child of the pure unclouded brow
And dreaming eyes of wonder!
Thy loving smile will surely hail
The love-gift of a fairy tale.

The dedication of the *Hunting of the Snark* reads:

Inscribed to a dear child ...
Girt with a boyish garb for a boyish task.

Shy with adults, he easily established contact with little girls, whom he amused with storytelling and mechanical toys. Generally, he seemed kind in his contact with adults; but he was extremely pedantic concerning the illustrations for his books and did not get along very well with his illustrators. He was interested in photography. He had a considerable gift for mathematics and wrote several books on the subject under his real name, which although not outstanding, won considerable acclaim. He was dry and uninspiring as a teacher. He was religious. He intended to write down some of his sermons, of which one on eternal punishment was dearest to him. The material available to us is scanty. We have, therefore, to turn to his work if we want to get deeper information.

In his pleasant fairy stories, one is astonished to find the expression of an enormous anxiety. Alice, in *Through the Looking Glass*, is standing bewildered. She does not know what to do; she does not even know her name. She cannot find the word "tree." When she wants to repeat a poem, another poem comes out, to her distress. She moves and comes back to the same place.

Most of her anxieties are concerned with a change in her body (body image). It is either too small or too big. When it gets too big, she gets squeezed or she fills the room, as for instance in the last scene in *Alice in Wonderland*. She feels separated from her feet. She does not find the gloves of the rabbit. She is frightened when she continually hears "cut off their heads." She is threatened by the Duchess and the Queen of Hearts. Time either stops (*Wonderland*) or goes in the opposite direction (*Looking Glass*). She has not the right ticket on the train. Animals pass remarks about her. The mutton she wants to eat starts talking. The food is taken away from her and the banquet scene ends in an uproar, in which she is threatened by the candles, the ladle, and the bottles which have become birds. These are indeed nightmares full of anxiety. We are accustomed to find such dreams in persons with strong repressions which prevent final satisfactions. Alice, although bewildered, remains passive. Things happen *to* her. Only toward the end does she revolt against the King and Queen of Hearts, and she even shakes the Red Queen, who turns out to be the black kitten.

It is remarkable that she is never successful when she wants to eat. When she eats or drinks she becomes merely bigger or smaller. Although she would like to cut the cake for the lion and the unicorn, she encounters great difficulties and finally she has no cake for herself. There are severe deprivations in the sphere of food and eating. Alice does not get anything at the mad tea party in Wonderland. Oral aggressiveness is found everywhere. The poem of the Walrus and the Carpenter is of astonishing cruelty. The lobster is cooked. Alice herself frightens the mouse and the bird by tales of devouring. There is also an owl to be devoured by a panther. The crocodile devours the little fish. Father William, as an old man, eats the goose with the bones and the beak since his jaw got so strong by arguing with his wife. It is remarkable that the little girls invited to visit Carroll also got very little food.

We also find oral-sadistic trends of cannibalistic character. There is no dearth of other cruelties. The Queen of Hearts wants to chop off almost everybody's head. There is a serious question as to whether one can cut off the head of the Cheshire Cat when it appears without its body being visible. It is this fear of being cut to pieces which comes again and again to the foreground. The head of the Jabberwocky is cut off (*Looking Glass*). The prisoner (the messenger) is threatened with death, as is the Knave of Hearts. Thus, there is, generally, a continuous threat to the integrity of the body.

In a paper on "Psychoanalysis of Space" (Schilder, 1935a), I have shown that extreme aggressiveness finally distorts space. The loss of the third dimension plays an important part in Carroll's work. In *Sylvie and Bruno,* the warden's brother calls a boy a nail which stands out from the floor and has to be "hammered flat." In a letter, written to a little girl, about three cats who visited him, he relates how he knocks the cats down flat as a pancake, and that afterwards they were quite happy between two sheets of blotting paper. It is, perhaps, in this respect remarkable that many of the figures in *Wonderland* are taken from cards and are reduced to cards again in the final scene.

The stability of space is guaranteed by the vestibular apparatus and by postural reflexes. The stability of space is continually threatened in *Wonderland* and in the *Looking Glass*. Alice is going through the rabbit hole, which functions like a chute. The White King and the White Queen make rapid flights through the air. A wind blows and carries the Red Queen. Bottles start to fly. Candlesticks elongate. A train is jumping over a river. It is an uncertain world. In addition, right and left are changed by the mirror. The King's whole army tumbles and falls; so do the Red and White Knights (*Looking Glass*). Father William (*Wonderland*) balances on his head. There is not much certainty in such a world. One does not wonder that Alice is rather afraid that she might be a dream of the Red King.

Time is also distorted. It either stands still (*Wonderland*) or goes in the opposite direction (*Looking Glass*), although it is difficult even for Carroll to persist with such a distortion for a very long time. One of the letters he wrote to one of his little friends starts with the last word of the letter and finishes with the first; a complete reversal. After all, Carroll was a mathematician. It may be that ruthlessness toward space and time is a characteristic of mathematical talent.

One may ask whether there was not a somatic basis for Carroll's pleasure in mirror writing (the first part of the Jabberwocky ballad is printed in mirror writing) and reversals, since he was a stammerer. Samuel T. Orton, especially in his Salmon Lectures (1936), has pointed to the organic basis for such combinations. However, left and right disorientation and reversals are very often symbolizations for the inability to find a definite direction in one's sexuality, and for a wavering between the hetero- and homosexual component impulses.

There is inexhaustible play with words in both the Alice tales. "Pig" is understood as "fig." As counterpart to "beautification," the word "uglification" is introduced. The shoes in the sea are made of "soles" and "eels." The "whiting" makes the shoes and boots white. No wise fish would go anywhere without a "purpoise." The tale about the fury and the mouse is arranged in the form of a "tail."

We know this phenomenon very well. It occurs when the word is not taken merely as a sign, but as of a substance of its own. What the word signifies (the referent) diffuses into the sign. The sign becomes the object itself, quite in the same way as Pavlov's dogs react to the signal alone with salivation, which should be the reaction to the actual food. The word is handled as a substance, as any other substance. A "rocking-horse-fly" is invented; it is made of wood. Humpty Dumpty can therefore say very well that he lets the words work for him. Humpty Dumpty is furthermore right when he says that the words have the meaning that he gives to them. Whenever one starts playing with words, the problem of negation and the problem of opposites will soon emerge. Alice, in the *Looking Glass,* sees nobody, and the King admires her because she can see nobody at such a distance. Humpty Dumpty prefers "unbirthday" presents since there are 364 days in the year when one can get "unbirthday" presents. The Red Queen says that she could show hills, in comparison with which the hills seen could be called valleys.

The Jabberwocky poem uses new words which remind one of the language of dreams and of schizophrenics; slithy-lithe and shiny; mimsy-flimsy and miserable; waby-way before and way behind; gyre—to go around like a gyroscope; gimble—to make holes like a gimlet.

The Jabberwocky ballad's first few lines were published about ten years before the appearance of the *Looking Glass,* with a slightly different interpretation. Five years later, in the *Hunting of the Snark,* Carroll explains the principle of "portmanteau" words. These are words which combine two words, by what we today call condensation. We find these condensations when the forces of the system of the unconscious come into play. This is a rather ruthless treatment of words. They are handled without consideration. It depends "who is the master," says Humpty Dumpty. Words are cut in pieces and the pieces are arbitrarily united. Such an attitude toward words is found in early stages of mental development. In childhood, there is an experimental stage in which the child tries to become clear regarding the sign function of words. In schizo-

127

phrenia, such a treatment of words signifies the wish of the individual to give up definite relations to the world, which is, after all, a world of regular sequences and of meaning.

Lewis Carroll is considered to be a master of nonsense literature. One of his biographers even calls him the founder of nonsense literature. The Red Queen said, after having made nonsensical remarks, "But I have heard nonsense compared with that which would be as sensible as a dictionary" (*Looking Glass*). The Walrus and the Carpenter "go out into the sunshine when it is night." The White Knight delights in nonsensical inventions. He carries a little box upside down so that the rain cannot come in, but the clothes and the sandwiches have fallen out (play against gravitation). He has a mousetrap on horseback (play with spatial relations); anklets against the feet of the horse protect against the bite of sharks (contraction of space). Freud says, justly, that nonsense in dreams and in so-called unconscious thinking signifies contempt and sneering. We may, therefore, expect that nonsense literature is the expression of particularly strong destructive tendencies of a very primitive character. No wonder that persons faced with so much destructive nonsense finally do not know whether they exist or whether they are part of a dream and will vanish. Many things vanish: the fawn, the beard of a passenger, and, in the *Hunting of the Snark,* the baker disappears, faced by a snark which is a "bojum." The scene in the story of the sheep changes suddenly. The figures in *Wonderland* taken from cards become a pack of cards again. The figures in the *Looking Glass* are in reality inanimate chess figures.

This is a world of cruelty, destruction, and annihilation. Alice, constantly threatened, still emerges bland and smiling. The kings and queens, the duchesses and knights, are reduced to "nothingness." Perhaps it is this final outcome which is gratifying to the child and to the adult reader and listener.

The child experiments continually with the qualities of space, with the shape of his own body, with mass and configuration. This is particularly obvious with children who are between three and four years old, as studies of Bender, and myself have shown. But it can also be observed in both younger and older people. In this respect, it is interesting to compare some of the Mother Goose rhymes with Lewis Carroll's writings. There we find a crooked man who went a crooked mile, a crooked cat, and a crooked mouse. The cats of Kilkenny disappear. A woman loses her identity after a part of her skirt is cut off. Bo Peep's sheep leave their tails behind them. The King of France merely goes up a hill and down again with 20,000 men. Elizabeth, Elspeth, Betsy, and Bess are four persons and still one person. The similarity is obvious. Saintsbury (1903) has also stressed this similarity, and remarks about Carroll, "There is something of the manipulations of mathematic symbols in the systematic absurdity and the nonsensical preciseness of his humor." It seems to me that the destructiveness of Carroll's nonsense goes further than the experimentation of the Mother Goose rhymes.

What does all this mean? How does Carroll come to this queer world? It is a world without real love and the queens and kings are either absurd or cruel or both. We would suspect that Carroll never got the full love of his parents. In large families, children often feel neglected. We suspect that Carroll, who often shows guilt in his diary and who wrote the sermon on eternal punishment, had been educated rather strictly. He must have looked with suspicion at the many children who came after him. Are the kings and queens symbols of his parents? Alice also very bitterly complained that the animals order her around so much. Are some of the animals also representatives of parents?

All kinds of disagreeable animals appear in the two tales. Carroll, in his childhood, liked to play with toads, snails, and earthworms. Alice is in continuous fear of being attacked or blamed by the animals. Do the insects represent the many brothers and sisters who must have provoked jealousy in Carroll?

We have, at any rate, the hypothesis that the demands of Carroll, concerning the love of his parents, were not fully satisfied. He may have found consolation in one or another of his siblings, especially his sisters. It is notable that Alice does not repeat her adventures to her mother but to her sister. It is also notable that Carroll, talking about Alice's future, refrains from picturing her as a mother who tells stories to her own children. He lets her merely gather about her little children who are strangers. (It is, by the way, also reported that Carroll showed jealousy when one of his former little friends married.) We may suppose that Carroll expected the love that he could not get from his mother to come from one of his sisters. The biographical material at hand is not sufficient to finally decide this question. Furthermore, we suspect that he did not feel sure that he could get this love as the oldest brother, but felt that he might get it if he could take the place of the parents, especially the mother. It may also be that he identified himself with one of the older sisters. He particularly resented the impersonations of females by males on the stage. Is this a defense against the unconscious wish to play the part of a woman, especially a mother and sister?

What, anyway, was his relation to his sex organs? Fenichel (1934) has pointed to the possibility that little girls might become symbols for the phallus. Alice changes her form continually; she is continually threatened and in danger. There may have been, in Carroll, the wish for feminine passivity and a protest against it. He plays the part of a mother to little girls but the little girl is, for him, also the completion of his own body. The little girl is his love object substituting for the mother and sister. These rather complicated discussions are not really fully justified, since we do not know enough about the fantasy life of Carroll and probably never shall. But, on the basis of other experiences, we are reasonably sure that the little girls were substituted incestuous love objects. Beside this kind of object relation, there must have existed a strong tendency to identification, especially with females in the family. As in all forms of primitive sexuality, the promiscuity in Carroll's relation to children is interesting. Seemingly, he tried to get in contact with a great number of children and to seduce them in this way.

It is obvious that such object relations, loaded with insecurity and feelings of guilt, cannot remain satisfactory and must be accompanied by hostile and negative tendencies. These hostile tendencies did not find an open expression in Carroll's life—a strong superego and a strong moral consciousness protected him. The strength of the repression may be partially responsible for the depth to which the regression took place. All the hostile tendencies therefore had to come out in the particularly severe distortion in his work. It is possible that his mathematical ability and constitutional difficulties, previously mentioned, may have had something to do with the type and depth of his regression. Since we do not know enough about the early history of Carroll, we cannot appreciate fully the relation between the constitutional and individual factors in his type of regression, obvious in his work and in the structure of his love life. Most of his biographers stress the difference between the official personality of Carroll and the personality expressed in his literary work. Carroll, himself, has highlighted this, through choosing a pseudonym and keeping Charles Lutwidge Dodgson strictly separated from Lewis Carroll. We can understand his motives for doing so; however, his stern morality, dryness, and mathematical interests were not separate parts of his personality, but were the reaction and basis of the tendencies which he expressed in his work.

I suspect that nonsense literature will originate as long as there are incomplete object relations and a regression to deep layers involving the relation of space and time on the basis of primitive aggressiveness.

To this writer, Carroll appears as a particularly destructive author (I do not mean this in the sense of literary criticism, which does not concern us here). We may merely ask whether such a literature does not increase destructive attitudes in children beyond a desirable measure. There is very little in *Alice in Wonderland* or in *Through the Looking Glass* which leads from destruction to construction. There is very little love and tenderness, and little regard for the existence of others. Maybe we can have confidence that children will find a way to construction for themselves. At any rate, the child may be led to a mental experimentation which, although cruel, may sooner or later lead to a better appreciation of space, time, and words and so, also, to a better appreciation of other human beings. Problems of this type will have to be decided by experience and experimental approach.

What do children do with Carroll's work? We know very little about it. Preliminary impressions of adults who have read Carroll's books in childhood make it probable that the child uses Carroll's nonsense verses and anxiety situations in a manner similar to the way he uses Mother Goose rhymes. Children take them as a poorly understood reality, to be handled better after one has played and worked with it. In comparison with other fairy stories, the dissociation resulting from extreme cruelty is more obvious in Carroll's work. Without the help of the adult, the child may remain bewildered and alone, and may not find his way back to a world in which he can appreciate love relations, space, time, and words.

131

## CHILDREN'S ATTITUDE TOWARD DEATH[9]

Philosophers have tried to demonstrate that human life is lived under the shadow of death, or that human beings live under the continual threat of annihilation. But if one observes human beings without preconceived ideas, one notes that while some are very much concerned about death, the majority do not give much thought to it throughout the greater portion of their lives. Superficial evidence speaks against the assumption that the average person's attitude toward death plays any fundamental role in his everyday psychology.

But one may raise objections to the method of naïve observation and comparison between different human beings. Modern psychology, and especially psychoanalysis, has taught us that we know comparatively little of what goes on in ourselves, and that the actions and utterances of human beings are very difficult to understand unless one investigates them systematically and with special methods. One of these methods is systematic self-observation. However, experience shows that the data obtained with this method differ with different observers, and that the data are not always reliable. Husserl (1913), taking cognizance of these difficulties, believed that the limitations of self-observation may be overcome by the use of what he called intuitive insight, by which one gets immediate access into the essence of logical structures. He believed that the data so obtained constitute a fundamental science, phenomenology, which, he thought, goes far beyond mere careful psychological description. This claim has not been substantiated. Husserl's phenomenology is just psychology, and as such, an empirical science.

The introspective psychology of the lone observer is misleading. The phenomenologist must check his results with other empirical methods, otherwise he is in danger of seeing the facts of inner experience in a distorted way. Phenomenology which presents its findings as evidence has not always escaped the danger of claiming evidence for mere beliefs and prejudices.

Heidegger (1929), who used the phenomenological method in order to discover what he termed the essence of human life, stated

[9] From Schilder and Wechsler (1934).

that death and absolute nothingness are constantly before the inner eye of man, and that life gets its inner meaning only through the ever-present knowledge of inevitable death. He was even of the opinion that the fact of death enables us to perceive time. As proof for these assertions, he offered certain data of introspection, which formed the basis of his philosophical generalization. But all this is merely unverified subjective introspection. No "inner" evidence can take the place of empirical proof.

If we want to know something of how human beings feel about death and what their attitude toward death is, and in what way the conception of death influences their attitude toward life, the only effective method is to make a systematic inquiry among a great many subjects. It is necessary, furthermore, to observe their reactions toward death and to record in detail what these reactions are. These observations must not be limited only to the reactions of adults, but must also include those of children. Finally, they must include observations on individuals of different cultural strata and, if possible, on human beings of different racial origin. Again, it will be necessary to employ all the methods of psychology—those making use of unconscious, as well as conscious, mental processes. Intuition alone cannot but be an unreliable method. We must replace it with empirical observation and add to it all the methods which the psychology of the conscious and unconscious offers us.

When we observe the conscious life of an individual or limit ourselves to a study of his conscious thought processes, we observe only a small part of his total psychic life. In addition to a conscious life, there is a very full and elaborate unconscious life. Freud has shown how greatly this part of psychic life influences our whole behavior. He has also shown that this unconscious life follows laws peculiar to itself, which are very different from those of conscious thinking. Symbolizations and condensations play an important part in it, and much of the mentation is determined by infantile strivings and desires, which are always present in the unconscious. There is a difference of opinion as to whether the unconscious has an existence all its own, apart from the rest of psychic life, or whether it is made up of experiences existing in the background of consciousness. The "unconscious" of Freud differs little from the "fringe of consciousness," as described by James (1902). It constitutes a special province of psychic life, which he has called the "sphere"; it is in this "sphere" that he believes the germs of thought originate.[10]

Whatever the nature of the unconscious may be, it is clear that there *is* such a phenomenon as repression, which hinders psychic experiences from coming into consciousness. Psychoanalysis is a scientific method by which these experiences (unconscious thoughts) may be brought into consciousness. It uses the method of free association, in which the individual is required to say everything that goes through his mind. In this way, it has been found that the stream of associations, unimpeded by logical rule or social constraint, brings to the surface, and hence into the full glare of consciousness, thoughts and wishes which have for various reasons been repressed. Among these are frequently thoughts pertaining to death. From such observations it appears that persons who are consciously unconcerned with death are very frequently preoccupied with it in their unconscious life. The earlier psychoanalytic literature has, in fact, shown that people in general are more concerned about death than they are willing to admit. Freud has always insisted, for example, that death symbolism plays an important part in dreams, and he definitely proved that the unconscious contains death wishes, against beloved persons, of which we are not only unaware but which we are also unwilling to consciously admit. There is, however, no doubt that psychoanalysis is correct in its insistence that human beings are much more frequently preoccupied with thoughts of their own death, as well as that of others, than they are conscious of.

In the light of the above, we may ask what meaning the word "death" can have, in the sense of unconscious thought, and what the idea of preoccupation with death may mean, from a psychological point of view. Freud believed that there exists such a thing as a "death instinct." According to Freud, all human beings seek to "live out" their life energies and thereby revert to the inanimate state from which life supposedly began. Every individual wants his own death, and, after the thermodynamic analogy, psychic energy is continually falling from a higher to a lower level. Freud seemed to think that this death instinct does not have any psychic repre-

[10] See Schilder (1924).

sentation anywhere, that is, does not even appear in the unconscious. Other analysts believe that there is a psychic representation of the death instinct. If the death instinct, as such, does not appear in psychic life, its existence cannot have very much interest from a psychological point of view. But Freud also identified the wish of the individual to die with the self-destructive tendency which he called primary masochism. He believed that the libido diverts this self-destructive tendency from one's own person to that of others. In this sense the death instinct and the aggressive tendencies become almost indistinguishable, although Freud still tried to maintain their separate identities. He did this by assuming that, in any concrete case, we are always confronted not by a simple situation but by a fusion of instincts, the fusion here being between the libidinous and death instincts. In any case, when Freud spoke about the tendency to self-destruction and the urge to destroy others, he entered again a field of psychology which he had left when he posited the pure death instinct, in the sense described above. Nevertheless, he nowhere gave a clear description of the psychic experiences connected with the word "death," of the self-destructive tendency. For him the word "death" merely indicates that life is at an end. That, however, is far from the only connotation it can, and does, have for different people. Actual investigation shows that, for different individuals, the word may have quite different connotations, and, above all, a variety of associations and connections which makes any single description entirely inadequate.

Human beings generally know that they have to die, but most of them actually do not seem to believe it. When they think about death, they usually think of it merely as a solution of their own life problem. The conception of one's own death is connected with the hope of securing things which one otherwise could not obtain, or with the idea that one will, by dying, obtain the desired love and affection that was, until then, kept back. Or again, it may be a means of punishing loved ones at whose hands one has felt oneself mistreated. People also derive pleasure from torturing themselves, and may even give up their lives in order to assure spiritual union with some cherished personality with whom they have strongly identified themselves. Such, at least, are the general conclusions of Bromberg and myself (1933), conclusions which, it should be noted, are not speculations of phenomenological constructions, but summarizations of introspective reports by ostensibly normal people. They were derived from descriptions of actual experiences, recorded in the responses of some seventy-five adult subjects to a questionnaire, and supplemented by data obtained by ten analyzed cases.

The paper by Bromberg and myself is one of the first attempts at an empirical investigation of the psychology of death. I had previously emphasized the necessity of such an investigation and called particular attention to the fact that this problem was especially involved with philosophical ambiguities and religious prejudices, which might perhaps be more easily avoided if the investigation were supplemented by a study of children's attitudes toward death.

In looking about for a method of investigation, the use of a systematic questionnaire was the first that suggested itself. The questions used by Bromberg and myself for adults were available for this purpose, but while these seemed satisfactory as a point of approach, it was very soon apparent that not only their form but their content would have to be radically altered before they could be used with children. The reason for this is apparent if one examines the individual questions. One sees at once that what the questions ask of each subject is not that he state his actual beliefs or opinion about any particular fact, but instead that he report what his introspections about the facts are. Such questions cannot be used at all with younger children and only to a very limited degree with older ones. In order to get answers from the young child it is necessary to give one's questions an objective and logical turn. One cannot, for example, ask, "What ideas or mental pictures do you have when you think of death?" Instead, one must ask, "What happens when a person dies?" "What does the corpse look like?" or, "Would you like to die?" "Does it hurt to die?" etc. In other words, our questions must be so formulated as to enable us to find out what the child's actual experiences concerning death have been. It is only in this way that we can find out what conception of death the child actually has, and what role it plays in his mental life.

When these investigations were started, the discussion method was the principal means of obtaining our material, although much attention was also given to our subjects' spontaneous utterances concerning death, as well as their spontaneous attitudes toward, and manifestation of, aggressive behavior. Later on, this method of obtaining data was supplemented by still another technique. A series of eight pictures was shown to every child and, as these were successively presented, the child was asked to tell or describe what he saw. After he had finished his spontaneous remarks, the child was then questioned about one or another detail of the picture and his answers, in turn, made the basis for further discussion. The pictures (see Figure 3) shown were the following:

(1)   A girl fainting. One man standing, another trying to revive her, bending over her.

(2)   A woman dying. A man in the foreground weeping. Three girls, half clad, who have just entered, very frightened.

(3)   Vaudeville scene. The magician thrusts a swordlike needle into the body of his assistant who holds up his hands without showing any signs of distress.

(4)   A ghost (the ghost of Edgar Wallace), directing the fingers of a female typist who has her eyes closed. Supposedly he is dictating detective stories.

(5)   A man reaching out of his tent in the desert sees with horror a skeleton half covered with sand. A bit of cactus is nearby.

(6)   A ghost (supposedly that of Sir Arthur Conan Doyle) visits his sleeping wife who has a tender expression on her face.

(7)   An old woman who has just fired a shot from a pistol at a younger woman, who is collapsing.

(8)   Russian spies hanging from gallows. Some people nearby watching.

The subjects in our investigations were seventy-six children on the children's ward of the Psychiatric Division of Bellevue Hospital, in 1933-1934, between the ages of five and fifteen. Sixteen were under eight years; twenty-four were between eight and ten years of age; twenty-three between ten and twelve; and thirteen between twelve and sixteen.

Two of the younger children and four of the older group were hyperkinetic, with an organic background. Three were children who suffered from epileptic fits and nine were mental defectives. The remaining children were, for the most part, children who had been classified as behavior problems.

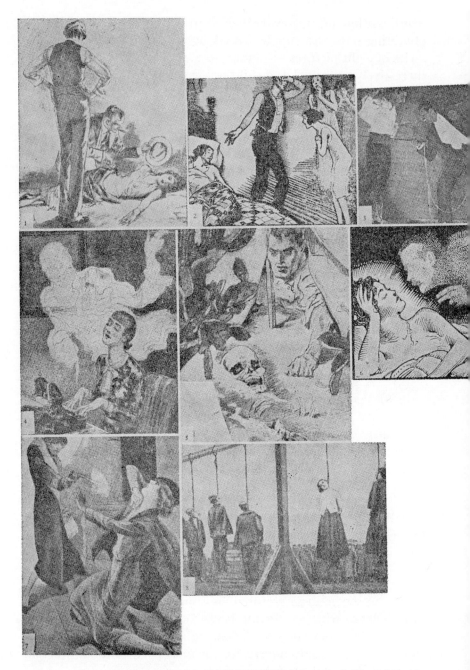

FIGURE 3. Pictures Used in Studies on Children's Attitude Toward Death.

Patrick, a six-and-a-half-year-old boy with an IQ of 99, was an orphan who had been with many foster mothers. He was generally amiable, but from time to time was moody, with outbursts of temper. He had a lisping speech. "I have three mothers. They were my mothers. Yes, I like them. I don't bite mothers. I don't kick mothers. If I kick anybody I say 'I didn't mean it.'" Do people die when they are sick? "I never die when I am sick. I stay. I have felt like 'pendicitis' [appendicitis]. My sister had it. My sister almost died in the hospital." What happens when a person dies? "The funeral comes." Can you come back after death? "A boy came back after he died. He did not die. He was in the funeral with his mother. The mother was in the casket. A little boy died. I saw the casket." Where is he now? "He has much fun with God. When you are bad the devils put you on the fire that harms you. I don't like to go into the fire. Do you? I am not going to die. I get old. They take the soul out of the body. The soul is in the heart. The soul is with God. God made me. God makes everything." What do devils do? "They don't do anything, they kill. They kill God on the cross. The devils have big green ears." How can one kill? "They stick a sword right into you." Would you like to be killed? "I would not like to kill anybody. I help the ladies. I had a real mother. She died. My father didn't. When you go out in the rain you can die. The baby got it. She died almost. Poor little thing. We saved him. We brought him to the hospital." He talked rapidly, spontaneously. When the pictures (see Figure 3) were shown to him, he gave the following answers:

(1) "A lady and a man." What happens to her? "They killed the lady." Why? "Because they did not like the lady. Some man can kill a lady. A bad man kills a lady."

(2) "Three ladies. One sleeping. Another lady is up." Why is she in bed? "Tired."

(3) "Two men. A man sticking something in. Anybody can do that. They are killed. They kill you. He can be put in the electric chair." Where do they put him afterwards? "They put him into a big hole and cover him up. If anybody stepped on it, he would fall down."

(4) "A lady. A man." What kind of a man? "A white man." What does he do? "He takes the lady away. Kidnaps her, puts her into a cellar and kills her. I would not kill. I would be put into jail for it."

(5) "He is going to kill him. Because he is mad at him. He kills him and he will kill him." Can he move? "Yes. He don't like him. Nobody likes a bad man who kills." What's the matter with the skeleton? "He does not know what he is doing. He has no eyes, he can't see." Is he alive? "Yes. Maybe he killed him in the night. Sometimes I am afraid that a bearded man will come and kill me."

In the doll test, he did not knock the doll down and said that it was not right to do that. Then he said that he would like to kill the doll. When it was offered to him he took it and kissed it.

\* \* \*

Alfred was eight and a half years old, with an IQ of 128. He was a behavior problem, restless at night, but generally amiable and attractive.

"I once saw a dead girl in an undertaker's parlor." What does it mean when one dies? "You never open your eyes again. You go up to heaven. Wait till I get there and find it out. It is bad. I do not want to mention the word [hell]. God wants them to die. He just wishes them to die and they die. The soul goes up and not the body." Can one see the soul? "No." Does the soul feel? "No. When you are in the ground you dream that you are in heaven. A sick spell comes over them. Somebody kills them." Is it right to kill? "No." Afraid that you may die? "No, they make me mad, mothers and nurses, so that I want to die because in heaven they do not make you mad." How would you like to die? "By sick spells. I want to get sick and die." How long will you live? "Sixty-one or sixty-two years. That's when most people die. The man across the street just died." Would you not miss something if you would die? "I would miss meanness, I don't care." But he adds, "I would look around the world and see everything before I die. I do not want to miss it."

These were the reactions of an intelligent and aggressive child, who considered the behavior of others as meanness. One can see the difference between his answers and those of less intelligent and younger children. He thought that death was an immediate act of God, but was, at the same time, aware of the fact that one may die from disease. He generalized by saying that most people die at sixty-one or sixty-two. His solution of the problem of life after death was unusual for a child and showed his high intelligence.

\* \* \*

Marian, eight years old, IQ 104, was brought in because of sex delinquency, about which she spoke calmly and openly. She had had two epileptic fits at long intervals.

What happens to dead persons? "They burn them." Is it bad to die? "No." How do they die? "By eating poison things." What do they feel before they die? "I don't know." Do they feel something after they are dead? "No. They put them in a graveyard." Do they come back? "No." Did you ever hear about the soul? "No." What about life after death? "No." Did you ever hear about heaven or hell? "No." What is hell? "A place where all dead people go."

(1) (See Figure 3.) "She is dead. A man is looking with his hand on the hips."

(3) "He is getting killed." Is he hurt? "Yes." Is it right to kill? "No. You won't see them no more." Did you ever see a dead person? "No." Would you like to? "Yes."

(4) "A shadow. It's her and her shadow."

(5) "A skeleton, face and hands. A man is scared." Why? "The skeleton will kill you." Can I become a skeleton? "No."

(6) "She is in bed. He is coming down to her."

(7) "This lady is shooting her."

(8) "These ladies are getting hanged up."

Do you think you will ever die? "No." Will I die? "No." Live forever? "No." In playing with tin soldiers and tin cars, she knocked down a soldier after a period of hesitation and said the car killed him.

While on the ward, she told the nurse and some of the other children that bad people are taken from the grave and sold at the market.

This was an unimaginative child with little inner or outer activity. But in the world which she knew, the idea of violence played an important part, death occurred by poisoning and dead bodies were sold on the market.

*   *   *

Ramirus, nine years old, IQ 109, was a Puerto Rican child, amiable and chivalrous. He stole money from his parents in order to buy something for his friends and to distribute candy among other children. He was very generous on the ward.

Is it nice to die? "No, I want my life." What happens after death? "They take the things out of the body and stuff it with cotton. They bury him." Does he feel? "No." What happens after he is buried? "They burn him. The man who takes things out of him keeps the stuff." What happens with the corpse in the grave? "They leave him there where he is buried." Can one come back after death? "No, because he is all stuffed with cotton and is dried up." Does he feel anymore? "No." Can he go to heaven? "Yes, because God sends him up. He sends angels down when the person is buried. They take the whole dead person. After they take him the grave is empty." What does a person do in heaven? "He remains with God. God takes care of him." Is he dead? "Yes." Does he feel? "No." How does the Lord take care of him? "He stays in a box." What happens with a dead person? "He never gets back to life." Does a good person come back to life again? "Yes." Is there a hell? "No." Where is heaven? "In the sky."

141

(1) (See Figure 3.) "A girl dead. They killed her." Why? "Because she was bad." Is it all right to kill? "No." How do persons die? "Because they kill them. Sometimes they get sick. They die." Will you die? "If I get sick." Do you think of death? "Yes, because I am bad. Then I go back to hell."

(2) "A lady is dead. Her sister."

(3) "A man who killed a boy."

(4) "The girl is dying in the fire. Flames. It's a head or person."

(5) "A skeleton." What is a skeleton? "When you die he turns to be a skeleton."

(6) "God. He makes the girl sleep."

(7) "The mother killed her with a gun. She got no right to kill her."

(8) "People choking. People hanging. They got no right to hang them."

This boy had difficulties in uniting the nonobservables with his correct observations of the facts. He was ready to believe in the death of others and readily inclined to believe in violent death. He was caught in a network of superficial moral connotation, due to punishments received from a severe father.

\* \* \*

Vincent, ten years old, IQ 92, was brought into the hospital because he couldn't get along with his mother; he had fainted when he was told that he had to stay in the hospital.

Did you ever see a dead person? "My uncle; I was about eight, he was in the coffin, it was not so nice." What happens afterwards? "They go six feet under, then they stay in the ground. Then after five or six years they are only bones." Do they feel? "How can they, they are dead. I would not touch one. It is not nice to kiss a person who is dead. You might connect with the germs. There is a certain kind of powder on them, and something is liable to happen to you. They can fine you." Why? "They may think that you want to attack a dead person, to go in and take the rope and try to hide him." Why should one attack a dead person? "For instance, he knows the dead person's grandmother or somebody, and he does not like them, so he says he will attack them and steal the dead person and hide it." What will happen? "If a cop catches him with the smell of the dead person he will ask him questions, and will send him over the water for ten years." Who told you this story? "I just make it up." Are you afraid of dying? "No, I shall die a natural death. I am afraid of shooting and being shot. I shall be about thirty, thirty-five or fifty, when I die. I might die at that age." Can you die earlier? "When you are eleven or twelve; you can die at any date." When do you think you will die? "I can't tell. You go on a certain time. You live after, if you are created afterwards and if you are in the next world." Is there a next world? "Maybe there is one. There is another world made already." Is it right to kill? "If he does something which he is not supposed to do." Did you ever wish that somebody should die? "No. But if you hate somebody, what is the use to wish." What is an angel? "It is a pure spirit. The Catholic Bible says so."

(1) (See Figure 3.) "Somebody shot this lady."
(2) "The family or something. She died."
(3) "He is putting the sword into another man but he is still alive. In a show they do that."
(4) "A woman is typing. She is dreaming of a man who is over her."
(5) "This man owns the tent. He has been dying. He seems to be a skeleton up from the ground."
(6) "She is sleeping. The man looks old, you can see his bones."
(7) "A woman shooting a woman. It is against the law to shoot."

This child, generally very rational in his attitudes, still had an exaggerated fear of death connected with infection, and his idea of death was fantastically related to crime.

**Some children deserve particular attention. One of these is a mental defective, who reveals, in especially striking fashion, uncritical acceptance of conventions and lack of distinction between observables and nonobservables.**

Frederick, ten years old, IQ 68, was brought up in a convent; he was a behavior problem.

"When a boy dies he goes to heaven. The soul goes up." What do people feel when they die? "They feel lonesome, they want to see their people again." Why do people die? "They eat things they are not supposed to eat. They pull things up from the ground and eat them." Do you know other causes of death? "Killing persons, murdering people. You shoot him—he dies. Murderers do that, they want the money." Did you ever kill? "No." Did you ever see a corpse? "No. All the bones are separated." Would you like to see it? "No. I saw a dead cat, I felt sad. The poor cat wants to live like us." Would you like to die? "No." Does it hurt? "Yes. When you stab a person it hurts the person." Must all people die? "No. Some people don't die." Do they live forever? "They might die, some of them live." Do you think that you will die? "Yes, I shall die, I don't know why."

(1) (See Figure 3.) "A girl. She is dead, I think." How did she die? "She killed herself."

(2) "She wants to go to heaven."

(3) "He got shot by the other man. Maybe he did something wrong. He feels sad. He stabbed him through the heart." What will happen to him? "He will die."

(4) "A shadow of a man. A wall shadow. She is playing. He kills her. He is a bad man."

(5) "A skeleton from the dead people." Does it feel? "No." Can he move? "He is coming up from the grave, he wants to kill that man."

(6) "A mystery man. He kills people."

(7) "She is shooting. She is a bad lady." The other one? "She is a good lady. She did not do nothing to that lady." What will happen to her? "She will die. She is a good lady. She goes to heaven, the other don't." What will she do in heaven? "She will be happy." Would you like to die? "No."

(8) "People who get hanged. They did something wrong."

In this case, the belief in an uncritically accepted convention was particularly strong. Also, his moral connotations were very outspoken. But violent death and death by poisoning were considered by this boy as rather natural events. He was a child of little impulses and slow processes. Many of the principles met with in younger children were particularly strongly expressed in this defective boy.

The outstanding feature in this case was the strong tendency to cling to convention and tradition. There was no integration of the contradictions between experience and convention. Mental deficiency shows itself in the answers; but the formal characteristics of the replies are similar to those we found in the answers of normal younger children. On the other hand, in the case of many mental defectives, one gets the impression that obtuseness toward contradictions generally and, in particular, the contradiction between the observables and nonobservables, is greater than that in normal younger children of the same mental age. In this connection, it might be pointed out that whereas the mental defective conforms readily to tradition and convention, he nevertheless continues to manifest a primitive cruelty.

Mere clinical experience shows a marked difference not only in the behavior, but also in the conversation of children with hyperkinesis with marked motor impulses, as compared with children of diminished or even normal motility. The hyperactivity of the former expresses itself not only in the form of increased motor action but also in an increased mental activity, especially as it concerns the child's fantasy life. The two are not wholly unrelated; the increase of the child's motor activity leads him into a closer contact with objects, which in turn becomes a stimulus for further fantasies.

The increased motility of the hyperactive child may be of two kinds. The first, connected with the more primitive drives, leads to a ruthless handling of objects and often to their destruction. In the second, the drives are less powerful and may be directed to a more or less useful activity. For convenience, we use the term "hyperkinesis" for instances in which the child's activity is dominated by the more primitive drive, and the term "hyperactivity" for cases in which the increased activity has been turned to more purposeful uses. The best examples of pure hyperkinesis are furnished by postencephalitic children.

Lawrence, eight years old, IQ 101, was a postencephalitic child with hyperkinesis, who told fantastic stories.

"My uncle was run over. He was crossing the street and was hit by a car. There was blood coming out of the mouth. He was half dying. About fifteen doctors came and saved him. He would have died. They put him into a grave and in a coffin." Here followed a complete and detailed description of what happens when somebody is buried. He said dying does not hurt, his father told him so. "Don't think I don't know anything about dying. They are dead, they never get out. When they go to heaven their soul becomes alive. No, I would not like to die." He said, "I like to shoot but I would not like to shoot people." He shot the doll in the play experiment. He reported the following dream. "I dreamed that George Washington killed Doctor W. with a big sword, bigger than this. Doctor W. did something to him. Doctor W. punched him in the jaw. If I dreamed it, he must have killed him."

\*　　\*　　\*

Other children with hyperkinesis showed the same type of psychological reaction. Robert, nine years old, IQ 96, when playing with the doll, said:

"She is dying. I shot her down now myself." What happens when a person dies? "I don't know. The funeral comes and they go up to heaven." Is it bad to die? "Yes." Does a dead person feel? "No." See and hear? "No." Do you think you will die? "I'll die sooner or later." Afraid of it? "Yes." Why? "I don't know that." Why do people die? What makes them die? "They are bad. He does not want them to live any longer." What makes them die? "Somebody kills them." But if nobody kills them? "It may happen during the sleep in the nighttime." Is it right to kill somebody? "God does not want you to kill anybody. That is His command." What happens after death? "They bury him with shovels. Then they take him out, then put him in, and then cover him up again. They put flowers on, and the funeral goes away." And then? "The people go away. They put flowers on, and then the funeral goes away." The body? "Stays in the grave forever." Does it change? "No." Heaven? "Everybody who has been good. The angels come to take the soul." What happens to the body? "They make another little baby out of it." Bad people? "They go down into the ground. The devil gets the body." What does he do with it? "He burns it." Does the body feel? "No." And did you ever see a dead cat? "Yes, I don't like it. It smells. In 1932 I saw a coffin with flowers in it. A little boy about eight years old was in it. He died on his birthday." Why did he die? "I don't know." Did you ever kill a cat? "No, it is cruel. God made the cats." Did you ever wish that somebody would die? "No."

His responses to the pictures were as follows:

(1) "A man, a woman dead on the floor." How did she die? "From a sword. He looks that way."

(2) "A man is sick. The other man is crying, don't want to look at him. The ladies are scared."

(3) "Stabbing another man in the stomach. He will die. The other man will go to jail."

(4) "She is typewriting. That is the wind. She is dying."

(5) "He sees a skeleton. He has no skin, only bones. He is in the desert." Can a skeleton walk? "Yes, it kills you."

(6) "That is the bad man who tries to kill that woman. She is good. He is bad."

(7) "This is a man in woman's clothes. He shoots the lady." Why? "She is good, and he is bad."

(8) "They hang people because they are bad." What does one feel before dying? "One feels cold."

This is a case of hyperkinesis of nonencephalitic origin. But his cruel interpretation of death and cruel play are of the same type as in postencephalitic children.

Hyperkinesis is connected with sadistic attitudes which manifest themselves in a specific attitude toward death, irrespective of whether the hyperkinesis is due to encephalitis, other organic brain diseases or constitutional makeup.

There is no definite borderline between hyperkinetic and hyperactive children. Hyperkinesis and hyperactivity very often lead to actions obnoxious to adults. Their negative reaction and the accompanying punishment of the child only serve to increase the child's sadistic tendencies.

In hyperkinesis, we deal primarily with an increase in the amount of impulses; in the hyperactive child, the motility is closely related to emotions and the increased motor activity is allied with the patient's general attitudes and interests. But, in addition to these two types, there is the aggressive child whose aggressiveness is due to some specific mental and emotional problem. The following cases are illustrative of this type.

Thomas, ten years old, IQ 106, came from a bad home environment, where a drunken father threatened the family. Death, for him, meant mostly violent death.

"Everybody dies if they take poison. That makes you die. I saw a man on the street, who was drowned." Would you like to die? "No, I'll wait until it is time for me to die." How does one die? "Some die from being in jail and being kicked by the cop, or on the electric chair, some get shot, hung, some get killed when they are fighting. Some get drowned and die. They can't swim. They can die also when they know how to swim. They can die in airplanes. People take poison, and throw themselves out of the window." Why should they kill themselves? "They have wives. When they are drunk they do not know what they are doing. They get drunk and kill themselves with a knife." How else can they die? "Struck by lightning." Can one live forever? "When it is time for them they get burned or they fall off a building." On another occasion he said: "They die when they need to die. God wants them to die. He takes them, strikes them with lightning, or makes them kill themselves." What did your mother die from? "She was too fat. One may get a poisoned needle." On another occasion, after having enumerated seven ways of violent death, he was asked if he knew of any other way and he answered: "Sometimes they get sick; they eat the wrong stuff; when it is your time to die, God

**147**

does magic stuff, he moves his hand and you die. They all have to die."
Why? "God needs them sometimes when he needs angels."

The aggressiveness of this patient came out only in his fantasies
and his attitudes toward them. Otherwise, he was very wise and
moral; on the ward, he was friendly and sociable; he was not at all
destructive in his play. His attitude toward death and his theoretical
ideas about it contained the only open expression of his hatred of
his father. The attitude toward death is the common pathway toward which all aggressive tendencies converge. It does not make
much difference whether sadism is derived from organic layers,
from a general hyperactivity, or from a particular libidinal constellation.

Our motor equipment, as well as our experiences, determine our
attitude toward death and allied subjects, and our judgments about
them. To inflict death upon another person is to dismember him;
also to show our power over him. But it may also be for the purpose
of inflicting pain on him and, eventually, for removing him from
our midst. To the child, his own death, so far as he can believe in it,
is merely a deprivation, an infliction of pain, a destruction of his
body by an external force, at the hands of an enemy.

Three of these children, ages ten, eleven, and fourteen, had been
in serious accidents. In all three cases, the children said that at the
time of the accident they thought they would die. They were run
over by cars and they looked upon the vehicle as a symbol of unlimited power of destruction. In the case of an adult with masochistic tendencies, psychoanalysis revealed early memories in which
running after a car was motivated by the wish to come into such a
masochistic situation. Masochistic tendencies may therefore lead a
person into accidents. This was not clearly apparent in two of the
cases, and in the third case, in which the accident seemed to be
psychologically unmotivated, the case history of the child definitely
revealed that he was terribly afraid of his father and in constant fear
of being attacked in a cellar. In the first two cases, there was a
marked hyperactivity with bravado feelings, of the type which leads
youngsters into dangerous situations. They were evidently under-
rating the dangers of the external world. One of the boys was an
unusually spoiled child, the only boy in a family of three adult

women; the other child was a narcissistic aggressive boy, though without any self-destructive tendencies. Both had met with a number of accidents.

The most effective way of presenting our basic findings seemed to be through a summarization of the protocols obtained from our sixteen youngest and approximately normal children. These will be given in the form of general principles, illustrated by examples from individual protocols.

The first strong impression one gets in discussing the problem of death with young children is that these children deal with death and its paraphernalia in an utterly matter-of-fact and realistic way. Thus, Edward, six years old, IQ 120, answered the question "How does one know that someone has died?" with, "One listens to the heart. I saw my father and mother dead. They were good people. I think they are still under the dirt. Do you know that the man who put my father and mother under the ground got a lot of money?" What else? "Anytime somebody dies they put flowers under the door." What did your father die from? "Pneumonia. When my mother died everybody said, 'don't cry,' but I know better." (The child's mother had died suddenly in a doctor's office, while receiving antiluetic treatment.)

Edmund, six years old, IQ 115, answered the question "What does a dead person look like?" with, "At first they look like they looked before, afterward they are a skeleton." How do you know that a person is dead? "They do not move. I touched them when they were asleep. When they are alive they move, when they are dead, they don't move." Louis, seven years old, answered the question "What happens when a person dies?" thus: "It goes in a big box into the ground; nothing else. They put flowers on top." Can they feel? "No, they don't feel nothing. When they feel they are not dead." Miriam, eight years old, gave a matter-of-fact description of how a dead person looks, of a funeral, etc. She thought that the dead were exhumed. What does a dead person look like when dug out? "Dirty like a pig." Angelo, seven years old, IQ 98: What happens when a person dies? "They bury him and put him in a coffin and they put him in a deep hole. They put flowers there." Does he stay in the coffin? "He goes to a cemetery; they make a funeral." Does he

149

stay there? "Sometimes they go see him and put flowers on him. He stays there."

The children may clearly distinguish between their own observation and what they have been told. Edward said, "A kid told me about devils. I don't know whether it is true. How should I know that they are in heaven? I am not a fortuneteller. I heard somebody say the angels take the soul. But I am not sure about it. They read it out of the Bible. I did not see it myself but I am sure that they are lying under the ground. I saw it." Elliott, seven years old, IQ 85, when asked "What happens with a dead person?" said, "He stays in a box." Hell? "I have not seen it in school." What do you think about God? "I have never seen God in school." There is marked skepticism concerning the nonobservables.

Children do not always show such a critical attitude; often they accept the conventions. Patrick, six years old, IQ 99, said, "A little boy died—I saw the casket." Where is he now? "He has fun with God—when you are bad the devils put you on the fire."

When there is a contradiction between convention and observation, the child often shows no tendency to solve this contradiction and remains insensitive to it. George, six years old, IQ 103, said, "Dead people go down in a big hole and then they put a lot of sand on. Then they don't feel anything. When we are good we go to heaven. We don't feel nothing up there. The hole that they put people in is near to heaven, right next to it. If you are bad you go to hell and burn up. Nobody can help. It hurts but you don't know if you are burnt or not. It's better to go to heaven and to be good."

Naïveté in solving problems is closely related to this insensitivity to contradiction. What does a dead person do in heaven? Angelo: "He flies around with wings." What else do they do? "They eat whatever God gives them." Can a dead person feel? "No." But when he goes to heaven? "Yes, he can feel."

All children emphasize the immobility of the dead. They can't walk, can't see, and can't feel. George, six years old, said, "He can't eat." Another child says, "A dead man never feels." The child therefore looks upon death as a deprivation.

The devil punishes orally, by withdrawing food or by devouring. Richard said, "The devil does not give food." Edmund, six years

150

old, said, "The devil eats them all up." Do they feel it? "Not when they are dead."

Children do not believe in their own death. Said Louis, nine years old, IQ 118, when asked "Do you think you will die?" "No, I don't know." And George, when asked "Can a child die?" "No, boys don't die unless they get run over. If they go to a hospital I think they come out living." Patrick: "I never die when I am sick—I stay." Edward: "I shall not die—when you are old you die. I shall never die. When they get old they die." But afterward, Edward said that he will also get old and die. One's own death is therefore either frankly negated or appears as such a distant event that one does not worry about it. Old age, in the minds of most children, is like a far-off land, so remote that even speculation of ever reaching it appears as an idle, useless thought.

To the very young child, death seems to be a reversible fact. Seymour, six years old, IQ 90, said, "When a man comes and says magic he can get up again after he gets dead. They put him in a grave; he stays in the grave until Saturday, then he may come out." Patrick said, "A boy came back when he died. He did not die; he was in the funeral with his mother. His mother was in the casket." These two children were the ones we found giving actual expression to this belief. Patrick, who seemed most positive, occasionally said things which caused one to suspect that, after all, he did not actually believe that the dead become alive again. However, most children, when asked whether the dead can come back, answer "No."

Death may be the result of disease. Patrick said, "When you go out in the rain you can die. The baby got it. He died almost—poor little thing. We saved him; we brought him to the hospital." Seymour said, "My uncle never gets sick. They get sick by ammonia [pneumonia]. When somebody gets sick they take him to a rat cellar and kill him." Why? "Because they say he is a crook." This shows how difficult it is for a child to believe in natural death. But Edward said, "They die by throat disease." Miriam said, "By pneumonia." Richard said, "When they get old." James, five years old, said, "My grandfather died by eating too much dinner."

The knowledge which the child has about these topics seems to depend almost wholly on what he hears by chance and is, therefore, rather haphazard and unreliable. But the child does not hesitate to generalize his limited knowledge; the child's tendency toward undue generalization.

Death as result of violence is a connotation which children form very easily. Seymour said, "Uncle died one year ago—his head has been cut off." How do people die? "They stick a knife in their heart." George said, "Dogs die when they get run over." Angelo said, "A lady died from fire." Edmond: "When they starve—when they get poisoned—when anybody stabs them." Seymour made a compromise by saying that sick people are killed. Patrick said, when picture 1 was shown to him, "They killed the lady." Why? "They did not like the lady." As a compromise, Edmond said, "God makes them die. He strikes them dead."

Fear of death was rare. Only Patrick was afraid that an old man with a beard might come and kill him.

Our children said almost unanimously that they did not want to die, even when they had just declared how nice it is in heaven. To the question "Would you like to be dead?" there were such answers as, "No, because I don't want it." The word "death" is seemingly a hollow shell which points to something agreeable or disagreeable, although its exact content and meaning are not known. But while the word is only a shell, still it lends a general direction to the thinking of the child; the child gets this direction from the attitude of adults.

Distinct suicidal ideas may be entwined with the idea of death. Such ideas were in the foreground in the case of Edward, who felt very inferior because of his antiluetic treatment. Both his parents had died in short succession, his mother during an antiluetic treatment. His wish to die was a wish to escape inevitable discomfort and also to escape from the feeling of inferiority. "I'll kill myself if I am a court case." The word "court case" here is also an empty word-shell.

A ten-year-old boy said, "When I cry I want to die." Alfred, an intelligent boy, eight years old, IQ 126, said, "They make me mad —my mother, the nurses. I want to die because in heaven they do not make you mad. I want to get sick and die."

On the other hand, children are always ready to believe in the death of others. The transition from life to death seems to be simple to them, when others are concerned. Almost all of our subjects responded to the first picture with the remark, "She is dead." For instance, Edward said, "A lady died, maybe somebody killed her." The death which children are ready to believe in is generally violent death.

Children are ready to kill. Harold, six years old, IQ 96, generally an amiable child, said "I'll sock you. If I had a stick I would stick it in your . . . [points to the genitals of the examiner]. I'll cut your head off." John, seven years old, an aggressive child, said while he tried to hit, "I kill you, I break your neck." George said he did not like the kids who called him by the nickname "Moonshine" and, therefore, would have liked to kill them. The content of the word "killing" may not be fully grasped. But the empty shell of the word carries more meaning with it than one is generally ready to concede. Thus, the last named child, questioned again three days later, protested, "I am not killing nobody," and when relieved of the fear that the examiner entertained such ideas, answered the question "How would you kill?" by saying, "With a gun, spear, knife."

The tendency to kill may come out only in play, as in Edward, who denied strenuously any wish to kill and who also did not make any spontaneous remarks which would show such a wish. But if one let him play with the doll, or with the soldiers, he indulged in repeated play killing. This is important from a methodological point of view. The answers of children are directed to the examiner, who is feared as authority and a substitute father. The child is therefore liable to repress aggressive tendencies, to hide them, and not to talk about them. One must give the child opportunity to express himself, and to show these tendencies without fear of being punished. The additional methods of showing pictures and the play technique afforded such an opportunity.

How much the child is filled with the idea of violence and death can be seen by the way in which children react to ghost pictures. Iona, seven years old, IQ 109, said of picture 6, "He kills people—the skeleton kills." Angelo said of picture 5, "He is a Frankenstein, he is trying to kill this man—he is coming out of the dirt." He said of picture 6, "A girl asleep—a man comes to kill her." Why? "She is a crook who steals money; she wants to buy clothes. They have her picture in the paper."

153

The killing ghost is a natural part of the world. God appears as a stage magician. Edmond said, "God makes them come up by magic. He puts his hand down—he comes up. The chair goes and gets the dead person who does not lie. If they lie, the devil comes up—he makes the magic. When you say 'presto' something comes up. When God says 'presto' they come up to him."

Appearance and reality are not sharply differentiated. Edward said of picture 3, "A show. This is a bad man; this is a good man. I like him. This man sticks something in him—he will die. I can see it is a show—there is a stage. Maybe he will not die." (But this was an isolated instance.)

The child feels the urge to pass a moral judgment on every person and picture. Edwin said of picture 3, "He is bad because he is fighting him." Patrick says of picture 1, "A bad man kills a lady." Seymour said, "They kill him—they say he was a crook." Every protocol contained instances of the urge for moral orientation. However, the professed morality is utilitarian. The child fears punishment. To the question "Would you like to kill?" Edward answered, "No, I would not like to go to jail. Maybe somebody gets the cops after me and puts me in jail." This is a typical answer. Religious morality relatively rarely enters into the child's attitude toward death. Only one case, Richard, said, "God would not like it," when asked "Would you like to shoot somebody?"

Before considering the principles just enunciated and the material from which they have been derived, it will be of interest to call attention to some of the more formal aspects of the child's thought processes, particularly those aspects pertaining principally to the significance of words as used by children, a subject which needs special attention because of the fact that so large a part of the child's education is verbal.

When an adult uses words, whether singly or in a sentence, the words, apart from any general meaning which they may have, point to some specific content. This content is usually not fully conscious, at least not at the moment when the words are spoken. Word meanings are generally vague, and it is only rarely that a given word has a specific content or bears upon a clearly singularly defined object. People nearly always give us connotations, rather than definitions in the scientific sense. Nevertheless, when used in sentences or ordinary speech, words do have some definitely circumscribed meaning or part meaning. The speaker wishes to point out some specific fact or particular attribute, and this is especially true of words as used by children.

In addition to expressing meanings, words also incorporate some emotional content which pertains not to the word itself, but to the attitude which the speaker has toward the object referred to. For example, when one says, "This tree is tall," the content of the sentence goes beyond mere statement as regards the size of the object. It also carries with it, unconsciously to be sure, the individual's attitude toward it. "This is a tree" also says, for example, "See, this is an object which does not have a very great influence on your life. There is no reason for getting very much excited about it. Still, it ought to give you some pleasure to look at it. Why don't you?" Most statements directed toward others have some sort of affective implications, and these implications often form the essential part of the statement's content.

We have digressed a bit, on this somewhat philosophical discussion of the meanings of words, because the meanings which words have for children are very much more complicated, if not more complex, than those which can be found in dictionary definitions. The emotional content which he has learned to associate with various words is particularly important for the child, because, very often, it is the emotional attitude of the speaker rather than what he says which is impressed upon the child's mind. Many of the words which the child hears for the first time are used in demands, warnings, admonitions, and exhortations from adults. Words used this way, generally do not so much define things as situations; they do not recall particular objects, but, rather, experiences associated with them.

The child lives in a world of verbal uncertainties and mysterious implications full of threats and dangers. He tries to escape from these verbal mysteries by seeking refuge in concrete experience, which explains the principle of the child's realistic attitude and the principle of undue generalization from a single concrete experience, which, for the child, is sufficient to shut out uncertainty. The process of development from the concrete to the abstract mode of

155

thinking consists, in part, of the incorporation of the experience of others into that of our own.

At first, the child makes use of words without their full meaning being at all clear to him. What he does understand is the emotional implication of words. Hence, one may speak of the word as a "husk." The word is a sort of shell which at once encases both a cognitive and a conative core. But these two cores are not equally substantial; the conative one is by far the stronger. The conative aspect of a word is the first to impress itself on a child. It is only later that the child is able to associate more definite meanings to words; when he does so, he may be said to have made his first important step toward a rational use of language. These first rational connotations, it must further be observed, are the meanings which children attach to concrete terms.

Initially, the child tends to believe everything he is told. Insofar as the assertions of an adult pertain to an observable fact, the child finds no difficulty in accepting them. But since much of what adults tell children does not pertain to things which children directly observe, they have a constant need to explore for themselves, and explain in the best way they can, the ideas behind the nonobserved objects. Children do this in one of three ways: they may doubt or entirely reject the nonobservables; they may accept the conventional meanings without asking for their real contents; or they may be altogether insensitive toward contradictions between observables and nonobservables, a situation which is achieved by incorporating the nonobservable uncritically into the bulk of their already acquired experience. The task of bringing the observables and nonobservables into a consistent whole is, of course, never completely solved, even by the adult. This is particularly true regarding his ideas of death and life after death. In the case of the child, the integration is even less complete, but a portion of his ideas about death is based on sound observation. Thus, the dead are deprived of motion and feeling and, what is especially important for the child, do not eat. The paraphernalia of death are noted in detail, although, very often, the child makes no connection between the fact of death and its symbolic appurtenances.

The child has no special urge to synthesize or unite impressions received at different levels of experience. Thus, his experience is never completely organized. On the contrary, he has a tendency to rely almost exclusively upon immediate sense impressions. For example, this is illustrated by the attitude of one of our children who identified acts of God with the actions of a magician, and for whom, accordingly, resurrection became a matter of mere observation. For such children, stage trickery and reality are almost identical.

The child is primarily not concerned with his own death, though having observed the death of others, he is ready to accept his own as a possibility. Nevertheless, he very strongly disbelieves that he will die. Even when he does consider his own death, the child projects it into a future so remote that it has very little reality. This is, in part, due to the fact that only the immediate future has any reality for the child. The next meal, the next day, and possibly the next month's outing are the only events which have anything knowable about them; anything beyond that cannot be appreciated. Old age exists for the child only as an intellectual possibility.

The child knows through his own experience or through information received from others that human beings die. This knowledge he generally accepts. In fact, he is very ready to believe in the death of others, possibly because death for the child primarily means only a kind of deprivation. The person who dies is deprived of his possessions and the affection of those near to him. And since he has no objection to depriving others of these things, he shows no revulsion against the idea of killing. Possibly because the child has no reason to fear complete deprivations, the idea of his own death is largely excluded from his beliefs. He thinks that the only way he can die is through some act of violence. Lack of observation of the dead and what happens to them, as well as the fact that he is himself alive, leads the child to believe in the reversibility of death. Death through violence is much easier for the child to understand than death through disease. Because of his special interest in food, the child also believes that death may come from overeating.

The idea of death through violence is closely ingrained in the child because of his own aggressivity. The young child, especially the aggressive young child, is constantly destroying things. The ability to destroy gives the child a sense of power, and is, accordingly, a source of pleasure. Children are afraid to express their destructive desires verbally, but these wishes readily appear in their play actions.

To the child, anything that is unexpected and unusual may kill —ghosts kill and so do the dead. This may explain a belief in the ability of a murdered person to come back and take revenge on his murderer.

The child's idea of hell in part reflects the attitudes of the adults about him, whose ideas on the subject are usually very childish. Morality concerning death is derived from fear of punishment, and, in this connection, it is interesting to note that some children report that the punishment for killing a person is incarceration. This morality may also have a religious character; but even there it is connected with ideas of punishment. This is, no doubt, due to the fact that the child's morality, whatever its nature, is derived from a system of education based on reward for being good and punishment for being bad.

The child thinks about death only when other kinds of deprivation seem unbearable. Death, however, seldom has the character of something definite and final. Death does not seem to be something that lasts, because the child's own deprivations are usually not of a permanent or lasting kind. This fact, too, seemingly makes it easier for the child to wish the death of others, and to speak of killing people without any conscious-stricken feeling.

The connotations of death, for children, consist primarily of the idea of deprivation. The dead can't move. This connotation is comparatively empty since there is a scarcity of experience which could give it a full content. The child's experience of death concerns the death of animals and of other persons, and the disagreeable sensations they get by the sight, touch, and smell of a corpse. The attitude of adults adds, to this connotation, the vague atmosphere of disaster. The child is ready to believe that this deprivation is, like any other, reversible. His own death does not lie in the field of probability. The child does not think about it. He does not expect complete deprivation, and the mere fact of existence contradicts such a possibility. The idea of death does not enter into the child's fundamental conception of life, does not form part of his concept of human existence. It does not appear that the appreciation of time is in any way linked to the notion of death. The child lives in a comparatively foreshortened world of time, in which the present is what is outstanding. Life goes neither far into the past nor far into the future.

Children are ready to believe in the death of others, which they primarily conceive as occurring through some form of violence, particularly with dismembering. To the child, dismemberment is the most obvious means of deprivation, and, since he knows deprivation primarily as a consequence of the ill will and hostility of others, he does not hesitate, when he wishes to punish others, to entertain violent ideas of death toward them. Furthermore, it is to be noted that the child lives in a world full of fear and threats. He sees violence everywhere and is ready to emulate this violence himself. Accordingly, his ideas and attitudes about death are inevitably connected with his sadistic tendencies.

The sadistic attitudes of children are closely related to the primitiveness of their motor impulses and the degree of their hyperactivity. Organic factors increase the original impulses and, correspondingly, the sadistic character of their conception of death. Constitutional factors also determine the amount of the child's activity, and this activity again influences his attitude toward death. The experiences of life may in and of themselves stimulate the child's native sadistic attitudes and give them a direction and form similar to those associated with primary hyperkinesis. Accordingly, in clinical practice, it is sometimes difficult to differentiate between a sadism derived from environmental (psychological) factors and one which reaches deep down into organic layers.

Death does not appear as the natural end of life: it is the result of the hostility of others; it is a punishment meted out for wrongdoing (by extension, the punishing agent may be God). Death by disease and old age has no reality for the child. He therefore does not fear to die, but does have a fear of being murdered.

The body image of the "ego" and the "thou" are intertwined. Accordingly, aggressivity against others is easily converted by the child into an aggressivity toward his own person. The child checks his aggressivity primarily because he fears punishment. He accepts the morality of strength. Tendencies toward self-punishment and self-destruction are in close relation to the creation of the superego. The superego, the moral consciousness of the child, is built up

159

through imitation of the parents (identification). Tendencies toward self-destruction have little importance in the younger child. Suicidal ideas are, for the child, an escape from deprivation, in which death appears as the less difficult solution.

This investigation being a study of children's attitudes toward death, the aggressive side of their behavior has come to the foreground as a matter of course. But, of course, there are also other sides, other things which the child manifests besides aggressivity. He has, for example, a very genuine interest in the well-being, integrity, and completeness of the bodies of his fellow human beings, etc. There are friendly adults who are constantly giving him something, especially food, and the child early becomes aware of such things as kindness and mutual aid. But because of the very nature of the subject of death, these aspects of the child's behavior had little occasion to come to the fore.

The teachings of adults concerning life after death are mostly accepted by the child, though generally made concrete. The connotations and judgments derived from the adult are taken by the child as part of his immediate reality. He is not bothered by contradictions. He does not feel the need of making a unitary whole out of the different parts of his experience. Generally stated, the child is an outspoken realist. God's influence in actions is taken to be similar to that of a stage magician. Ghosts are usually accepted as having factual existence, though classed among the things of life that are dangerous, just as all unusual phenomena are thought to be dangerous. In general, the child finds it hard to incorporate conventional, metaphysical, and religious conceptions into his experience, and he only succeeds in doing so when he decides to accept these conventions without analysis, however contradictory to experience they may be.

# V

# Motor Development and Motility — Psychological Implications

## PSYCHOLOGICAL IMPLICATIONS OF MOTOR DEVELOPMENT[1]

The observations of Gesell, McGraw (1935), and others, show that there is a distinct development of motor patterns from birth to maturity. These patterns develop in lawful progression. "The trend toward an erect head station, the trend toward upright body posture, the tendency toward combining objects, the progressive dominance of the radial digits, the emergence of the index finger for exploitive and prehensory adjustments, the increasing responsiveness to demonstration, and a host of other behavior patterns or behavior modalities might be reviewed for evidences of maturational mechanisms [Gesell and Thompson, 1934, p. 310]."

However, these patterns undergo changes in relation to the environment and the state of the organism, including the exercise of functions and the emotional factors. We may call these the influences of the situation. These influences are partially of a psychological type. There are other influences which act directly on the organism, such as those in the field of pathology. The sequence of behavior patterns might be disturbed because of a constitutional inferiority of the organism, especially of the central nervous system. Disease processes may affect the brain in intrauterine life and after birth, and every pathogenic influence on the organism may affect the central nervous system directly and indirectly. Behavior pat-

[1] From Schilder (1937).

161

terns are correlated to form and function in the central nervous system.

What is a behavior pattern? Let us consider, for instance, grasping and the attitude of the infant toward the rattle. The newborn child moves his hands continually in a choreoathetotic fashion. Whenever an object is put into the hands of the newborn he closes his fingers around it. However, this grasp is not persistent unless the fingers are extended or tension occurs in the flexor muscles of the arm. Watson (1930) found that the majority of babies were able to support their own weight with either hand, up to the age of three weeks. In later development, the grasp reflex does not seem to occur in such direct relation to a simple sensory situation (touching of the palm and stretching of the fingers). It appears when the child is in danger of losing his equilibrium and clutches toward his support, the mattress, or toward the body of the mother. In further development, such grasping comes in connection with a specific object and is in close relation to the child's attitude toward the situation. It is very probable that one deals with a motor apparatus which at first serves a very primitive situation which cannot be differentiated into its parts, and which can later on be used in the service of more complicated situations which can be better differentiated into the whole and its parts.

We deal in some way with the development of a situation in which the motor answer is an integral part. One often hears about reflexes. However, it is an erroneous assumption that such grasp behavior can be understood by such simple responses. Grasping is regularly increased during sucking. It seems that the grasping serves at first as a help to equilibrium and only later on becomes a method of approaching desirable objects with the final aim of incorporating them into oneself. It is interesting to see that in children in whom the lower part of the body has been paralyzed or weakened, the function of the grasp as a help to equilibrium again makes its appearance. Grasping was present in the case reported by Gamper (1926), in which the brain was found to be functioning only from the level of the nucleus ruber downwards. It reappears in persons with lesions of the frontal lobe or where there is diffuse damage to the brain. It also appears in alcoholic encephalopathy in which lesions are chiefly periventricular (Bender and Schilder, 1933).

In such cases, the phenomenon is obviously in close relation to a cerebellar asynergia in which the patient is in danger of falling backwards, and tries hard to maintain his equilibrium. It is further observed in paralysis agitans cases, in which retropulsion is outspoken. Even then, it does not remain an isolated function. When the grasp reflex has been elicited on one side, it is easier to elicit it on the other side. Even in so-called one-sided premotor area lesions, the tendency to such a transfer can be observed. We may draw the conclusion that a differentiation of action into a left and right action is not a complete one, and we see, indeed, that in primitive forms of activity, symmetrical bilaterality of action is common. In the child, in the first few months of his life, the asymmetrical mechanisms of gait and creeping vie with symmetrical flexions and extensions. The pathological grasp of the grasp reflex reverts to a motor symmetry, characteristic of the earliest stages of development.

This is not to say that all primitive activity is symmetrical; however, the primitive organism does not have the choice of changing the symmetrical pattern. Furthermore, in the pathological grasp reflex, another total pattern is revived. In the infant, there are close relations between sucking and grasping, insofar as they reinforce each other. In the pathological case, this interdependence between sucking and grasping is revived. We come to the conclusion that the fully developed organism has by no means lost the primitive patterns, but they may reappear in other connections, become adaptable to serve other functions, and no longer function as units which cannot be differentiated into parts. Pathology revives the various aspects of these patterns and it is hard to believe that they should not play any role if the pathology were not present.

It seems that with the development of this pattern, the grasp, which primarily occurs only when the palm is touched and the fingers stretched, later reaches into the distance. It seems that the pointing of the index finger is one of the first steps in this direction. The nearness of grasping and groping is also proven by the pathological material. Patients in whom the grasp reflex is elicited, also start to grope even if they did not do so before. This groping may even be unilateral and may be considered a local psychic phenomenon. There is no fundamental difference in the psychological attitude concerning grasping and groping. It is hardly possible to come to a full insight into the many organic structures which are involved in such a simple reaction, which some are inclined to call a reflex. In cases of alcoholic encephalopathy, one can observe, step by step, how the tendency for groping finally diminishes as the patient recovers. However, there is still the tendency to grasp things without any apparent reason and the situation finally ends in a particular pleasure in handshaking, a modified grasp. Rabiner (1935) points to the tendency to an increased grasp reflex in panic. The psychological implications of such a simple "reflex" are, in this respect, rather appalling.

The rattle behavior has been studied in detail by Gesell and Thompson. They found that up to the age of sixteen weeks, possession of the rattle had no influence on the child's observable behavior. Opening and closing of the fingers on the rattle handle, and mouthing, were increased, but otherwise the patterns of manipulation and exploration were much the same whether or not the infant's hand was empty. The authors draw the conclusion that we often wrongly ascribe a stimulus function to outward objects. The movements become only slowly associated with visual auditory components. Consistent optic attention to the rattle is highest when the child is about twenty-eight weeks old. The rattle in the hand is also most appreciated at this time. Visual and tactual presentation of the rattle may provoke general body activity, specific arm activity, and hand extension and closure. It cannot be ascertained what the behavior with the rattle actually means. It is difficult to ascertain what a sound means to the infant, but it does mean something; however, it is difficult to say whether even the older child brandishes the rattle in order to produce the sound.

The motor behavior of the child often determines his sensory capacities and approaches. Young children often lose objects out of their sight, obviously in connection with an underdevelopment of the visual motor apparatus. It is difficult to ascertain generally what constitutes an object for the child. The investigations of Rubinow and Frankl (1934) make it at least probable that it takes a long time until the bottle is recognized in its configuration. It is in marked contrast to this fact that the recognition of a face takes place very early. The rattle behavior, the reaction to the bottle, and the relation to the human face obviously put the child into a rather complicated situation. We are not able to analyze the situation from a pathological point of view as closely as we are able to recognize the mechanisms involved in the grasping. The recognition of form obviously has a development of its own, closely related to the fundamental urges and needs of the child, which also express themselves in motility.

Motility is always a part of the total behavior situation. Perception is also a part of the total behavior situation. The separation is artificial; however, perception and motility may be in complicated correlation to each other. Furthermore, it is obvious that the emotional attitudes are not merely determined by the sensory motor-vegetative unit, but are a part of it and influence the sensory motor experiences as well as they are influenced by them. Before we try to discuss this aspect, let us turn our attention to a group of illustrative pathological cases.[2]

Three-year-old Charles is a child who lies in a supine position and cannot sit up. His spontaneous movements consist in turning his head and eyes from one side to the other. During these movements, wide openings of the mouth occur. The head is mostly pulled backwards and is more often turned to the right than to the left side. The arms are in continuous movement, especially the hands and fingers. There is no definite regularity in these movements. The movements remind one of a choreoathetotic play. The hands mostly drop at the wrist. The right arm is more often flexed than the left one. There is an irregular sequence in the legs consisting of stretching the one and flexing the other. However, symmetrical bending and stretching of the legs are very often combined with a spontaneous Babinski position of the toes. The right leg has a greater tendency to go into flexion. The right arm is usually flexed at the same time. When the head is turned to the left, the left arm and leg are extended and the right arm and right leg are held persistently in flexion. The tendon reflexes are present. There is an outspoken Babinski reaction on both sides, which combines with flexion in the legs.

When an object is held before his eyes it is looked at attentively. During the act of looking, the spontaneous movements stop. When the object is suddenly brought toward the face, the child blinks and smiles

[2] The children were observed in 1937, at the Children's Reception Hospital of New York City, which, for a short time, cared for a group of the more helpless defective children committed to State care.

or opens his mouth. He reacts vividly to the sound of keys. He turns his head and smiles, opens his mouth and starts licking his lips. A touch in the middle of the upper lip and at the sides of the lips immediately results in the opening of the mouth. A touch on the skin on either side of the face stimulates mouth opening. The effect of a touch on the arms is less outspoken, while touching of the legs has no effect on mouth opening and smiling. Every passive movement of the head causes mouth opening. The child struggles actively against any passive turning of the head. Only an incomplete turning of the body follows the turning of the head. During the struggle, rhythmical opening of the mouth occurs. The same struggle goes on when one tries to change the posture of any limb. There is an active resistance against any stretch. This is also very outspoken when one stretches his finger. A powerful grasp reflex occurs. When one tries to extend the arm at the elbow against the resistance of the child, not only the fists are clenched (the thumb is closed into the fist) but the legs are extended and the feet go into a grasping position, the soles turned inward. The posture of the legs has no influence on either the posture of the arms or of the head, and the posture of the arms has no influence on the posture of the legs. However, as the previous description shows, Magnus and DeKlein neck reflexes are present. They can be observed more easily with spontaneous movements of the head than with passive movements against which the child struggles. The struggling has obviously two components; a more primitive negativistic countertension and a more deliberate struggling with many qualities of an active movement.

When the mattress upon which the child lies is suddenly shaken, the arms are extended symmetrically and abducted. The legs show symmetrical flexion. The arms remain abducted for a short time. Rhythmical movements of the right leg follow. Sudden noises have similar, but less outspoken, effects. The child cannot keep his head in an upright position when held in a sitting posture. When he is elevated into a prone position, the head is held upward and the legs are stretched. When the head is bent downward the legs remain stretched. When the child is held with the head downward the legs go into a flexor contraction. When the child is held in the air supported on the chest, the legs go into a complete extension.

It is obvious from this description that one deals here with a motor picture which corresponds, in an exaggerated way, to the motility of a child of two or three months of age. Standard mental testing gave the child a mental rating of this age.

We do not know what causes such an arrest in motor development. In such children, the following fundamental characteristics can be seen: This is an organism which reacts to almost all stimuli with opening of the mouth. This is obviously an incomplete sucking mechanism. The other activities of the organism consist in adaptations to positions. The Magnus and DeKlein neck reflexes are important regulatory mechanisms in this respect. The child also reacted in a decisive way to changes of the head in space, although the examination performed was incomplete, using merely a rough clinical examination. There is further countertension and struggling, in close relation with the tendency to maintain the posture of the body and the free movements of the limbs. The grasp reflex is in very close relation to these functions, although, in the case observed, its true biologic value could not be determined. In such a case, we may suspect that fundamental apparatuses for motility and behavior are involved. The maintenance of the posture by postural and righting reflexes and by grasp is obviously a preliminary necessity for the reception of food. The tensions of resistance are a part function of this stabilizing mechanism. However, impulses are going on continually. There are the rhythmical impulses akin to walking and the choreoathetotic play in the arms and legs. The child makes only a few noises. One does not err in seeing, in these impulses, the tendency to spontaneous adaptation.

During the last few years, the so-called Moro reflex has found great interest. Its description varies. Moro (1918), himself, emphasizes that a concussion of the support on which the child lies, results in raising of the arms which are abducted afterward as in an embrace. Freudenberg (1921) says that the arms are extended at the elbows and abducted. Later on, they are brought nearer to the midline. The subsequent adduction can be absent. The fingers are spread and halfway flexed. The legs are mostly extended and abducted. The feet supinated, the big toe abducted. The reflex is most outspoken in the first three months, but can persist, in a weaker form, up to the fifth and sixth month. Almost any stimulus can provoke the reflex. However, Moro's method is the most efficient one.

In our case, as mentioned, the reflex was connected with flexion in the legs. McGraw (1935) emphasizes that the distant phalanx of the index finger is flexed and that the thumb is flexed and abducted on the palm of the hand. Whatever the movement may be, it is likely to be bilateral and simultaneous, and connected with an extension of the spine. She states that instead of extension of the legs, flexion can be observed. This reaction is also called the "body startle reaction." According to my observations, it almost always starts with blinking and the startled expression of the face. McGraw reports that the reaction is very often followed by crying, but this takes place obviously only when strong stimuli are applied.

If the stimulus is not too strong, the Moro reflex is followed by mouth opening and smiling. If one analyzes a greater number of observations, one sees that children who show the Moro reflex use practically the same motility pattern on a variety of other occasions, and the so-called Moro reflex appears more or less as a pattern which shows great variations and is the motor reaction to danger, especially postural danger. If the danger is very great, crying occurs. If the child is immediately reassured by postural security, smiling takes place.

The defective child just described gives us insight into fundamental behavior patterns which obviously are not merely motor problems, but problems of attitudes.

Organisms have to be secure in their posture. They have to be secure concerning their freedom of motility. They want to have the possibility of overcoming dangers, and they want to be fed. All these psychological reactions are performed in patterns of motility, which can be preserved for a longer time in retarded children. If one has once given attention to these problems one will easily find them in the play and the reactions of children, concerning equilibrium and security in posture. Many games of children consist of a mild danger to equilibrium which is afterward regained. The primitive patterns provide for a continuous play between restless activity (choreo-athetosis) and postural patterns, and the attempt to secure the position of head, trunk, and limbs against changes arbitrarily imposed. Although direct proof is difficult to give, one very often finds, in extensive analyses of anxiety neurosis, experiences of insecurity, from earliest childhood on, concerning the equilibrium.

Many of my cases complain of difficulties in walking on inclines or on smooth surfaces, and of early experiences of dizziness. As children, they did not have the moral (erotic) and physical support from their parents. One may draw the conclusion that children's experimentation concerning posture and equilibrium should be guided and supported from earliest childhood on. The child should not be exposed to threats concerning his motor security without having reassurance. It is not possible to go into details in this respect. Only a few of the functions which are of importance for this problem have been discussed so far. Further discussion would have to go not only into the problem of postural and righting reflexes, the Moro reflex, grasping and sucking, but also into a deeper study of tone and the vestibular apparatus.

In spite of the deep retardation of motor development in the child just discussed, one finds fundamental activities. It is difficult to determine whether there is any specific lesion or a general retardation in development.

Very much in contrast were the observations of two-year-old Owen, who lies quietly with arms and legs flexed. Only rarely does one get the impression that he shows any attention to his surroundings. When objects are shown him he does not give them any attention. When an object is brought toward him quickly, there is blinking and a slight tendency to mouth opening. Sudden stimuli (Moro reflex) merely increase flexion of the legs slightly.

The child follows noises with head and eyes. He reacts only occasionally to moving objects. There is no reaction to slight touches on the body. Turning of the head has no effect, and the child is merely resistive and starts crying, which is stopped by acoustic stimuli. There are changing rigidities all over the body which occur mostly against resistance. Grasping occurs only when rigidity is present. There are no reflexes of posture.

This is a child in whom motor activity is diminished to the utmost. There are no adaptations, and the child is merely quiet and resists muscular change. We may suspect that pallidar lesion plays an important part in this case. In other cases, even the grasping may be missed and no resistance is present against the change of the predominant flexor posture of the legs.

There are many transitions between the cases of these two groups —cases with primitive motor activities and strong impulses of a very primitive type, and cases in which even the so-called reflex activity is diminished to the utmost. Sucking reflexes, choreoathetotic movements, the Moro reflex, and grasping may be present only to a

169

minimal degree or they may be absent altogether. Resistance, crying, and mouth movements remain—but activity is diminished to the utmost.

The next three cases to be discussed, lead us into further problems.

Five-year-old Veronica has severe central cataracts and is almost blind. She shows irregular jerks all over the body. Her movements are jerky and mildly asynergic. When one supports her arms she walks in an asynergic way. There is a combined flexion of the hips. There is a bilateral Babinski reaction but no other signs of pyramidal tract lesions. Her vision is obviously severely impaired; however, she reacts to strongly lighted, large objects. She has no speech but makes inarticulate noises.

The child is in continual motion, with tremors all over the body. Her motion consists chiefly of crawling on the floor. Very often, she holds her mouth wide open. When one lets her lie on her back on the floor, she turns around and walks on all fours. Occasionally she pulls herself up to larger objects. She grabs after objects and tries to gnaw at them. For instance, she gnaws at the rim of the wash basin or at the leg of a table. She puts the wastepaper basket over her head, crawls out again, puts it on the floor with the bottom up and sits on it. However, she cannot sit there very long because of her tremors. Again she crawls into the wastepaper basket, and finally sits on its edge. Half-crawling, half-supporting herself with her hands, she navigates from one object in the room to another, using her arms in a continuous search for the next object. Her movements are jerky. She very often uses the persons around her for support. She crawls between their legs and hides her head between their legs. She likes to push her head into holes. She seeks to crawl into something. Every object is something worth grasping, to get hold of, and use for equilibrium. Then she pulls the object with great force.

Considering the severe impairment of her vision, and her obviously cerebellar impairment of motility, her agility and efficiency in moving around are astonishing. She uses human beings from the point of view of equilibrium more than from any other point. It is a case of increased tactile and motor experimentation and exploration. She grasps for objects in order to get hold of them. It is in no way a grasp "reflex." This is the fully developed motility of a five-year-old child who also has cerebellar lesions. However, we must note that there is an enormous increase in motor impulses. These motor impulses, in close relation to form and perception of form, are no longer the primitive impulses of the Moro reflex and the postural reflexes. An individual handicapped by visual defects and intellectual underdevelopment is continuously driven by motor urges, which drive an apparatus which is well developed, but disturbed by localized lesion. We have reason to believe that such impulse disturbances can be in connection with lesions of the substantia nigra and the striatum. A changed impulse here uses a motor apparatus of comparatively high development. We meet the same problem in the next two cases.

\* \* \*

Richard is a three-year-old child who can stand alone. However, he is much concerned with his equilibrium. He does not want to be moved from the spot where he is standing, and resists every attempt to move him. Occasionally he puts his fingers into his mouth. He very often supports one arm with the other. He moves his head while looking around and moves his trunk with the head. When he moves a little more, an extension of the index finger occurs. When one tries to turn his head passively he resists. The resistance, in this case, is in ascendancy over the postural reflexes. It is difficult to make him lie down flat on his back. He lies on his back for a short time and gets up rapidly without any particular turning. He reacts to sounds by turning his head in the direction of the sound. Even when he stands still in one spot, his arms are in continuous motion. He grasps objects, but when he gets them in his hands he keeps them for only a short time and then throws them away with an expression of pleasure. After the activity has gone on for awhile he starts to move around, but pretty soon he again stands in one spot which he does not want to leave. When sitting, he makes movements with his legs which remind one of walking. This continuous activity of the legs while sitting is in sharp contrast to his tendency to stand in one spot, when his soles touch the floor. When he gets excited (sitting) all extremities are flexed. He pulls the hand of the examiner toward himself in a playful way, but then immediately pushes it back. When the examiner pinches him, he pushes his hand away, but this defense remains more or less local. There is no display of hostility and his attitude remains playful.

There are no gross neurological disturbances. There is obviously a particular distribution of impulses concerning standing and activities in the arms. It is furthermore obvious that this impulse distribution is in close relation to psychological problems.

\* \* \*

Two-year-old John walks a few steps, with a broad base, when left to himself. However, his arms are in slight extension and in cataleptic position. He is interested in his surroundings, smiles, and turns his head with jerky movements toward the person in whom he is interested. The cataleptic posture of the elbows is not changed when jerky movements occur in the shoulders. He protests with grunts against any passive movement. Symmetrical movements in the arms and legs are common. There is no definite muscular resistance; however, the child tries in active movements to counteract everything which is done. When one takes his hand he tries to withdraw it. When the hand is let loose, he makes flapping movements with his arms. When a doll is brought near him, he becomes frightened, screams, and covers his eyes. When the chair on which he sits is balanced backward, the child makes desperate movements in order to keep his balance. He sits rigidly on the chair and has difficulty in getting up. When he walks, he often points to objects with one arm and reaches out for persons. When one tries to approach him, he turns his back, or walks some steps backward. The fingers are mostly in movement, with a great tendency to spread them, and the little finger is very often abducted. When he gets frightened, he very often makes gait movements. He is extremely careful before he grasps an object, but afterward uses the object to retain his equilibrium. When he is lying on the floor, flat on his back, arms and legs are flexed and he does not make any attempt to get up from this position.

Although there is a history of epileptic fits, it is obviously a developmental disturbance, in which a lack of impulses blends with a general attitude of rejection, which is partially based on the fear of losing his equilibrium through the approach of other persons.

It is simple to supplement these observations by observations of children with akinetic and hyperkinetic phenomena of a postencephalitic type. We are merely interested, here, in pointing out that the flow of motor energy is determined by general developmental factors and by the state of specific apparatuses in the brain. The state of the motor apparatus, especially the motor apparatus concerning the equilibrium experiences of security and insecurity, further determines the way in which motility is used. The flow of motor energy is partially determined by comparatively primitive apparatuses (like countertensions, grasp reflex, and sucking reflex), but also by the state of the higher levels of motility. These, in turn, are fundamentally influenced by the state of specific parts of the brain. From this point of view, we shall consider three definite types of organic lesion of the brain: (1) Lesions of the cerebellum; (2) Lesions of the striopallidum—substantia nigra apparatus; (3) Pyramidal tract lesions.

The psychological state of cases with cerebellar lesion has been studied by Bender. Children with cerebellar lesions (my experience also contains instances of this type) very often show a deep attachment to the persons around them. They are clinging, full of love, and show great insecurity when left to themselves. Although, when in need of support, they cling predominantly to their parents, they turn easily to every person around them. One cannot understand the attitude of these children, if one does not take into consideration that the cerebellar lesion, by provoking asynergia, especially in the trunk, makes balance difficult. At the same time, the primitive postural and righting reactions are not only preserved, but increased.

Of extra-pyramidal diseases, we shall consider, chiefly, the so-called Anton Vogt disease in which there is a striopallidar lesion, in which the striatum lesion predominates. The choreoathetosis is in the foreground of the picture. However, cerebellar signs are very often present. In most of the cases observed there is also an intellectual underdevelopment. The disease may be familial.

So in the case of Anne, fifteen months old, and Mary, six years old, who are sisters. Anne cannot sit upright, and shows a tendency to sucking when the lateral side of the mouth is touched. There are choreiform movements in the trunk, pointing in the fingers, and a continuous tendency to get hold of the rail with her legs, in order to escape the uncertainty in posture. There are no grasp reflexes. The movements in the arms and legs are choreiform. She continually tries to turn around. When held upright, supported on the chest, gait movements start after extension of the legs. The picture is dominated by general restlessness and resistance against any passive movements.

Mary walks with asynergic movements, is in danger of losing her balance but recaptures it with the help of primitive postural reflexes, which appear exaggerated. This child is also decidedly hyperkinetic. The child laughs often, and almost every perception provokes mouth opening, but not of the primitive type. However, this mouth opening can be very easily provoked by conditioning, and stimuli (such as touching the skin of the extremities) which are otherwise not efficient, provoke the mouth opening. It occurs also at sudden noises.

\* \* \*

Rose is eleven years old, and shows considerable mental retardation. She is in continuous movement of the choreoathetotic type. A great part

**173**

of her voluntary activity is directed to the suppression of the choreo-athetotic movements which dominate the picture. No sustained attention for action or perception is possible under these circumstances. This is an individual dominated by a wealth of motor impulses of primitive type.

In the so-called Hallervorden-Spatz disease, the lesion of the substantia nigra and the pallidum system leads to tensions, often of passing character. This tonic picture, in comparison with the tension of resistance which I have described in the developmental group, is of a more neurological character and has less close relation to the general psychic attitude of resistance.

Fourteen-year-old George grasps playfully, but very soon afterward pushes away the object which he has just grasped. Very often, tonic innervation occurs in muscles which are antagonistic to the movement which was intended. When he is ordered to make a movement, a movement in the opposite direction may occur. This is a neurological counterpart to catatonic negativism. However, as a person, he is not negativistic. He takes great pleasure in grasping whatever comes near to him and pulls it to himself. Sometimes he goes into rhythmical movements with his arms when he has an object in his grasp. When an object is put into his hand, he handles it almost correctly. A strong tone pulls shoulders, arms and hands into queer postures. The shoulder girdle is hypertrophied. In the pauses between the tonic contractions, the hands and fingers are hypotonic. The tone contracts the legs in flexor posture. The left toe then goes into Babinski posture. The patient is retarded mentally. He does not talk spontaneously, but tries to answer questions. He counts, but his articulation is so bad that it is almost impossible to understand him.

This individual is bothered, in a most severe way, by the motor disturbance, which even makes it impossible for him to express his intention to movement in the right direction. His general tendency to motility is rather increased, but he has to check it in order not to become still more disturbed by the motility which functions in an arbitrary way. An almost identical observation can be made in a boy nine years of age.

It is obvious that cases of this type cannot express themselves because the lower impulses have become autonomous. These autonomic impulses occasionally force the individual into actions not otherwise intended. Human contacts remain restricted, since the motility absorbs too much of their attention, and, very much in contrast to the cerebellar case, the help given is of no fundamental importance.

Cases with extra-pyramidal rigidity which is not changing, who are impaired in the use of their extremities, show a completely different picture. They have learned to adapt, can make use of whatever is left of their motility, can utilize the help of others, and may finally gain a comparative independence. If their motility gives way, they are not similarly a prey to gravitation, and they are therefore less clinging. In many respects, they are not different from individuals in whom a peripheral or muscular lesion has impaired the power of motility.

Eighteen-year-old Peter is very amiable. He shows extra-pyramidal tension all over the body and exhibits the picture commonly described as Little's disease. He is impaired in his intelligence. A single conversation gives sufficient insight into his attitudes:

The patient says he could not walk since he was a kid. "I never walked. I get around places and help my mother and father." What do you want to do yourself? "Trade." Three wishes. "I want to walk." Whom do you like? "Mother and father because they put me into this world." Do you like to be here? "Yes." Why? "You get a lot of things, you go around places. There is play and football." Why do people kill themselves? "They have some reason. I don't like to hit anybody unless they start first." Do you like to kill? "No . . ." When asked about masturbation he became shy and reticent and denied it. Why do people die? "God wants them to die." Why? "Nobody knows. You can't live all the time. The power of God wants it. That's God's way that I'm paralyzed." Are you happy? "Yes." Which food do you like best? "Home food; macaroni—lot of people eat it, like my mother does it." What is the nicest time of the year? "June and Spring—there are trees and flowers." The patient has a mental age of seven years and one month.

Since I have found the same basic attitude in cases in which pyramidal tract lesions prevail, no further illustrations of this type of motility disturbance and its influence on attitudes are given.

It is obvious that, in the majority of cases found in institutions, one does not deal merely with motility disturbances in reference to the one or the other motility apparatus. Most of the cases discussed

175

here also show a more or less outspoken mental retardation. However, basic psychological trends are determined by the state of motility. One should make it clear that motility is built up in various levels. There is a primitive level, with grasping, sucking, and changing rigidities, and particular problems of insecurity and equilibrium. There is a type of motility which is in closer relation to definite object structures and definite human relations. There are the general problems of impulses of the various levels. The impulses can be increased and decreased. The distribution of impulses concerning gait and arms might be irregular. Localized lesions of the brain, like cerebellar lesion, might have an influence on general attitudes. Lesions in the striopallidar system and the pyramidal tract offer further instances of this principle. In every stage of development, the motor reactions are in close connection with general psychic attitudes. It is well to bear this in mind, even if one talks about the grasp reflex and the Moro reflex.

It is obvious that in some stages of development the mother or the father is something to hold on to. Objects might be those which provoke startling and fright, and an approach might be something to resist. It is furthermore obvious that comprehension of these fundamentals is necessary for the understanding of the behavior of individuals, since motility is not merely a neurological phenomenon, but is closely interrelated with behavior from a general point of view. Study of motor development in children is of fundamental practical importance, and its correction is the indispensable basis for progress in psychological treatment. From a theoretical point of view, the relation of these phenomena to so-called catatonic phenomena and schizophrenic negativism is obvious. One also sees that fundamental problems express themselves in a different way at different motility levels. Further, the analysis of anxiety neurosis cases has led me to the conviction that motor behavior in early childhood very often has a fundamental influence on the further development of a neurosis.

Hermann (1936) and Rotter-Kertesz (1936) have made similar observations. I have, furthermore, pointed to the fact that organic impulse disturbances play an important part in some forms of obsession neurosis, and it is very probable that an insight into such early impulse disturbances can be of fundamental importance in the prevention of obsessive neurosis. Every step of motor development influences the libidinous and aggressive general attitudes. A child with disturbed equilibrium needs the mother (father) more for support and help, and will appreciate at the same time the libidinous attachment of the mother (father) to him. Hyperactivity may lead to greater sexual exploration or to an enormous psychic aggression and may cause counteraggression. The study of these cases may become fundamental for a deeper study of the tendencies of the ego in relation to libido.

A few remarks about more complicated cases:

Albert is seven years old, and is the second child in the family who is afflicted with progressive deterioration and severe spastic pyramidal signs, but without Babinski. There is also an asynergia. He does not talk spontaneously, but answers questions and continually makes noises. He answers "yes" to almost every question. There is enormous activity, in spite of the fact that he can neither sit nor stand. He wriggles around continually. There is obviously a familial disease, probably an encephalitis periaxialis diffusa, in which impulse disturbances are present in spite of the severe "mechanical impairment" of the motility.

\* \* \*

Two children with amaurotic idiocy were observed from a similar point of view. In three-year-old Hugh, who has an IQ of 20, rhythmical movements of opening and closing of the mouth occur. The trunk is moved rhythmically. His postural reflexes are very outspoken. The whole body is in continuous movement. He can turn around. There is little tendency to grasp, but there is continual babbling. There is no sucking reflex. Bilateral Babinski is present. Sudden noises provoke crying. Rhythmical clapping is answered by rhythmical synchronous movement of his right arm. The brother, Francis, six years old, shows outspoken pyramidal tract signs. He can speak, but with bad articulation. When he is ordered to repeat, he is able to repeat simple sentences of about three words. When he gets orders to do something he mostly says "no" at first and does not do it. However, when one says "yes" to him forcefully, he repeats "yes" and obeys the order. It is easier to make him do something when he has to imitate a movement. His spontaneous speech is restricted to "I want to get up" and "in the bed." He clings to the nurse and puts his arms around her. Wants to be taken up by the nurse. Cries when he is put down in the chair again. Continually turns to the nurse, and pre-

177

fers the posture in which he sits with his knees flexed. Shows a decided preference for the nurse. Is resistive toward strangers.

It is obvious that on the basis of his impaired vision and motility, primitive psychological attitudes have become paramount. It is true his IQ is only 46, and it may be difficult to prove which influences have been emotional and which influences are in connection with a motor inability and his intellectual retardation. However, his resistive attitude does not come out in a motor attitude but in a verbal resistance, which can be overcome verbally. In such cases one can see how the motor difficulty blends with the general emotional situation, and one sees the line which leads from muscular countertension to resistance and finally to verbal resistance.

It is interesting to approach the more complicated problem of Mongolian idiocy from a similar point of view. When the idiocy is extreme, one sees a predominance of symmetrical movements, very often connected with a tendency to fetal hyperflexion in the legs. There may be restlessness, the tendency to turn, and some general resistiveness, although the tensions mostly are not so outspoken because of the basic hypotonia.

In the cases I have so far examined, the Moro reflex was absent, obviously in connection with the fact that the general motor energy in these cases is not very high. Rhythmical movements in the mouth may be observed. There is little initiative, but the tendency to imitate was observed and the movement, once found, may persevere. It seems that in the behavior of these children, the hypotonia plays some part, the resistiveness is comparatively limited and the tendency to imitation may be increased. However, further study is necessary. It is obviously not possible to consider this group merely from the point of view of motor arrest.

The psychological and neurological picture in hydrocephalic cases is similarly complicated. The following short protocol of a three-year-old child will illustrate:

The child gets very much frightened when eye grounds are examined. As far as one can see, the disks are pale, but there is no irregularity of the borderline. The child makes rocking movements with her trunk. She is aware of what is going on in her surroundings. She can sit up alone, but is obviously very much scared of falling. Clings to the examiner in order not to fall, and grasps very vigorously in order to keep her equilibrium.

Her difficulty in maintaining her equilibrium is, as far as one can ascertain, chiefly cerebellar. The tendon reflexes are lively. No Hoffman. Meyer reflexes absent. It is almost impossible to find out if the child has a Babinski, since she is very resistive to every approach. No Rossolimo. Her defense movements are rather asynergic, but not in a very outspoken degree. There is no exaggerated reaction to the turning of the head. Grasping for objects is asynergic, too. The attitude of the child is dominated by fear concerning every approach; at the same time she clings when she needs better support in her equilibrium. From time to time there are choreiform jerks in her trunk. She takes objects in her hands and uses them as if rhythmically hitting. Grasps the object and is unwilling to give it up. Wants to put a quarter in her mouth. Obviously sees objects approximately clearly. Follows objects with her eyes. When the examiner shows the thumb she grasps it, tries to touch the examiner. This is a case of hydrocephalus with very outspoken retardation and chiefly cerebellar signs. All her psychological reactions, and her attitude toward objects, are characteristic insofar as she does not use the objects according to their structure, but either uses them for rhythmical movements or tries to put them into her mouth. However, she differentiates between the touch of a person and inanimate objects.

In this case, one sees the general signs of primitive motility due to the general retardation. At the same time, there are decided psychological signs, pertaining to motor helplessness due to the cerebellar lesion.

Finally, a hydrocephalic case may be discussed which points to new problems, which can only be indicated. This is a six-year-old girl, who is generally fearful when approached, but quiets down very quickly. Her reactions to pain are very outspoken. There are not many neurological signs. The hydrocephalus is of medium degree, the disks are pale, the tendon reflexes are lively. She has an outspoken Rossolimo on the left side, but there is no Babinski. There is a general awkwardness in motility, but obviously she does not know how to use her motility. When the examiner tries to test her diadochokinesis, she takes the hand of the examiner as if she wants to make him continue. When the examiner stretches out one arm and orders her to do the same she stretches out both arms. When she is ordered to imitate a long nose, she does not do it. When the examiner pats her on her cheeks, she does the same herself. Very often she makes helpless rotating movements. She obviously does not differentiate between the movements of the examiner and her own

179

movements. Such difficulties may arise after cortical damage. At any rate, her problem is to coordinate movements with definite purposes, and the use of motility for definite tasks is impaired in a specific way. Such problems express themselves in her speech, which shows interesting characteristics. A shortened protocol is now quoted:

Patient: "Do you want a book?" What kind of a book? No answer. Names correctly a pin, key and glasses. Says "Do you want the glasses?" Names a knife correctly. Is not able to name parts of the knife and nose and eyes. Calls her hand a nose and is also unable to name the eyes. When one points to her eyes she says, first, "nose," and then, "tongue." Where is my nose? She points to her ear. Where is my nose? "Gone." Say "the nose is nice." She repeats this, only after repeatedly being told to do so. How many fingers have I? No answer. Say "the hand has five fingers." She repeats the sentence correctly, "the hand has five fingers." Her articulation is good. Afterward, when one points to her nose and asks "what is that?" she says, "five fingers." When one points to her thumb, she again says, "five fingers." Where are your five fingers? "Gone." Where is your nose? "Gone." Where are the eyeglasses? "Gone." She perseveres very much. When the hand is shown again, she says, "five fingers," and when the nose is shown she says "nose," but she repeats this when one points to her ears. She also does not know the name for hair. She shows a great interest in the glasses. Goes into the pocket of the examiner and says "Do you want the glasses?" She obviously does not know what it means when she asks "Do you want the glasses? Do you want the book?" This is obviously a remembrance of a sentence or repetition of dialogue which is in some way taken out of its natural context. When the hand is shown, she says "five fingers." What do you have inside here? "Belly." What is inside of belly? "Gone." What is inside of here?—pointing to head. "Want the book?"

Here is a tendency to persevere, to stick to a solution once found— and this tendency to perseveration also expresses itself in language. She very often takes sentences which she has heard and repeats them without clearly understanding what the sentences mean. The problem of imitation and of the use of imitation emerges. Furthermore, she does not differentiate between her actions and the actions of the examiner. One sees fundamental problems arise in this case, but they are no longer in connection with the primitive motility patterns in which we are here interested.

## Conclusions

The child's motility has the function of maintaining the posture as the basis for subsequent action. The mouth, an organ with a fixed posture in the face, has specific functions. However, there is, at least at an earlier stage of development, reaching of the mouth for objects and rhythmical sequences of mouth movements. The child needs security in posture and freedom of action which brings him in relation to objects, and to the world. The tasks of posture and action are, of course, different in the different stages of development. Furthermore, the child does not want any passive movement to be imposed upon him. He guards himself, with resistance, against postures imposed upon him. There are many apparatuses serving these fundamental functions of motility. Grasping, at first a function in the service of the maintenance of posture, later on serves for relating to objects. Pointing is derived from grasping. There is a muscular tension as expression of the resistance against imposed postures.

There is, furthermore, a psychic resistiveness in close relation to the muscular countertension. The motility which counteracts the tendency for safety is, in the beginning, dissociated and continuous (choreoathetotic). At first, symmetrical movements and primitive rhythmical movements (gait) prevail. Unilaterality and arhythmicity follow. The further development of motility is guided by contact with the world. However, the basic problems of equilibrium, posture, grasp, freedom of movement, and efficiency of movement remain the basic problems. No child is satisfied merely with security. There is, continually, the urge to experiment (continuous freedom of movement). The motility is dependent on impulses and the energy of impulses. The impulses may flow into the postural apparatus, in the grasping, in the free movement, and in the resistance. The energy of impulses will be of fundamental importance not only in the approach to the world, but also in the utilization of the apparatus of posture in the equilibrium.

Further problems originate from the tendency to imitate and from the tendency to persist in motor and psychic solutions, once found. Every step of this development is in closest relation to the

181

world around the child, especially the adults. Every step of this development is closely connected with emotional problems. The love of the mother (father) does not merely consist of stroking the child, but also in protecting the equilibrium and posture of the child, without impairing his freedom of motor expression, and without imposing postures on the child which he does not want. The emotional problems connected with motility blend with the intrafamilial libidinous problems. The help the child needs is also motor help.

Pathological cases show the mechanisms involved, in a clearer way. In pathological cases, we find general motor retardation sometimes combined with impulse disturbances. The lesions of specific apparatuses in the brain, which are concerned with specific phases of motility, lead to specific psychological attitudes and to characteristic psychological problems. The psychological attitudes of children with cerebellar lesions, striopallidar lesions, and pyramidal tract lesions are fundamentally different. In many pathological cases, the problems of motor retardation and the lesions of specific motor apparatus are combined, as, for instance, in some encephalitis cases and in hydrocephalus. It is an unsolved problem whether the hypotonia of Mongolian idiocy does not offer specific problems. Children who are impaired in their motor development need the specific motor help which cannot be given if these fundamental problems are not understood. Also, children who do not have specific motor disturbances, have motor problems in no way less important than the so-called psychological problems in the narrower sense. It is very probable that unsolved motor problems, concerning the security of equilibrium, may be one of the factors in the later development of anxiety neuroses, and unsolved impulse problems in childhood may have a more or less outspoken connection with compulsive and obsession neuroses in later life.

Play, concerning posture, which the child loves so much, is often not handled in the right way by the adult. It is obviously correct to let the child experiment with any posture and action. It is justifiable to rock the child, to raise him in the air and then let him drop, provided that the danger situation does not become overwhelming to the child. He should learn that after experimentation and danger, he can regain security with the help of others. He may finally learn to rely on his own capacity to regain postural security. He should never be brought into a panic of equilibrium or, more generally, into a motor panic. Furthermore, he should not be thrown into postural situations which he resists more than necessary. He should not have the feeling that motor restrictions are imposed upon him which are lasting.

It seems to me that the motor education of a child is a preliminary step in all education and carries with it important emotional and libidinous implications. We may suspect that mere knowledge on the part of the parents will not be sufficient to handle the problems of equilibrium in the child in a correct way. The parents will need, besides their motor equipment and their will to help the child in his motor expression and security, an emotional inner balance.

Equilibrium is not merely a motor and vestibular problem, but also a moral one.

### Clinging and Equilibrium[3]

Hermann (1936) has quite rightly called our attention to the significance of clinging in the mental life of man. I here propose to adduce certain facts which confirm his ideas and amplify them. Bieber (1937) and I have carried out tests with newly born infants which have shown us that the act of sucking is, in fact, always accompanied by a heightening of muscular tension, especially in respect to grasping. Insofar as grasping can be voluntarily initiated, it enables sucking to proceed more easily. Hermann quite correctly comments on the amount of energy involved in the act of grasping.

According to Watson (1930) and Richter (1931), newborn babies and monkeys are actually able to maintain themselves suspended by the strength of their grasping reflex. Richter has shown that the grasping reflex in monkeys regularly disappears in the process of development. The fact that the grasping reflex makes it possible to cling in defiance of the law of gravity, and subsequently diminishes, further points to the probability of there being a connection between grasping and sucking. A child must feel securely perched against his mother's body while sucking.

A very interesting finding of Bieber's, which I can confirm, was

[3] From Schilder (1939a).

that sucking reinforces the grasping reflex and vice versa. For example, in cases with severe lesions of the brain, we very often find that it is, at first, only possible to activate the grasping reflex. If we reinforce this, we elicit the sucking reflex too. The reverse can also happen. It follows that we are dealing with a function forming a single whole. The child sucks as he clings to his mother. But this original association of the functions is not maintained.

At the next stage in his development, the child must learn to stand upright and walk. Clinging is still very essential to him, but it is now needed to enable him to stand erect against the forces of gravity. In alcoholic disturbances, one can observe that the grasping reflex becomes especially marked when the subject is in danger of falling backwards. In cases with paralysis agitans with retropulsions, I have very often noticed that forced grasping was present and became especially marked while retropulsion was taking place. Here, the grasping reflex aims at securing support in the struggle to assume or maintain an upright position without loss of equilibrium. It is not so much contact with the mother's body which is sought, as her help in dealing with dangers of gravity. Especially in cases of paralysis agitans, there is often no sign of the sucking reflex. Grasping has become an independent function.

In the course of the child's later development, grasping undergoes a further change in aim; the child seizes the object and brings it to his mouth (taking nourishment). But the relation between grasping and sucking has now become something entirely different from what it was in the newborn infant. In the original sucking clinging function, clinging served to secure the child's equilibrium (protection against being dropped) and physical warmth (proximity to the mother's body), especially when absorbing nourishment. At a later stage, clinging helps him to preserve an upright posture. In either case, we may say that it helps to counter the forces of gravity.

We may go further and say that it is one of the functions of a mother to safeguard her child against these forces. Bender (1940) has been able to show that children suffering from defects of the cerebellum develop an especially great need for support and tenderness. They require their mother's (parents') support against the forces of gravity. These problems merge into the great problems of posture and preservation of equilibrium, which anatomically is related to the apparatus regulating this (the vestibular apparatus) and that concerned with the stance and postural reflexes. It seems that children respond with anxiety and panic whenever they feel uncertain of their ability to maintain their position. This panic may be compared with the sensation brought on by turning around and then suddenly making a movement of the head (Purkinje's falling phenomenon). Adults react to such a situation with a feeling of dizziness.

I do not hesitate to say that this powerful apparatus constitutes one of the nuclear formations of the ego, in an analytical sense. It is, in the first place, only indirectly connected with grasping, holding, and mastering, although, as Hermann rightly points out, such connecting links do undoubtedly exist. But I think it would be more correct to assume that the act of taking hold, which is involved in the grasping reflex, is not simply to be accounted for by reference to the erotogenicity of the hand, just as we assume that an ego component is also present in the act of sucking. Both ego functions, by their very nature (ego and id have their roots in the same soil), form a natural starting point for oral and tactile libidinal functions. A more important point is that sucking and clinging, and being supported, lead to a union and a fusion, or one might say to a reunion with the mother's body, and thus they enter directly into the main stream of the libido, as Rotter-Kertesz (1936), especially, has shown so well.

Clinging may take place by way of the mouth to the nipple and other parts of the body or by means of the hands to the breast, hair, and other parts of the body; but its aim is always support and union. It is a matter of posture and position (tonic) and leads secondarily to a momentary act (phasic) which may be rhythmic (sucking) or arhythmic. Attacking and mastering are phasic. I am convinced, therefore, that these manifestations are only indirectly related to sadomasochism.

These considerations have a direct clinical bearing on our conception of the anxiety neurosis.

One of my cases, a thirty-year-old woman, found it especially difficult to walk on an inclined surface. Similarly, it was only with difficulty that she could walk across a marble floor; the reflection seemed to play havoc with its solidity. In her fifth year, she often felt giddy, and vomited when traveling on the subways. During her childhood, she would run to her father and put her arms around him only to find her advances coldly repulsed. At four, she was unable to sit on a swing. She was perpetually afraid that somebody might trip her up. She had been warned by her mother against sliding down haystacks. Her mother never went out, and before her death was unable to walk alone any more, suffering as she did from a pernicious anemia, accompanied by disturbances affecting her equilibrium. During the patient's anxiety attacks, it was impossible for her to walk and she would hold on to a chair.

All of these factors only acquired significance because neither her father nor her mother had ever afforded her the erotic gratification which she had not the courage to demand of them, for fear her mother might tear her to pieces. She was also possessed of a fear of being burst asunder from within, by a child or by some coveted object (perhaps her father's penis). But this anxiety would appear to have been directly concerned with instances of aggressive behavior on her part and by a mother and a nurse toward animals, which occurred in her fourth year. Her dread of being left alone and powerless to maintain her equilibrium, and her dread of being torn and burst asunder from without and within, did not apparently stand in a genetic relation to one another, although there were doubtless connections between them. Her fear was that she would be punished for masturbation and this fear activated her other anxieties. Her dread of being dismembered was closely bound up with her own aggressiveness, which was sustained by exceptionally strong feelings and aimed at dismembering other persons, especially her mother.

It is far from my intention to ascribe to this mechanism a decisive role in every anxiety neurosis, although it seems to be almost invariably present. But we can frequently demonstrate its existence in other cases as well. We find numerous dreams of flying and gliding, leaping across difficult passages or steep inclines, or floating over precipices, almost always accompanied by a feeling that the parents (father and mother) have not been sufficiently generous with their love (contact, support, embraces).

Hermann contrasts "clinging" with "going exploring" and believes that he has here found an important pair of antithetic instincts. I feel more disposed to contrast "clinging," in the first instance, with "maintaining one's position." It is a fact that children are uncommonly proud of every advance they make in physical equilibrium. They are insatiable in their demands to be swung, thrown, caught or lifted in midair. If, however, they do not feel sufficiently secure in their love of adults, these games, as I was able to observe in one case, are accompanied by increased feelings of uncertainty. In favorable cases, the child acquires the necessary confidence to enable him to maintain his posture and to avoid being left completely at the mercy of gravity. Thus we see that the child strives to make himself independent of others, in preserving his equilibrium, although he does not find it pleasant to renounce the libidinal gratification afforded by support and contact with his mother. In the next stage, this satisfaction in securing his equilibrium leads to the child's running away from his mother, which makes possible the acquisition of new objects to lean upon (love objects).

Dependence in the matter of posture is, sooner or later, felt as a matter of compulsion, as an obstacle to the individual's freedom of movement, and he reacts with rage and destructiveness. But behind this mechanism, which must be regarded in the first instance as being imbued with libido, we once more encounter the ego apparatus which clamors for postural independence, in accordance, also, with the evolutionary laws. Children conduct endless experiments to test their equilibrium, as anyone can easily see by observing them. Every anxiety neurotic experiences the bitterness of the restrictions which his illness imposes. Helene Deutsch has pointed out that the victim of agoraphobia hates and punishes the person who protects him from his anxiety. At the same time, the presence of that person acts as an assurance that he is still alive. Death wishes against the person to whom one clings and looks for support are unmistakable. According to the peculiar libidinal structure of each patient, the death of this supporting figure may simply be experienced in terms of his removal or, as in the case just mentioned, of his dismemberment. The fear of insanity, so often present in anxiety neurotics, corresponds to their fear of their own destructive rage, especially insofar as this is directed against the supporting figure. In this connection, it should be mentioned that all cases of agoraphobia reveal a wish to embark on distant travels, to run away, to explore. Here again, I believe that the desire for, and progress toward, postural independence is to be ascribed to the nuclear structure of the ego organization, but that libidinal postures of great significance are coordinated with this part of the ego structure. Fundamentally, they are postures which free one from dependence on a supporting figure, lead away from it, and deprive it of its libidinal significance or finally bring about its destruction (by dismemberment). At this point, we may once more recall that proximity, approximation in space (to a loved object) and, finally, contact, are indispensable conditions for a positive erotic relationship, whereas remoteness in space is incompatible with any close libidinal attachment.

## ORGANIC PROBLEMS IN CHILD GUIDANCE[4]

Every perception and apperception is something going on in the sensory field, but which brings forth motor responses of varied types. These motor responses go on at different levels. There is a mass response of the whole body, as Goldstein (1934), and Hoff and I (1927) have shown. This response is mostly of a tonic type. At least half of the body is involved at any time. The tone of the body is changed as a result of hearing or seeing. Besides this change in tone, there are also actions and movements which are reactions to the stimulus. These reactions do not involve half of the whole body, but serve a particular function of a particular organ. On the other hand, motility also influences perception. Vision, for instance, would be very incomplete if there were no movements of the eye or of the head. It has not been sufficiently emphasized that motility, as such, has a very close relation to perception, and that every motor action has a tendency to bring with it specific impressions, ideas, and fantasies.

This discussion may start with the so-called hyperkinesis of children. Hyperkinesis can be of very different levels. There is a hyperkinesis in chorea and athetosis which is a more or less primitive type of hyperkinesis. It is not an excess of action, but merely an excess of more or less fragmentary movements. There is another kind of hyperkinesis, in which a general restlessness prevails. This restless-

---

[4] From Schilder (1931a).

ness may be unpatterned, without any particular purpose. But there may also be continuous grasping and groping, taking objects and dropping them, running from one person to another, clinging to a person, pinching, pulling, breaking, and tearing. We know this type of hyperkinesis well, from our experience with postencephalitic children. This type of hyperkinesis is due to a lesion of either the striopallidal system or the substantia nigra. The observations of Holzer (1926) and A. Meyer (1927) point to the importance of the substantia nigra. In the cases of Meyer, especially, there were no changes in the cortical region.

Some of these hyperkinetic actions appear to be senseless, if the hyperkinesis is something that has nothing to do with the individual's personal aims and tendencies. But there is a synthesizing tendency in the organization of the mind. When the hyperkinesis decreases, the individual will take it into the personality in some way and use it for his own purposes. He will be hyperkinetic and still know, in the hyperkinesis, what he wants to do. So he may organize his wild impulses. The impulses of postencephalitics not infrequently lead to antisocial or criminal behavior. There is a case, in the literature, of a postencephalitic who murdered because he heard that this would cure him. This superstition alone would probably not have been sufficient, without the help of increased subcortical impulses. One patient, who was usually in an akinetic state, tried to strangle another patient on a sudden impulse.

It is a remarkable fact that, according to the statistics of Engerth and Hoff (1929), a great number of postencephalitic children became criminals (in Austria). One of them organized a gang and committed many burglaries. Bond's (Bond and Appel, 1931) child patients, in the Franklin School of the University of Pennsylvania, also became delinquent. From our point of view, we say that the surplus of impulses has been synthesized into the whole personality. The surplus of impulses has another important significance. It may lead to the destruction of objects, also to sadistic actions against animals. The surplus of impulses will lead to the handling of the object and will often lead to increased curiosity and to cruelty. There will be a close relation between the surplus of impulses and sadistic attitudes. Every strong muscular or motor exertion tends to force the outer world to submission. Destruction is only a short step

189

further. The violent motor explosion of the epileptic fit is often followed by violent aggressiveness. Epilepsy is mentioned in order to show that there are hypermotilities of different types and each hypermotility probably carries a special psychology with it. For example, hyperkinesis in the region of the mouth, according to observations by E. Strauss (1930) and me (1927), leads not only to spitting, biting, and devouring, but also to tendencies to curse and use profane language. Motility then determines specific psychic content. It may also be mentioned that the attitude of clinging, persistent mischief, and pestering, in children, can also be connected with some kind of hyperkinesis.

Naughtiness and aggressiveness are among the leading problems encountered in child guidance. Problems of sadism may be associated. It is a question as to how often hyperkinesis, in the sense discussed here, is at the root of misbehavior. The slighter degrees of hyperkinesis, especially, may be synthesized with the personality, and the neurological foundation of naughtiness, aggressiveness and pestering may be overlooked. It is therefore of importance to know what signs may be expected in mild encephalitic cases.

Difficulties in convergence of the eyes, and a phenomenon that Hoff and I (1927) have called the convergence phenomenon of the arms, are the most sensitive symptoms. The convergence phenomena of the arms consist of a slight flexion of the elbows, which appears when the arms are outstretched with the eyes closed. The tips of the outstretched fingers then come closer to one another, due to a slight flexion in the elbow joint. Another reliable, but less sensitive, sign is the tendency to step backward when the head is passively bent backward.

But it is not only encephalitis lethargica that produces hyperkinesis in children. The child is already hyperkinetic in comparison with the adult, and it is one of the peculiarities of the infantile and juvenile brain to react with hyperkinesis to a lesion to which the adult brain would react in a different way. Localized chorea and athetosis are much more common after brain lesions in childhood, and even Sydenham's chorea minor chiefly occurs in childhood. We are less interested in this more primitive hyperkinesis, although we often find a more generalized hypermotility, especially in chorea minor cases. Almost every infectious disease of childhood, every

190

childhood encephalitis, may provoke such hyperkinetic states. Sometimes they are connected with signs of mental deterioration. It may be said that, in general, hyperkinesis is one of the reaction patterns of the underdeveloped brain. It is not known exactly where the lesions that provoke hyperkinesis are located. Probably striopallidal lesions, as well as lesions in the substantia nigra, may provoke them. I have often pointed to the importance of cortical impulses. The frontal lobe and the temporal lobe, and probably also the parietal lobe, have to do with the regulation of the impulses.

There is another factor of great importance. The investigations of Schwarz (1924), in particular, have emphasized that birth is chiefly not a physiological event, but a pathological one. It is often a trauma in which lesions of the brain substance occur. The lipoid cells are scavenger cells, and are signs of destruction of the brain substance, either by hemorrhage or by contusion. The striopallidal system is probably often involved, due to its vulnerability and peculiarity of blood supply. It is still not known in what way the impulses are changed by the birth trauma. Besides these lesions due either to a trauma or to encephalitis, we have to reckon with constitutional differences in those organs which regulate the flow of the motor impulses. Thus, it may be seen how many organic motor factors may determine what is usually called naughtiness, aggressiveness, and sadism.

It cannot be denied that hyperkinesis and sadism may arise in connection with psychic problems, and that even hypermotility may be psychically determined. I have (Schilder, 1924) often spoken of "the two-way principle," meaning that an organic function may be changed by psychic causes as well as by somatic ones. An additional problem is in relation to the development of motility, as Homburger (1922), for instance, has pointed out. We know there is a very complicated process in maturation from the primitive motility of the child into the graceful motility of the adult. Postural reflexes and the Moro reflex change in the course of development. The Moro reflex disappears completely after the first few months. The motility of early childhood reminds one of chorea or athetosis. At the time immediately before puberty, motility shows many mannerisms and ticlike movements and may have awkward, almost ataxic character. In different individuals, the development of motility

191

proceeds in different ways, due either to constitutional factors or to infectious disease and trauma. But awkward motility will also express itself immediately in the whole psychic attitude of the child. He may become self-conscious and shy.

In addition to the primary changes in motility, there are influences on the character and habit formation of the child, and the feelings and impulses that accompany changes in motility; but motility is usually connected with strivings and instincts, and is a part of instinctive or volitional behavior. Thus, many organic processes contribute to the behavior patterns in children. Their endocrine glands also play some part. The cretin shows a lack of impulses. The same is true of myxedema in adults, and hyperthyroidism changes sex behavior, motility, and, secondarily, the emotions, in the adult. Hypomanic pictures are very common. It seems that an increase in the higher motor impulses is usually connected with elation and other manic features. Motor aphasia shows psychic and motility features similar to depressive conditions.

It is of great interest to study, from this point of view, the diencephalic lesions which make such deep changes, not only in sex (dystrophia adiposa genitalia), but also in hunger and thirst. The restlessness of the sleepless person, in connection with lesions in the sleeping center, especially in children, may be mentioned. Every change in the instincts will immediately change the thought content also. Little is known about the strength of the impulses or drives. It is not known why, in one child, sexuality reaches an extreme so easily; but the possibility must at least be reckoned with that the increase in sexuality, in such cases, may originate in the organic sphere. Witness, for example, the attitudes of people with tumors of the pineal gland.

Motor impulses and changes in the drives or instincts lead to very difficult behavior problems. Naughtiness and aggressiveness in boys, and sexual promiscuity in girls, certainly are the major problems in child guidance. Changes on the intellectual side and changes in perception resulting from organic brain disease, may also have an influence on behavior, of course. But mental deficiency, as such, generally offers a minor problem as long as it is not combined with changes in the emotional sphere and the sphere of impulses. It is true that mental deficiency changes the aspects of behavior problems. The emotional reactions of mentally deficient children are more difficult to understand, and it is more difficult to handle them.

Behavior problems that originate from the psychic side are problems that are better understood at the present time, and can be handled better than all the difficulties in connection with organic deficiencies and changes. It should not be forgotten that every disease in childhood also changes the whole libido situation in the family. The love of the parents or the parents' anxiety comes to the surface in a more open way. An acute disease, in this respect, certainly has a different psychology than a chronic disease, and the whole aspect of the child's life may be changed accordingly.

We must also consider that we do not yet know in what way pain and itching influence the attitude of the child. Itching will change the attitude of the child toward his own body. The same thing is true of pain. The organ that suffers will attract an enormous amount of attention, not only from the child, but from the people around him. The problem of organ inferiority, first discussed by Adler, can be mentioned in this connection. Every organic disease and deficiency is, in this respect, also a psychological problem of enormous importance. In the analysis of adults, it is often seen that a disease in childhood was a turning point in the development of the child, although sometimes it may be difficult to find out how much was due to organic factors and how much to psychological ones.

The events of life, the environmental influences, the psychic attitudes, and the mental and emotional problems of the child, all take place in an organism. The motor instinctive and sensory constitution will always be at the basis of the reaction. This somatic basis may be changed by diseases, but behavior will finally be shaped by the problems of life, which are, after all, problems of the personality as a whole.

## PSYCHIATRIC ASPECTS OF CHRONIC NEUROLOGICAL DISEASE[5]

When we speak of "disease," it should be clear that disease results in an impairment of function. The individual cannot act as he otherwise would. It is not merely a structural defect, but an impair-

[5] From Schilder (1934a).

193

ment of function, and this makes new adaptation necessary. The organism has to adapt and, especially, the sick individual has to adapt anew. We do not deal with diseases, finally, but we deal only with sick individuals and we have to care for these sick individuals who have to make this new adaptation. Adaptation goes on in the somatic sphere as well as in the psychic sphere. Disease is always a personality problem. Even in acute illness, the attitude of the person will not only shape the symptomatology, by determining the amount of pain and suffering, but will also influence, more or less, the course of the disease. In chronic diseases and in stabilized defects of the organism, the adaptation to the environment becomes the paramount problem. The organism has to fight against infection or against toxic influences, but, even in acute disease, it is very important to know what attitude the individual takes. The way in which pain is experienced depends very largely on the attitude of the total personality.

There is practically no symptom, in any disease, which is not finally modified by the attitude of the personality. This attitude influences not only the subjective aspect, but also the changes in the organism which are under the influence of psychopathological processes going on in the individual. When he is well adapted and well balanced mentally, the final outcome will depend on the patient's attitude toward the disease. In chronic disease, the personality factors play the outstanding part. Human beings live in society. They can have goals and aims only in relation to other human beings. Greater freedom in moving around becomes senseless when an individual does not know what to do with his freedom.

Mechanical treatment becomes really therapeutic only when imbued with the spirit of social helpfulness. In every step of somatic treatment, the problems of the total personality have to be considered. This is the psychiatrist's approach to every chronic organic disease, whether or not it affects the central nervous system.

In chronic neurological diseases, specific problems arise due to the fact that in encephalitis, birth injury, and epilepsy, organic changes in the brain not only cause neurological signs, but also psychic changes. The organic process may impair intellectual capacity. After encephalitis in infancy (other than encephalitis lethargica), and birth injury, we may find all types of intellectual impairment, from borderline deficiency to idiocy. In epileptics, a specific deterioration is often observed, which may include slowing down of mental processes, perseveration, circumstantiality, and impairment in the memory function. But the terms "mental deficiency" and "deterioration" are misleading. There is no such thing as an isolated intellectual function in the human mind.

Intellect and emotion are closely coupled with each other, and, in all degrees of mental deficiency, we find more or less outspoken emotional deficiencies and disturbances. We are inclined to overlook them when they have the aspect of quantitative diminution or insufficient depth and organization. But the incidence of manifestations generally considered as psychotic is, as Greene (1933) has shown, rather high. Wide emotional outbursts, fargoing withdrawals, seclusiveness, paranoid trends, and even hallucinations are not uncommon. Are these disturbances, and the mental deficiencies, the immediate expression of the lesions in the brain? It is well known that emotional blocking may play a great part, and that mental deficiency may be absent in spite of insufficient intellectual functioning. The level of defects is always dependent on the emotional situation.

Generally speaking, modern psychology no longer believes that any symptomatology is the direct result of a defect. The symptomatology is the expression of the function of those parts of the brain which are preserved. Or, in other words, even in low-grade idiocy and imbecility, we deal with a personality with specific problems, reacting to the environment, the social situation, and the persons around him. As long as there is life, psychological adaptation and reactions continually take place, modifiable by psychological approach. This does not hold true only in the emotional sphere, but also in the intellectual field.

It should not be asked which are the problems that the deficient person cannot solve, but, rather, which are the problems that he *can* solve, and in what way can he be educated to make social use of his faculties, whatever they may be. Investigations by Bromberg (1934), on the children's service of Bellevue Hospital, show that children with borderline intelligence or mental deficiency of minor degree are often susceptible to emotional situations, and many form symptoms, on such a basis, which may even resemble schizophrenic pictures. Neurotic habits, often impulsive, compulsive or obsessive in nature, may assume such importance in the life of the mentally deficient child that other activities may become impossible. If such behavior can be understood as the child's attempt to solve a particular emotional problem and if he is permitted free expression, then he may also be able to proceed to the use of his less impaired abilities. Mentally deficient children, with exaggerated verbal and intellectual capacities, in whom intellectual training has been over-stressed, have an increased consciousness of their maladaptation, which may lead to panics in which sexual preoccupations are, in some instances, predominant.

The problem of the physician, the social worker, and the teacher, in all such cases, will be to find out the proper level of performance on which emotional adaptation is still possible. Otherwise, the child will react like Pavlov's dogs, who lost all their conditioned reflexes when too complicated differentiations between similar forms were demanded from them. Careful handling of all emotional problems, especially the sexual ones, in all cases of intellectual impairment, will be of utmost importance. Contrary to widespread opinion, intellectual deficiency often goes hand in hand with a particular emotional sensitivity, and the emotional reactions of such persons are often more violent and longer lasting than the emotions of intellectually well-developed individuals. A case with intellectual impairment, due to an undefined encephalitic process, who reacted to the absence of a beloved companion of the same sex with a violent outburst of excitement, sleeplessness, rage, and flight of ideas, subsided only when the companion returned after an absence of two weeks. Sedatives in high doses proved ineffective.

Clark (1933) has shown in several studies how much amentia can be helped by the psychological approach. Epileptic rages and violence are justly feared by everyone who deals with such patients. The organic background of these conditions is beyond doubt, but the point of view that the organic emotional disturbance defies a psychological approach cannot be justified. The final shape of an emotion is never determined by the organic factor alone, but by the activity of the total organism and the total personality. In many cases, it proves possible to lead destructive impulses into useful channels and to make a social adaptation possible. Epileptic aggressiveness is often directed against those who have made mistakes in social approach to the patients. Cases with mental deficiency, intellectual deterioration, and organic changes in the emotions need, therefore, all the psychological care the normal and neurotic child needs, and often more. Their individual problems must be recognized and brought into their consciousness as much as possible, to liberate emotional energies, which are bound by neurotic conflicts, and make them free for social activities. But this will not succeed if the individual cannot be convinced of his social usefulness and if he cannot be given a life plan which has meaning for him.

Intellectual defects are uncommon in patients who have suffered epidemic encephalitis, but even in the milder cases we find aberration in drives, impulses, and motility. Akinesis (lack of motor impulses) is common in adults in which the Parkinsonian picture, with rigidity and postural disturbances, prevails. Cohen-Booth (1935) has shown that a picture similar to Parkinsonism develops in persons of a specific type, the understanding of which helps the patients in the use of their motility, and even changes the strictly neurological signs. The psychiatric literature is full of instances proving the enormous influence of psychological factors on this seemingly purely neurological picture. To direct these activities, for the purposes of the personality and society, will not only make symptoms disappear, but will also give greater satisfaction to the afflicted individuals. The increase in drives, the hyperkinesis, observed in postencephalitic children is again due to the organic lesion of the brain. This drive is modifiable by outward circumstances. It can be directed; it can be made less destructive; it can be integrated into the total personality. Aimless sexuality can be prevented and, in a proper environment, the child can be an active, not a destructive, playmate. When he reaches adolescence, he will be socialized, and not become a criminal (as some cases reported in the literature). Modification of organic drives is a difficult, but not impossible, task. Organic drives are modifiable, just as emotions are. There is no definite borderline between the organic and the psychological aspects of human life. Whatever a lesion in the brain may be, we always deal with human beings reacting to an environment. Therefore, they can be educated.

The task is to give the chronic neurological patient his place in

197

society. He has to know that he is not excluded from this society, and that he can be useful in it. His social adaptation is, in many respects, the most important factor in his cure. This social adaptation must take place on a broad scale. The individual treatment of the patient is necessary, whether he is in an institution or not. Generally, institutions will be better equipped to give chronic neurological cases the specialized psychiatric treatment they require, and it will also be easier to provide, in institutions, the community spirit which will later enable patients, at least in some cases, to also find a social adaptation outside of the institution.

## Mannerisms in Organic Motility Syndromes[6]

Motility disturbances as manifestations of neurological problems and of psychiatric problems seem, at first sight, to be fundamentally different. In neurological cases, we are accustomed to think of comparatively stable phenomena, caused by lesions in the pyramidal tract or sensory tracts of the spinal cord, while in psychiatric cases, we find quite different pictures, such as the catatonic states of schizophrenia. However, Kahlbaum (1902), the first modern writer on schizophrenia, seemed to think that these catatonic tensions could be understood from an organic point of view, and Wernicke (1906), and his followers, especially Kleist (1923), have shown that one can approach motility problems which occur as manifestations of psychiatric conditions from an organic point of view. Kleist, himself, at first followed the footsteps of Wernicke, and Liepmann (1920), and was inclined to emphasize the similarity of catatonic manifestations to the phenomena observed in organic cortical lesions, and also studied the apractic phenomena. Later, under the impact of the new work of Wilson (1929), Vogt and Vogt (1920), and von Economo (1931), on the subcortical motor apparatus, Kleist stressed the relation of the striopallidar and subthalamic lesions to the phenomena observed in catatonic and other psychotic states.

Our own observations have included a group of phenomena observed in various clinical conditions, especially in children. Levine and I (Levine and Schilder, 1940) have described the rest-

---

[6] From Bender and Schilder (1941).

less motility of patients put into the state of anoxia by nitrogen inhalation. They move their legs, rotating them outward or bending and stretching them at the knees. These movements, and similar movements in the arms, look like voluntary movements; however, the patients obviously want to control them and one sees that they often hold their legs together to prevent these movements. The restless movements soon change into mild cloni of obvious subcortical origin. It cannot be said that these patients have a conscious wish to move their legs under the influence of subcortical impulses, but it seems that the total motor part of the personality has some share in such semivoluntary activities.

The phenomenon is similar to the behavior of some patients when they are under the influence of insulin, as described by Orenstein and me (Orenstein and Schilder, 1938). They start to move around in a manneristic fashion. It seems as though they play a rather crude game. They make grimaces and throw themselves around; they roll around and toss about. Some of these patients are amnesic, for what, at first sight, looks like a graceless prank. It is, of course, impossible to determine whether this clowning and manneristic play is due to a disorder of cortical or subcortical mechanisms, since both are disturbed in these cases.

A third group of cases, with disorders of this type, were reported in alcoholic encephalopathies by Bender and myself (Bender and Schilder, 1933). We have particularly found this picture in alcoholic Negroes (Parker, Schilder, and Wortis, 1939). In many of these cases, outspoken changes in the postural reflex were found to be present. Clinically related groups show clear-cut catatonic phenomena in the field of motility. These are cases in which neuropathological changes are found predominantly in the periventricular grey matter and adjacent structures in the brain.

The clinical picture suggests a subcortical mechanism as the chief cause of the phenomena. This also seems to be a possible approach to the pathophysiology of the manneristic and clowning movements of schizophrenics. The clowning of the alcoholics, mentioned above, is, in some cases, really difficult to differentiate from the clowning of schizophrenics.

This study presents a group of cases, several children and one adult, which may contribute something to the understanding of this problem:

Alice, of white Puerto Rican parentage, was the second of five siblings. In the summer, when eleven years old, she became very much alarmed during a lightning storm. Two months later, she became irritable and showed the symptoms of chorea, with which disease she was admitted to the pediatric service of a general hospital in February. For two months she could not talk and had to be tube fed. After six months, she was taken home, but had frightening visual hallucinations. She saw a man standing in the doorway, heard noises, and was generally unmanageable. In August of the second summer, she had a recurrence of rheumatic fever, endocarditis, and chorea. From time to time, she was in a psychotic condition, bewildered and confused, somewhat cataleptic in her motility, and tended to hallucinate, especially at night.

Then her elevated temperature receded, and there were no signs of endocarditis or arthritis. The choreatic movements in the extremities completely disappeared. When examined in December of the second winter, she showed disturbed motility phenomena, chiefly in the face. There were no choreatic movements in the face in the common sense, however the mimical expression seemed to be very manneristic. Whenever she made efforts in the extremities, there were no associated movements in other extremities, but associated movements in the head and face. When ordered to keep her eyes closed, she became restless, opened her eyes, and looked away. In connection with facial grimacing, there were manneristic movements of the fingers, which corresponded neither to choreatic movements nor to associated movements. The same movements appeared in her trunk muscles. However, the associated movements were much more outspoken in the head. Although the closing of the eyes caused the strongest reaction, there were similar reactions seen with the opening and closing of the mouth. Occasionally, she closed her eyes when she opened her mouth.

When counting, she made twisting movements in the trunk, rotating on her legs and making small steps. She would not continue counting, or any form of speech, for long. Her speech was halting, with uncoordinated respiration. It did not appear, however, that difficulty in breathing was the cause for the halting speech, rather, it even appeared that the halting speech caused the difficulty in breathing. When the arms were outstretched, they tended to pronate and sink down, both when the head was turned to the right and to the left. She often showed countermovements, in turning, with paradoxical deviation of both arms. Occasionally, a flexion also occurred in the arm toward which the chin was turned. She complained of pain in the neck when the head was turned. She also complained continually of paresthesia in the face, saying that parts of the face were sleepy and deadlike. There were no objective sensory disturbances. At this time, she had great difficulty in drawing or painting the human figure, while her natural scenes, though overelaborated and somewhat confusing, were esthetically satisfying to herself and others.

After this, she had a short remission followed by a recurrence of the whole picture for several months. During the third winter of her illness, she had a short episode of increased paresthesia in the hands and right side of the face, which progressed into an acute myoclonic picture. This lasted a few days. Afterwards, a second attack of endocarditis occurred, which left the girl with a cardiac murmur; but from that time on, she showed improvement in her chorea and associated phenomena. This was reflected in her human figure drawings, although the face was still unclear. Because of difficulties in the home, she was placed in a Catholic home, with her siblings, and got along satisfactorily there, until her late teens, when she became independent and was not heard from again.

There was no doubt that this girl suffered from a chorea, of rheumatic etiology. At the time of the above examination, the chronic stage was reached, in which the extremities no longer showed chorea. Even in the face there were no choreatic twitchings in the common sense. However, there were increased associated movements in the face and extremities, especially associated movements to other facial muscles, such as the mouth, on closing the eye. There were also associated movements from the mouth to the face, the eyes, and, also, the extremities. In connection with these associated movements, there was a considerable distortion of expression in the face, and even the movements of the trunk and arms had a manneristic character. She gave the impression of being manneristic in facial expression. It should be noted, however, that at this time she still showed deviation in the postural reflexes. Grimacing and mannerisms, in this case, were due not only to the associated movements, but also to a change in attitude toward innervation. This changed attitude was due to the patient's awareness that subcortical distortion would not allow an efficient innervation. We may suppose a fundamental change in motor attitude, which elaborates a phenomenon basically due to subcortical changes in the motor impulses.

In the next case, the clinical diagnosis of schizophrenia was pretty certain and subsequently confirmed. This was a patient in whom there were very definite disturbances in the postural reflexes, with a tendency to whirling around the longitudinal axis. The grimacing, mannerisms, ungraciousness, and clowning, all had the appearance of an organic touch.

Sherman's birth and development were apparently normal. He walked and talked at eighteen months. At the age of four, he had measles, followed by otitis media.

He was taken to a child guidance clinic, at the age of four years and three months, with the complaint that he had temper tantrums, and was unmanageable and destructive. He was so unstable and hyperactive, at that time, that it was difficult to arrive at a satisfactory estimate of his mental level. An IQ of 61 on the Merrill Palmer and Kuhlman test was regarded as minimal. However, two years later, the test was again given when he was five years, seven months old, and he rated the same IQ. The patient was admitted to the children's ward at Bellevue Hospital at the age of ten. In the two years preceding admission, he was said to have acted peculiarly. He had frequent spells of laughter during which he said "something makes me do it." He heard voices saying, "There is Shermy" or a man would say something to him and frighten him. A week before coming to the hospital, he complained of seeing a man coming toward him who terrified him. He voided on the bathroom floor and made no attempt to dress himself. He became irritable and the other children refused to play with him. His thought processes were rather disconnected. He was very much interested in the connotation of time. He was continually afraid that other children might hit him.

When interrupted, by a nurse, in his nose-picking, he said, "Shut up, you bastard, I should have jumped in the river. I'm sick. The boys hit me and pee on me and tell them to stay away from me. What is your name? Where were you born? What year, what day, what holiday, how long? Where's your mother? Were you here when you were a small boy? I'm hurrying—what does hurrying mean? Shut up, you mix me up. I'm talking to myself. January, December. Dark day in January, sunny day in December. What is a season? When will a season start? Will the sun move it? In the summer the sun gets slower. If it is winter, then the sun gets so that it comes this way—you can see the sun. When I went to sleep, I slept fast; yesterday when I went to sleep, I slept slow. That is the farthest time—slow. That is not a good rest when you are frightened. Oh, did you see a colored boy locked up in jail? All night it went on and on.

I couldn't sleep. When he got the gun he was calling, before he got the gun."

The patient showed decided deviations in his motility. The out-stretched arm showed movements which were partially choreatic and partially manneristic. There were also rotating movements in the trunk, which reminded one of the movements of Huntington's chorea. He walked with unequal steps. His movements were never of definite neuro-logical character and, like the facial expression, they were manneristic. The outstretched arms diverged widely, and when the head was turned there was a tendency of turning around the longitudinal axis. The arms increased their tendency to divergence. The chin arm rose. There were no associated movements in the common sense. When the head was bent backward, the whole trunk was bent backward too. The motility can be best described as an extreme degree of increase in postural reflexes. There were movements which were more organic in character than mere mannerisms and less organic in character than choreatic or athetotic movements. There were no disturbances in associated movements or al-ternate motions. His human figure drawings were crude, but still depic-ted his own body image problems quite well, as though body boundaries were not clear.

This boy was under treatment with us for two years, between the ages of ten and twelve. A minimal IQ of 73 was obtained in the early period and 80 after shock treatment. He had forty insulin shocks without ap-parent benefit and twenty-three metrazol B-erythroidin shocks, with con-siderable improvement in social behavior. However, his bizarre behavior and scattered thinking made it impossible to cope with him at home or in the public schools, and he was transferred to a state hospital.[7]

This was a clear-cut case of childhood schizophrenia, with an apparent clinical onset at four years, seen by us first at ten years and followed until he was twenty. The low IQ reported both early and

---

[7] He was in and out of state mental hospitals for four years and could never remain home long, because among other things, he assaulted his sister. In the hospital, he was reported to be episodically unmanageable, screaming, cursing, grimacing, catatonic, mute, or muttering. At fifteen years of age, he quieted down, and was transferred to a state training school for mental defectives; his IQ was reported to be 54. At seventeen, he returned home and has remained there for three years, though dependent, dull, and inappropriate in his behavior. Another examination, by our staff, showed at twen-ty, that he was tall, well built, handsome but stiff, manneristic, and occasionally grim-acing, with choreoathetotic movements of the hands and a doughy tone to his muscles. He was dull, empty, and had very little to say about his interests or inner fantasy life. His human figure drawing was remarkably like the one drawn ten years earlier, al-though somewhat more compact. (Reported more in detail by Cottington, 1941-1942.)

late in his career was no measure of his potentialities, which were best exemplified by a verbal score at the twelfth year level, when he was ten, and by the IQ of 80 obtained after his shock treatment. Throughout, his motility problems were quite typical of the schizophrenic child, and showed the expressions of personal problems, in part, and, also, a great similarity to motility disturbances of subcortical lesions. There were also changes in postural reflexes, and changes in tone which persisted into adulthood.

Patsy was a ten-year-old white boy of Italian extraction, referred to us from a pediatric hospital, where he had had a mastoidectomy for an infection which had been chronic since the age of two. It was thought that he might have a brain disease. For over a year there had been a striking personality disturbance. The chronic mastoiditis had been the focus of attention for consideration in diagnosis and treatment, but a diagnosis of juvenile schizophrenia was made on discharge from the pediatric hospital.

There had been bizarre, withdrawn behavior, with a constant flow of speech expressing his preoccupation with voices, his fear of being crazy and causing too much trouble and expense to his parents, and his inability to concentrate on his school work. There had been some compulsive bizarre motor play and posturing, sitting in corners with his head ducked between his legs and his hands over his ears. At times, he was self-assertive and excited, complaining of mistreatment, of bugs and dirt in his food. His thought processes were disturbed. He was incapable of any of the normal activities for his age. Intelligence quotients were between 80 and 90 on several tests.

The electroencephalogram showed deviations in brain waves on the right side, and an air encephalogram showed dilated ventricles, especially on the right.

When examined in March, 1940, he would not speak at first. Then he said, "Are you a doctor or are you a man? Where do you come from?" With eyes closed he let himself fall, it appeared voluntarily, mostly to the back or right but he could stand quite well on one leg. There was no nystagmus, asynergia or whirling tendencies. While stepping from one foot to the other, he said, "I draw a picture—no good—a picture—a man in the corner—I draw—I draw." There was some tendency to pronation in the right arm. Both outstretched arms showed a tendency to drop. The hands could only be held up with a compensatory lordosis. When the head was turned to the right, there was a decided tendency for countermovements in both arms. When the head was turned to the left there was a countermovement and pronation on the left. From time to time, he would enter into an exaggerated lordotic posturing with swaying. He said, "I hear a noise—a mystery cave man—I say it—thereafter it says the same thing—nobody said it—I made it up in my mind and after I think it, a man said it." During this conversation, he maintained a queer posture: his legs crossed, swaying his right arm and body, and with the little finger of his left hand in his mouth. "When people talk I still think they are talking. I still gotta put my hands like that. I still got it. I can't get rid of it. It's—it's like somebody talking. They say like stuff lotsa stuff. I dream something, and then next year I dream it again—like a storm, like a penny firecracker, like bullets like. I wasn't even happy yet. I don't bother with my father. When I was two years old I was nice to my father. I'm nice. I don't make people touch my father. I am so ashamed of myself. I don't take so many baths at home but my mother likes me. She says I talk too. I'm a clean boy, when I was one year old I wasn't clean. That doesn't make sense, does it? I'm a dope. I got brains but I don't know what. I do things nice but I imagine voices. But I don't really hear them. I talk in my mind about money—millions and millions. It is just a habit. I bother myself. Even if somebody is crazy, they don't got to talk about it."

He remained under treatment with us for six months, receiving twenty-two metrazol B-erythroidin shock treatments, and was somewhat improved. He returned home and was accepted in school, but was only tolerated for the rest of the year. During the next summer, he improved more rapidly and during the next school year was considered a satisfactory pupil. He was seen when he was twelve, and he appeared somewhat stiff and self-conscious in motility and facial expression, but otherwise seemed normal. He spoke objectively of his past mental illness, but appeared somewhat overanxious to make good at school, home, or during a clinical examination.[8]

[8] He continued to improve steadily during his early adolescence, attended school and did well there, and was no special problem to his mother or other members of the family. However, when he was sixteen, he suddenly became disturbed, unmanageable, went out on the fire escape nude, and attempted sex play with other boys. He was returned to the hospital with the help of the police. He was found to be hallucinated and deluded. He spoke of hearing unknown persons threatening to injure his wife and child (which of course he didn't have). A good part of the time he was amiable and compliant. A psychometric on the Bellevue-Wechsler scale scored at 80. The electroencephalogram was reported normal. There were no neurological deviations or other evidences of the old organic brain disease. He presented a classic picture of adolescent schizophrenia. He received twenty electric shock treatments, but did not improve sufficiently for discharge. He was sent to a state hospital. The diagnosis was dementia praecox. His IQ was reported at 64. He was given fifty insulin shock convulsions. He was frequently paroled home, but, as frequently, shortly returned to the hospital. When he was eighteen he was able to remain at home, dependent, dull, helping his

This was a case of combined organic brain disease and a schizophrenic psychosis, typical in all its clinical features, and which responded to shock therapy in the prepuberty and early puberty period, but later followed a typical dementia praecox course.

The next case to be cited was that of a thirteen-year-old Negro boy of light-brown color. He showed personality changes after his dog was killed by a car and he came home spattered with blood. Several weeks later, his hand was injured in a fight in school. He came home fully preoccupied with his body, and his talk in the hospital went as follows: "My teeth are crooked on the bottom. They are a green foghorn. I don't like it. Everybody keeps fooling around with cards. They play too much on my mother's table. They make fun of my breath that I have for years. I am the only one who knows how to clean my teeth. They say it smells funny."

His IQ was 70. He was manneristic, dissociated, and silly, and showed a clinical picture which was undeniably schizophrenic. He had motility disturbances which looked somewhat less organic than the motility disturbances in the previously discussed case (Patsy). His motor mannerisms were decidedly dissimilar from chorea and athetosis. Nevertheless, the patient showed outspoken changes in the postural reflexes. His arms diverged widely and there was a decided increase in the tendency to turn around the longitudinal axis. The phenomena in this case corresponded very closely to the phenomena, described by Hoff and myself, observed in adult catatonics. He was transferred to a state mental hospital where he ran a chronic course.

*   *   *

We may further mention the case of a fifteen-year-old schizophrenic girl, who, during an acute phase, showed abnormalities in postural tendencies, mannerism and motor awkwardness, but, in addition, also showed phenomena reminiscent of oculogyric crises. The eyes were con-

---

mother with the housework and doing small errands in a ritualistic fashion. He read books on psychiatry, it could not be determined to what benefit, and frequently went to talk to a local physician.

When he was twenty he was re-examined by our research staff. He was found to be well developed and tall, but with poor posture. He was generally untidy. He had no hallucinations or delusions except hypochondriacal ideas about mental illness and dying. He was anxious, but empty, and had no interests or aims; he was, at times, illogical and repetitive. He did not show any neurological or other motility disorders, such as he showed as a child, whirling on the longitudinal axis or poor motor tone. He did later admit to some feelings of apprehension that he might fly off into space. He was seen at intervals, until he was twenty-four, and the picture was the same, except that he was sometimes more anxious and restless and would then ask for an appointment to come and talk to the psychiatrist.

tinually directed straight upwards. However, this upward deviation of the eye had a much less organic character than oculogyric crises have.

The following case has different significance. The phenomena in this case were not manneristic and clowning, but gave the impression of motility of semivoluntary character, in spite of the fact that one was immediately aware of the seriousness of the condition and anticipated the fatal outcome. This adult case is included to emphasize the significance of the motility pattern in children.

A.L. was a forty-three-year-old white male. On the day he was admitted to Bellevue Hospital, he walked around the ward very much bewildered. His eyes were directed upwards, his gait was slow, and he assumed very grotesque postures. He seemed to seek support by feeling his way along the walls. At times, it appeared that his vision might be impaired, and he was unstable on his feet. On the following day, he assumed catatonic positions. He sat rigid, his arms flexed, his head motionless, staring out of the windows. He spoke very slowly, in a monotonous singing tone. He answered questions as though speaking into vacant space. He said, "This is heaven." He said he saw candles, and that he felt like a small, tiny little person. He called the examiner "father," and related the following dream: "I have had a dream that I gave second thought to it because it affected my immediate loved ones. It wasn't anything too lengthy. It concerned a neighbor living at the south side of the road of houses on Washington Avenue. The dream concerned two large cats. They were left in the house along with my boy and myself asleep. Being large cats I was sort of worried in the dream that the cats had been feasting their hunger on my boy's body and that gave me sort of a little shock. The shock was that I thought they were going to attack my boy's body and myself and I was not strong enough to protect ourselves. Then I woke up and I found that the folks were at home and I knew that my fears were an empty shell. The cats were like Persian monstrous-looking cats with large fangs of different colors, like tigers."

The third day after admission, he became negativistic and mute. He understood commands and made vague efforts to carry them out. His arms and legs were rigidly flexed and this flexion increased at the attempt at passive movements. Sodium amytal did not make these flexions disappear. A week after admission, the patient lay stiffly in bed, head partially lifted from the surface. All muscles were tense, with flexion prevailing in the arms. He responded to the stretching of muscles with strong countertensions. There was an atypical tendency toward grasping.

207

The abdominal muscles were contracted. Marked resistive tensions in the legs were present. There was generalized sensitiveness of the muscles to stretching and an occasional strong tendency to shortening reactions (paradoxical contracture). When he was taken out of bed, he flexed both legs maximally, as psychogenic cases do, and made no effort to walk. His speech was inarticulate. He appeared very sick and died two weeks later.

Cases of this type are difficult to classify from a clinical point of view. They correspond to the old connotation of "delirium acutum." However, this diagnosis is spurious, since we do not know what delirium acutum is. These cases start rather suddenly, with very violent manifestations, and are characterized by very severe regressions and dissociations in the psychological sphere. This patient had the fear that cats might feast on the body of his son and to this fear he added phenomena reminiscent of catatonia and far from typical. In many respects, they reminded one of phenomena seen in acute extrapyramidal diseases. There was a paradoxical phenomenon of Westphal's and the sensitivity to stretch, which reminded one of the sensitivity to stretch seen in some encephalitics. There was, on the other hand, some degree of resistiveness which looked voluntary. When the patient became worse, the organic character of the tension became more obvious.

Alice, the first case discussed in this section, had a definite subcortical pathology, with a residual chorea restricted to the face. Her grimacing went beyond a mere subcortical change in motility, although associated movements in the face were doubtless an important influence. It is important to note that the more or less immediate subcortical change necessitated a fundamentally different attitude toward the problem of movement. This adaptation was only partially conscious.

In the last case discussed (A. L.), a severe organic subcortical motility disturbance was welded with a change in the total attitude toward motility. Since the organic disturbance was more severe, in this case, the change in motor attitude seemed to be less prominent.

In the schizophrenic children, we saw the same problem, with the accent on the change in total motor attitudes, which also appeared closely related to life problems.

Sometimes it may be difficult to differentiate the parts played by the cortical or psychic and subcortical functions, in motility. The associated movements in the face, described in Alice for instance, are sometimes to be found in motor aphasia cases. There is no doubting that motor disintegrations, similar to those found in subcortical disturbances of motility, can be found in apraxias. However, it seems that, in general, the correlation of subcortical apparatuses to the total integration of motility is closer than to the cortical apparatuses. It is well known, for instance, how great an influence the emotions can have on choreatic postencephalitic pictures. It is true that phenomena due to cortical lesions can be influenced by psychological factors. However, as I have stated, these psychic factors do not have so much to do with the central personality problems as do the psychic factors related to the subcortical motor apparatus. We believe, therefore, that the subcortical motor factor is in particularly close relation to the total motility.

Clowning, grimacing, and mannerisms in schizophrenia, in organic conditions, or in normal persons under special conditions have to do with the function and disintegration of function of the subcortical apparatus in relation to the total motor personality. We should like to call such motor disturbances "paracortical," indicating the closer relation to the subcortical apparatus and the total motor organization. We find such paracortical disturbances in: (1) the restless movements in anoxia due to nitrogen inhalation; (2) the clowning movements of certain stages of insulin treatment; (3) the clowning and the mannerism of certain cases of alcoholic encephalopathy; (4) Sydenham's chorea in children; (5) certain badly defined cases of delirium acutum; (6) infantile and juvenile schizophrenias (though more rarely); and (7) adult catatonic schizophrenia.

In those cases in which there is an indication of a lesion of subcortical motor apparatus or of a change in the postural apparatus, there occur restless movements, clowning, mannerisms, and stiffness. It seems that these disturbances occur through an interaction of subcortical influences and the total motor personality structure. The name "paracortical" disturbances is proposed. Childhood schizophrenic motility disturbances are considered from a similar angle.

# VI

# Action, Impulsion, and Aggression

## ACTION[1]

In every action, the individual must start with an orientation toward his own body and the bodies of others. Every action is based on the body image. Action means a dynamic change in the body image, which is in a state of equilibrium before an action takes place. It leaves this equilibrium during action and reaches it again with completion of the action.

Objects are in a definite order in space. Space is psychologically not homogeneous. We do not act toward isolated points in space. There is a well-regulated system of geometrical coordinates of space, in which the vertical and horizontal planes play an outstanding part. Furthermore, there is a network of object relations and orders of manifold types. An object always has a definite relation to the body image. An object is the crossing point of many worlds. It is in the world of physics as well as in the world of practical and moral values.

The end of an action means not only a new equilibrium in the body image, but also a new orientation in space and morals. Physiological impulses of tonic, rhythmic, and phasic character, which are in such close relation to the impression of the senses and the formation of the object, determine space in its properties and the dynamic relation of the body image to space. The body image continually creates a new space equilibrium around itself.

[1] From Schilder (1942).

210

The investigations of Feuchtwanger (1933) are particularly important in this respect. In discussing space, it has been mentioned that there is a primitive tonic system of space and that the phasic system is built on this tonic system. Tonic and phasic systems build up the object, space, and also the basis of action. The tonic component, however, is already action. It means an adaptation to the outside world; tone leads either toward the object or away from it, when the object becomes too threatening. In this respect, it is of particular importance that the investigations of Magnus (1924) and DeKleijn (Magnus and DeKleijn, 1912), Quix (1924), and others, have shown that the orientation to gravity is important in tonic attitudes. The plane of action is emphasized in investigations of Bender and myself, which show that experimentation with different planes of action and gravitation are important functions in the primitive play of children.

Tone is not merely dependent on space, but is space-creating and correlates the fundamental directions of space. Tone is both an attitude and an action. The fascinating task of following this problem through the range of animal psychology and the tonic reactions of animals cannot here be dealt with in detail. Newer investigations have decisively shown that the tonic reactions of lower animals are not merely tropisms of mechanical consequences of physical-chemical influences, but are primitive actions. Actions might also be expressed in physical-chemical terms, except for the complexity of physical-chemical functions.

Space, action, and body image are not determined merely by tonic innervation, but also by phasic action. I have mentioned that the term "reflex" has been abused. The patellar reflex seems to be so simple that it looks almost mechanical; the older physiologists took the reflex as *the* unit, and, by increments of such reflexes, assumed final action is created. If there is any relationship between reflexes, of the type of the patellar reflex, and action, then the reflex is a product of schematization, simplification, and degeneration of action. One sees this particularly clearly in a reflex such as the scratch reflex. The scratch reflex is actually not a reflex, but an action with an aim: to restore the body image from a distortion which has taken place. The same may be said of reflexes involved in walking. Walking changes the situation of the body image in space, and carries the individual away from something or brings him closer to something. The individual retains his relation to gravity in his final outcome, but must experience rather decisive gravitational changes before coming to a new equilibrium. This constructive process is guided by continuous impressions from the soles, joints, and muscles. It is basically the expression of central tendencies.

Reflexes and tone are split-off parts of actions. The split may sometimes generate a more primitive unit of action, but we have no right to assume that the higher type of action is merely a summation of so-called primitive units. Sherrington considered the reflex as a biological unit, and did not ask what it led to and what its aim was. In the further pursuit of his study, a mechanical point of view became more and more apparent. The problem became one of flexor and extensor muscles, and their tone, rather than one of the actions to which flexion and extension lead and of which they are a part.

The stretch reflex seems to be much more mechanical than the scratch reflex. It is very questionable whether one should consider the scratch reflex as a rhythmical series of movements or whether it is not better understood as the removal of a disturbance to the body image. If we search for primitive units of action, we certainly shall not try to find them in a meaningless tonic contraction. Sherrington's work contains the important nucleus of further biological studies. Decerebrate rigidity can be understood very well when related to standing and orientation to gravity. Richter and Bartemier (1926) have found that the sloth's decerebrate rigidity is a flexor rigidity. This clearly shows that the central nervous system does serve functions. A function cannot be understood from the point of view of anatomy alone, but only from the point of view of environment and situation in relation to anatomy.

A dog's standing corresponds to the sloth's hanging from a tree, and the decerebrate rigidity merely exaggerates the basic orientation to gravity. Further elucidation can be gained from the investigations of Magnus and DeKleijn (1912). The postural and righting reflexes are dependent on the position of the head in space (otolith reflexes), the body's surface pressure, and whether the animal is in usual correct position or not. The animal tries to get into a position of comparative stability. The biological implications of these findings have been extensively studied by Goldstein (1934), who has shown that the problem of tone is also the problem of being directed toward, or getting away from, something. He has further introduced the concept of the "comfortable position," and the tendency to return to this comfortable position. He has pointed to the importance of the different planes on which motility takes place. One should stress the importance of gravitation and the comparative static phases in the body image. Without the concept of the body image, no deeper understanding of action can be gained.

Tone has something to do with the outer world and an adaptation to qualities of physics. The tonic individual considers the world chiefly from the point of view of physics, inertia, mass, gravitation, and also from the point of view of preparedness of the organism. In order to do something, one must at first adapt to the general situation of mass attraction. It is true, for instance, that for ctenophora, floating in the water, the orientation to gravitation and the physical qualities of water are almost all that is needed. Where finer qualities of the objects are involved, tonic adaptation becomes insufficient. Tonic adaptation is chiefly of importance when we deal with rather stabilized conditions.

We must turn, therefore, to more decidedly phasic actions. Grasping and sucking offer themselves as the first activities to be considered. Both have been the object of extensive studies by psychologists and physicians.

We begin with a consideration of sucking. Sucking has two phases. When an object is brought close to a child's mouth, the child turns his head and eyes, with open mouth, and the body follows. Sometimes, the head is withdrawn as if the child expected that something would drop into his mouth. When the object is finally brought to the mouth, the lips close around the object and sucking begins. We again deal with a rhythmic activity. It seems that the touch of the lips initiates the sucking movement. During the sucking process, the child clenches his fists and increases his grasp. Two types of lesions permit this activity to reappear: a lesion of the prefrontal area, and a lesion of the brain stem (especially seen in alcoholic encephalopathy). Sucking is not only cortically initiated in human beings, as proven by a case of Gamper (1926), in which sucking was present although the hemispheres were lacking and

213

only the brain stem was preserved (without optic thalamus). One is inclined to believe that grasping and groping are subsidiary to sucking. This is not correct, since, as we know, the child does not grasp the food which he needs, and in Troemner's (1928) case of anencephaly, grasping alone was preserved.

It is true that in later development the child puts objects into his mouth immediately after receiving them. Apparently, in development, grasping and sucking are independent of each other for some time. It is true that when a child is sucking, the sucking invariably provokes grasping. Functions which are independent in early development may be united in later stages of development. One might say that the unification which is in the plan of the organism has not yet been performed. This means that parts may take an independent course in development, or the development may unite two independent units in their later course (see Coghill, 1929, 1933). Development probably takes place piecemeal, and, in this respect, is comparable to eidetic imagery as described by Klüver (1934), and by myself.

Further information can be gained from study of the grasp reflex. In studying tonic perseveration in grasping and groping, Walshe and Robertson (1933) found that grasping and groping appeared only in lesions of the prefrontal area. They consider the tonic perseveration which can be elicited by stretching the fingers to be a true grasp reflex. It cannot be elicited by tactile and visual stimuli. This grasp is strong, cannot be voluntarily released, and increases as the muscles are stretched. They differentiate this reflex component from an associated volitional component for which visual and tactile stimuli are important. The grasp reflex disappears in coma. They differentiate psychic from physiological grasping. Grasping, in contrast to the grasp reflex, is merely psychic, according to their opinion. This, however, can easily be refuted. My own investigations with Bieber (1937) have shown that increase in grasping, by repetition of the stimulation, very often provokes groping in the same hand, and is often transferred to the other hand as grasping and groping. The unbreakable grip of one hand may be transposed to the other hand. The grasp of the contralateral hand may be released by conscious effort of the patient. During grasping there is strong tonic innervation in the arm, even if it were not present before. The tonic innervation is not grasp, for grasping and groping have directness and the tonic innervation is merely subordinate to this aim. Grasping and groping in the newborn monkey or human being is a fundamental action, and cannot be understood merely as a tonic phenomenon. Clinging pronate to the body of the mother is thereby achieved, especially during the act of sucking.

Tonic innervation, in the sense of Walshe and Robertson (1933), is a part function of grasping, and there is no justification for separating psychic grasping from the "neurological" grasp. In alcoholic encephalopathy, grasp may also become unbreakable. Usually, the patient can open his hand even when its muscles are stretched. The muscular changes, in these patients, resemble the changes observed in tonic innervation. In both groups, grasping, groping, and sucking are usually present at the same time. Very often, the sucking reflex, although otherwise not present, can be elicited by an increase in the grasp reflex. As mentioned above, sucking itself increases grasping.

The difference in tone after cortical destruction and after subcortical lesion is merely a greater variability of the tonic increase in the subcortical lesion. Grasping and groping is a unified function, which becomes tonic because tone is the sense and meaning of the function. As shown by Watson (1930) in humans, and by Richter (1931) in monkeys, the grasp reflex occurs when the individual tries to hold himself against gravity. We observed three postencephalitic paralysis agitans cases, in which grasping was particularly obvious when the patients were in danger of falling backward from retropulsion. This factor is mentioned also by Rabiner (1935). In alcoholic encephalopathic patients, we have found that the patient almost invariably has a tendency to fall backward. Grasping should not be considered as subservient to oral activities only. An individual with a frontal lobe lesion acts as if grasp were fulfilling its function in maintaining posture, although no objective need be present. One might call this motor preparedness due to dysfunction in equilibrium, or, if one wants to be paradoxical, a motor hallucination concerning the maintenance of equilibrium.

One of our most important functions is to maintain our orientation to gravitational forces. At first, grasp helps in clinging to the mother's body (Hermann, 1940). Later on, grasp develops other functions. The maintenance of erect posture is secured by tonic

215

influences on the first level and by grasping on the second level. The great importance of these functions can also be seen in patients with cerebellar disorders, who frantically try to maintain their equilibrium. Since the postural reflexes are not only preserved, but are decidedly increased, one sees that equilibrium is very often maintained against odds. Children with cerebellar agenesis show very important psychological trends, in addition to these motor disturbances. They cling to adults from whom they get support (Bender, 1940). The grasp reflex is only one line of defense in maintaining one's position against gravity; the other one is an attempt to get support by clinging. The mother is not only protection in general and an agency for food for the child, but she protects the child against the everpresent enemy: gravitation. Dependence also means the wish to have help in standing upright.

When grasping and groping appear to be futile, then pointing (which is functionally the same, in that one finger reaches for the distant object) takes their place. Another development leads from grasping to hand shaking, which is an attenuated form of grasping, gives mutual support, and hinders aggressiveness (the other person cannot hit you with his hand while shaking hands). One sees how many activities develop as a natural consequence of such primitive activity. Sucking also has inner developments. The opening and closing of the mouth, single phases of the sucking act, are used in functions different from the act of oral incorporation.

Indeed, if one considers grasping and sucking as the beginnings of human action, it seems that primitive human action expresses the urge to come into apposition to objects. Destruction of the object does not seem to be the primary aim. An important part of the psychology of grasping is dependent on the preservation of the love object. Closer approach to an object is likely to interfere with the structure of the object and to be destructive to the object, especially when the individual tries to put it into his mouth and devour it. It is wrong, however, to see only the physiological function of devouring. The relative functional independence of grasping from sucking, in spite of their interdependence, is of great psychological importance.

Just as imagination and perception can destroy objects as well as

216

build them up, so there are also destructive tendencies in motility. Experimentation with objects, and especially studies of their consistency, may sooner or later lead to their destruction. Action gives a sense of power over other objects, both animate and inanimate. Action, in itself, thus becomes a moral problem, which is outside the field of our discussion. I consider grasping, groping, and sucking to be the nucleus of the function of the ego and the ego instincts. In the psychoanalytic sense, no trace of a death instinct is to be found, and it is wrong to overemphasize the idea of destruction. Destruction is an important phase, but destruction is not the final aim and goal of human action.

It is not our task to follow the development of action. Reflex, instinctive action, expressive movement, and voluntary actions are merely phases of the general process of adaptation. Darwin has shown succinctly that expressive movement may be considered a derivative of voluntary action.

We have, thus far, neglected reactions of defense in our analysis of primitive functions and actions. There is, at first, a closing up (encapsulation) of the body (as far as possible); closing the eyes as in crying and secreting; closing the lips and even protruding them, as in pouting; pushing the tongue forward; and, finally, movements of closing the pharynx. The arm may be drawn protectively before the face and body. When defensive measures are not sufficient, pushing away occurs, in which abduction and extension movements play an important part. Grasping is chiefly a flexor and adductor function. It is important to consider the organism and its motility from the point of view of abduction and adduction, flexion and extension. One tears objects apart by abduction, and puts them together by adduction. Goldstein has developed similar ideas. Adduction and abduction are also very important for the construction of the object. Motility is not merely directed toward the object, but is concerned with the creation of the object. The resistance of objects to push and pull makes them objects. Push, pull, and the momentum of objects are object qualities closely related to the motility of the individual. Human action progresses by the creation of more complicated objects, which, in turn, gives opportunities for further development of action.

217

## IMPULSIONS: A SPECIFIC BEHAVIOR DISORDER[2]

Human beings have interests toward which they retain varying degrees of freedom. They may be preoccupied with specific thoughts and ideas; they may be specifically interested in one or another group of objects or data. A person may, for instance, have a great interest in railroads, pictures, landscapes, clothes, or flowers. These interests may appear to be theoretical. However, such interests never remain only in the sphere of contemplation. Sooner or later, they lead to actions. The person interested in landscapes will have to travel in order to see them, or at least will have to go to places where landscape paintings and pictures are exhibited. The person interested in technical problems will, sooner or later, start to construct, or at least to collect. Interests of this type may be worthwhile, and may even mean a life work or life interest. One is inclined to believe that persons should have such an overwhelming preoccupation with their work. However, it is understandable when a man does not live out these impulses in his professional life, but enjoys his hobbies or collecting in his private life. It is sometimes difficult to decide which of these interests are commendable and which are not.

Here, our concern is the direction of flow of the impulses of the individual person. He may be more occupied with sex than the average person, or he may collect stamps. He may be a gambler and feel that his life interest centers around the card table; or he may think that he should do nothing but hoard money. He may wish to do what he does and also feel completely justified in his attitude. It has been learned that persons who have neurotic symptoms also show definite trends in their impulses; that is, definite character trends are found to be connected with neurotic symptoms. Character trends and neurotic symptoms differ from each other, insofar as a man fights against his neurotic symptoms and suffers from them, but he accepts his character trends. In other words, the neurotic symptoms are rejected by the ego, in the psychoanalytic sense, and cause suffering, while the person suffers from his character only to the extent that society punishes him. These facts are well known in psychoanalysis. According to Fenichel (1934), the obsessional char-

[2] From Bender and Schilder (1940).

acter is always an anal character. Following the concept of Freud and Abraham, he mentioned stubbornness, defiance, orderliness, and parsimony as basic features. Anal characters are pedantic and punctual; they have a tendency to collect and to enjoy possessions. Winterstein (1921) has also written an interesting study on collecting.

We have made a series of clinical observations on children, which seem to lead to a deeper understanding of these problems. Billy, age five, showed an overwhelming interest in doors and door checks, so that it was almost impossible to remove him from the vicinity of doors. He looked at them, played with them, and was so preoccupied with them that one needed force to get him away from them. He was severely impaired in his social functioning. Larry, age eleven, was interested in numbers. He wrote down a long series of numbers and was preoccupied with counting. Before coming to the hospital, he had spent hours running in the streets noting the house numbers. In this way, he wanted to explore the longest streets in New York.

After having studied several such obvious disorders, we became aware that such behavior in children is by no means rare. We saw children who were preoccupied with the drawing of animals. They enjoyed their activities and interests, although, from time to time, they became aware that they were helpless to prevent them. The chief difficulties arose from the fact that their behavior led to a conflict with the surroundings. These preoccupations might casually be referred to as obsessions and compulsions. The children, however, felt that they had an interesting and fascinating occupation, and regretted merely the lack of understanding of adults. We propose the term "impulsion" for these preoccupations and activities. They do not represent merely a passing or fleeting impulse, which suddenly breaks through the defenses and fears to the surface; rather, they are preoccupations and actions which are in the foreground of the person's experience for weeks, months, or even years. Impulsions are not obsessions in the strict sense. They have something in common with the obsessive character trends.

The term "impulsion" has been used, in a similar sense, by Dewey (1934). Whitehorn (1932) called impulsion the signal of a biologic need and distress leading to action. Murray (1938) spoke of impulsion as the tendency to respond quickly and without re-

219

flection. Murray uses the word in a different way from Dewey and Whitehorn. We use the term to characterize a clinical entity.

Let us first consider a case in which impulsions and obsessions were present at the same time.

Marvin came to the mental hygiene clinic of Bellevue Hospital for treatment when he was about twelve. He was a tall, rather poorly nourished boy of Jewish descent. He complained about obsessions and compulsions. When he crossed the street he had to hit one leg, with the other, four times, otherwise he feared that he might be hurt or killed while crossing. He was also afraid that somebody might touch him on the street and kill him by this very touch. Later we learned that he had a vague idea that he might acquire tuberculosis by the touch. The obsession had become so severe that he had stopped crossing streets and would not go to school. These obsessions developed after he had heard his mother tell how interesting life might be in a Polish village in Europe. He had wished urgently to go there and to participate in all the fun. This thought had acquired an overwhelming intensity, and he finally decided not to think of it any more. But he found this impossible. Finally, he threatened himself with death if he did not stop, and started to kick himself in the shins. Even that was not successful and, from then on, he feared he might die while crossing the street.

His early history revealed a great amount of aggressiveness. With a group of boy friends, he enjoyed catching cats, tying them, and torturing them to death. Once they also tied up another boy; however, the patient said he disapproved of this. He finally gave up torturing cats after he had a nightmare in which an enormous cat sat on his chest. When treatments began, he was at the beginning of puberty. There had always been great sexual curiosity concerning his sister and his mother. His attachment to his mother was close; he was afraid of his father. He had a brother about eight years older than himself, who had been considered schizophrenic. However, in our opinion, the brother was not schizophrenic, but suffered from complicated aggressive impulses.[3] The whole family was a rather violent one. The father and mother fought incessantly and threatened violence to each other and the children. The children had outbursts of hate against each other; the patient, himself, had once threatened his sister with a knife. There cannot be much doubt that aggressive impulses

[3] This older brother of Marvin was able to maintain himself in the community, while he received group therapy with Schilder. After Schilder's death, he became progressively more disturbed, and was institutionalized. A diagnosis of schizophrenia was made, he was given shock therapy, and, later, a lobotomy, after which he deteriorated.

were of enormous importance in this case. However, characteristically, the picture started with an unfulfilled wish. The boy obviously felt that his wishes should not be denied him; they were of enormous urgency. "I hit myself in school in order to forget a desire to go to Europe. I hit myself four times on the left arm with the right arm and said to myself: 'If I don't forget I should get killed.' I know I don't want to die and I figured by threatening myself with death I could conquer the power that gains control over my reason." He hit himself on another occasion. "Only when I fought with a guy and hit him hard and I felt it was too much, I said, 'I hit myself now so that you get even with me.' " He was obviously afraid of the strength of his own impulses, especially the aggressive ones. He did not have the power to deny himself any wishes. He liked to hitch rides on trolley cars; he liked to go fishing, although he knew that it was against the law. He was very unhappy when he did not immediately get whatever he wanted. He usually succeeded in securing, either from his older brother or from his mother, the fulfillment of most of his wishes. In this way, he acquired a book on jujitsu, a bicycle, money to join the "naval reserve," and, finally, a bayonet. Under treatment, he gained insight and lost his symptoms; however, the urgency of his wishes remained. He still often asked his mother one question several times, preferably four.

Since the age of four, he had been interested in death, partially owing to the influence of his brother, who was continuously preoccupied with death and murder. "I used to think what would happen if my mother died." He also thought of the death of his father, when the latter went to a hospital for an operation. His father and mother were both aggressive toward him; they repeatedly hit him. The mother, in addition, was much attached to her children and tried to make them as dependent on her as possible. He was continuously fighting with his sister. He was also interested in seeing her undress. He began to masturbate at ten years of age, two years before he came for treatment; emissions started at this time, which made him feel weak and scared.

The treatment lasted for six months, when he was twelve. The next year he complained occasionally, and asked his friend, three or four times, not to forget to call him when he went fishing. His dreams were still of the following type: "One of my friends was run over by a subway train." He would like to have had a gun to shoot rats.

When he was fourteen, he broke his arm while jumping from a trolley car on which he was hitching a ride. He was aware of the danger of hitching rides on trolley cars, but he could not resist the impulse. The healing of the fracture was uneventful, but he became preoccupied with hypochondriacal ideas; for instance, that his arm was weak, that there was a red mark, and that the veins "stuck out." He felt like a cripple; he wished that everybody else would have a broken arm. His apprehensions expressed themselves in dreams. He also worried that his breasts were too large, and that his hand might fall off at the red line. However, these symptoms disappeared after he realized that his fears were punishment for his aggression. He wanted to kill people who pushed him in a crowded subway. He bought a gun to compensate for his weakened left arm, and then felt that nobody would touch him. At the age of fourteen, he had his first sex relations with a prostitute. He felt that he would like to go to a prostitute every day. He showed his penis to a woman looking out of a window. Both he and his family decided that he should be sent to a boys' institution for a while. When this was decided, he demanded of the physician that it should be done immediately. Meanwhile, he and some friends broke open a parcel post package in the hope of finding candy and money. He had continuous fights at home. He said he would like to kill his teacher, who had a grudge against him, or run over him with a car. He finally was placed in an institution, but he soon felt that he had to go home again, and he repeatedly ran away. He was discharged. He complained only of his strong sex urge, however he was fairly well adapted. His dreams were of the following type: "There was war in this country and they gave everybody a revolver in school. They gave me a .38 revolver. I felt very happy. Maybe I want a girl more than a gun."

When he was sixteen, he came to the clinic again, complaining that his brother was "butting in" on his girl friends, and that he also made him nervous by talking about spooks all the time. Marvin said that he was losing interest in school, and wanted to quit and join the army.[4]

This patient had very strong desires. He wanted to have his wishes fulfilled, and immediately. He also wanted to be reassured that his wishes would be fulfilled; his tendency to repetition was

---

[4] He did join the marines, just before Pearl Harbor, thinking he could get away from home, travel, and have a gun. When there turned out to be a real war, he became frightened and anxious, and got a neuropsychiatric medical discharge. He returned home, married, and had a son. He remained dependent on his family and his wife, and was neurotic, especially anxious and hypochondriacal. In July, 1953, Marvin, then a young adult, again came to us for psychiatric help, because his obsessional thinking was threatening to overwhelm him and ruin his life. He had become so increasingly absorbed with gambling on horse racing that he was neglecting all his responsibilities. Abandoning his schooling (under G.I. benefits), he became desperate for money, sold his home, and exhausted his wife's funds. She had consequently left him and taken their only child. Regretful over these results, he nevertheless was helpless to control his obsessional drives.

partially due to this. He could not stand disappointments. His wishes were chiefly of an aggressive type (with some exceptions; he wished, for instance, to go to Europe and to play with other children). There were also frankly sexual wishes. It is probable, however, that even the wishes which were not frankly aggressive had an aggressive element. He tried to keep himself away from these wishes by threatening himself with destruction. His wishes led him to actions which were more or less dangerous, such as hitchhiking, and fishing in forbidden waters. Once such a wish had occurred, he was completely preoccupied with it and did everything to fulfill it. He felt that he should be punished; when he finally broke his arm while hitchhiking, he said that he deserved it. One can only surmise the psychogenesis of these impulsions. One suspects that he felt overprotected, on the one hand, and threatened on the other hand. He reacted with a wish to kill, for which he felt that he deserved punishment. This case shows particularly clearly the relation of impulsions to compulsions and obsessions. It also offers elucidation of the psychology of accidents, and shows the close relation between hypochondriacal ideas and the fear of punishment.

Stanley, age nine, was seen first in the mental hygiene clinic. He was under observation on the children's ward the next year. In a Stanford-Binet Intelligence Test made in the clinic, his intelligence quotient was 104. According to the reports of teachers and agencies, it was impossible to discipline him. He went to movies once or twice a day, broke things, especially mirrors, and tore his mother's clothes off her body. He also liked to use cosmetics and wear his mother's clothes. He was inclined to show feminine mannerisms. The agency had tried to hospitalize him since his first contact with the clinic, but the mother did not cooperate until forced to do so by a welfare agency. She consistently denied that there was any problem. Her only complaint was that he was not 100 per cent boyish. On the hospital ward, he was restless and fidgety. He did not have much contact with other boys. He could not stick to any occupation. He made an effeminate impression and other boys called him "sissy." He sat and daydreamed, and did not do his schoolwork. He showed no evident anxiety nor any capacity for making attachments. He seemed completely preoccupied with his daydreams, except when he was drawing pictures of girls, mostly in vivid colors, with large heads and rather elaborate dresses. It was almost impossible for him to draw a man. Finally, when he was persuaded to do so, he also immediately drew a girl and

223

asked "Can't I draw a lady too?" Why do you want to? "I can't help it." He stated that all women and all men have testes and a penis; this, in spite of the fact that the year before he had said in the clinic, "I would die if my penis would be cut off, but I would look just like a girl then ... Only women have babies; I don't know why." He volunteered the information that his testes were "up" and that then they descended. He asked the examiner why his body looked like that of a girl. "See my waist comes in like a girl. The fellows say so. It should be straight." He said that he slept in the same bed with his mother because when he was alone he was afraid of "spooks." With regard to his earliest memory, he said, "My mother was in the bathroom and I went in and she shut the door on my finger; it hurt. That was before my daddy went away." At the age of six, he dreamed that he shot his father because he hit his mother. "I shot him through the heart; he was dead and I was scared. I awoke feeling scared because I thought I had shot my father."

Stanley's father suffered from tuberculosis for many years. From infancy until he was nine, Stanley was boarded with private families and in a boarding school. In the boarding school, he had an accident and the mother said that he had changed afterward. The mother was an aggressive, suspicious person who believed she had clairvoyant powers. She expressed devotion to the boy.

When the boy first came to the clinic he had undescended testes, and was short and obese, with a girdle type of fat distribution. His hands and feet were soft, small, and infantile in configuration. His muscles were flabby.[5]

This boy was preoccupied with the problem of masculinity and femininity. He seemed to have a fundamental doubt concerning his masculinity, partially based on the fact that his testes were undescended. His idea that women also have testes and a penis, although smaller, showed his deep reluctance to acknowledge that human beings exist without testes. That one indeed deals with a compensatory mechanism is proved by the fact that the boy previously acknowledged that girls have different sex organs. He appeared to be resigned to play the role of a girl, and paraded before

[5] The father died the next year, and the mother and Stanley became dependent on public welfare. Throughout the next several years, social agency records show the efforts that were made to help these two people. They became more and more dependent on each other, and refused any effort to give them any constructive help. When Stanley was seventeen, it was recorded that mother and son shared one bed, and that there were definite implications of an unwholesome relationship between the two. They refused to accept psychiatric help, which was repeatedly urged.

the mirror in his mother's dresses. He drew pictures of women in an impulsive way. His pictures usually showed long hair, a large mouth, and crude and unfinished bodies. In some drawings the breasts were emphasized. His drawings tended to become more and more schematic and distorted. At the same time, he showed a deep attachment to his mother and a tendency to identify himself with her, and strong hostility toward his father. He said that he could not draw a picture of a man. His first memory was that his father did not want to have him home, and the first dream he could remember was one in which he shot his father. He showed no manifest anxiety, although he often spoke of being afraid. The impulses were here directed toward an expression, in drawing, of a specific topic which was closely connected with his fundamental problems. There is no question but that his drawings did not directly express his problems. One does not expect impulsions to be direct expressions of drives. Also, as in the case of Marvin, it is clear that many of the patient's impulsions had a more or less symbolic character. In this respect they were not different from compulsions.

Although, in both Marvin and Stanley, the impulsions played an important part, they did not dominate the picture as completely as in Billy's case.

Billy was five and a half years old when he was first admitted to the children's ward of Bellevue Hospital. He was a boy of superior intelligence, the only child of parents with college training. His parents had not been entirely compatible; several times the mother had gone home with Billy because of jealousy, sexual incompatibility, or a so-called nervous breakdown. The birth was difficult, since the mother had a narrow pelvis and instruments were needed. He was born with an imperforate anus which was operated on the second day after birth. The function of the anal sphincter was impaired and he had to have dilations of the anus by his mother's finger almost daily, and by physicians' instruments from time to time until the age of two and at intervals thereafter. The normal course of his Oedipus complex was interfered with because of the relationship between the mother and father, and the frequent visits of the mother and child away from home. He openly expressed a hatred of the father, the desire for his death or removal from the home, and the wish to have the mother to himself. He wished to be like his mother. He wanted to sit down to urinate; he often denied having a penis.

At the age of two and a half years, when he was visiting with his mother in the home of his grandparents, he enjoyed automobile rides. He was fascinated by the "Stop" and "Go" lights, and seemed to believe that they made the cars stop and go. He would play in a little cupboard, where he could sit on a shelf and close himself in by a door, like the door of an automobile. He would take imaginary rides with imaginary "Stop" and "Go" lights to make the car stop and go. He then became interested in doors as such, in their knobs, keyholes, hinges, and finally in the door checks. Door checks became an impulsion with him, which occupied him up to the time of his admission to the hospital. He was preoccupied all day with doors and door checks. He was rejected from kindergarten because he smashed the fingers of other children in the doors. He could not play on the streets because he could not be stopped from playing with the neighbors' doors. He was very much concerned with the shapes of doors, doorknobs, casements, and hinges.

All his questions were concerned with how doors open and close. He expressed the belief that other openings were regulated in a similar way, by door checks. Thus, when told by his mother how babies are made inside the mother's uterus, he expressed the opinion that they got out by means of a door check. He would also occupy himself by the hour in drawing doors with door checks. He valued these highly and became extremely aggressive if an effort was made to take them from him or destroy them. It was highly important, in the drawing of these doors, that they maintain certain proportions, and that the place for the keyhole and doorknob, and the hinges, all be square or rectangular and turned so that the long axis was vertical. If they were drawn for him so that the long axis was horizontal, it disturbed him to the point of rage. Green doors and door checks were especially valuable, as they represented "Go," while the red ones meant "Stop."

So far as we could see, this child was much concerned with movement and the impetus for movement, with openings and the mechanisms of openings, and with the symbols for these things. When dealing with them as visual motor patterns, he demanded that they conform to his concepts of such patterns and he treasured such patterns highly.

After he was on the children's ward for a month, he was returned home and frequently came to the mental hygiene clinic for psychotherapy. During this time, there developed new compulsions. He resented his placement in the hospital, away from his mother, and was greatly preoccupied with the reasons for sending him there, and with his new experiences and associates. An effort had been made to direct his good intelligence along the lines that usually interest a child of his mental age. He was taught numbers and how to read. He then became preoccupied with the numbers, especially with the number 6. This is the number of the floor on which the children's ward is located. Much of the day was spent

in the schoolrooms and playrooms of the roof, or eighth floor. On returning to the ward by the elevator, it was Billy's habit to watch the mechanisms of the elevator, especially a slit in the wall whereby the elevator
mechanic could determine the number of the floor. The 6 was a large,
open-faced figure. It was this 6 which fascinated Billy for a long time. He
seemed to think that it indicated the arriving at and leaving of the ward.
He was preoccupied with the number for months, just as, formerly, he
had been occupied with door checks. He made 6's with paper, crayon,
and clay all day long. He experimented with all kinds of 6's and noted all
their characteristics. He compared other numbers with 6. Thus, he said
he liked 6 best of all because it was all closed up and sad. Next to 6, he
liked 2 and 5. He also liked 6 because it had an edge on one side of it, but
he hated number 1 because it was all edge. He did not like 7 because it
was almost like 1. He said the 9 was a 6 upside down, but he was not
much interested in it.

Owing to his increasing aggressiveness under treatment, he was returned to the ward about eight months after his first admission. On this
occasion, he became preoccupied with the dials over the elevator doors,
which indicate the position of the elevator and the direction in which it
is moving. These indicators had a clocklike face and nine numbers with,
as it happened, 6 at the top. At the time that he first learned his floor
number, he had shown some passing interest in the clock, with its numbers and moving hands. The elevator indicator, however, fascinated him
completely. He thought that the indicator made the elevator come and
go. He believed that the numbers on the indicator regulated the numbers on the floor, and since 6 was at the top, he concluded that all the
floors in the hospital centered about this important floor. He was occupied all day long with the spatial problems of the series of floors from 1 to
9 and the circular series of numbers on the indicator, with 6 at the top. In
addition, he was also preoccupied with the doors on the elevators. These
were sliding doors, with a little window in each of two partitions, so that
when the doors were wide open, by sliding on each other, the little windows were parallel. Thus, he was soon able to preoccupy himself with
nine sliding pairs of doors with nine indicators each, with the complete
series of numbers on their face, always with 6 at the top. It must be realized that he had been occupied with the philosophy of space, of sequence,
and, therefore, of time; with movements and the mechanisms of movement; with doors and means of opening; and with symbols for all these
things; and that, by this time, 6 probably represented himself. It was also
a feminine number, not being penis-shaped like 1. It was also a smiling
and open number, not completely closed like 8. At home, he often made

227

6's with clay, or paper and crayon, and gave them to his mother as a precious gift. He could not be induced to give them to his father, with whom by this time he was on fairly friendly terms. It is not possible for us to say what all the mechanisms were that related these preoccupations with his personal experiences—with the difficulties with his anal sphincter, his hatred of his father and his own masculinity.

His reactions to puppet shows allowed us a still deeper insight into his problem. Primitive oral and anal trends, and an enormous aggression came into the foreground. He was particularly preoccupied with a play called "Casper and the Devil." Day after day, he would play in an impulsive manner with the puppet characters, the devil and Casper. He played the following scene: The devil appeared with a pitchfork with which he stuck Casper. Casper whimpered and cried. The devil laughed, "I am going to take you down to hell, ha-ha-ha-ha." The devil took Casper down to hell. After that, both characters were held up again and the entire scene was re-enacted. Billy was observed to repeat this scene as often as twenty times in the course of one afternoon. During the play, Billy let the devil threaten Casper by saying, "I'll cut your eyes out. I'll chop your head off. I'll cut your stomach out." On a few occasions, the devil also took Billy's mother to hell. Frequently, Billy kept Casper down in hell and let the devil attack him with a pitchfork. When Billy was told that the devil was a bad character, he denied it. He said, "He is Billy's devil. I tell him to do these things."

Billy continued to have psychotherapeutic interviews, sometimes at long intervals and sometimes intensively. During latency, he was preoccupied with his father's car, which he called a jalopy, and which he fantasied would break down. Then, for a while, he fantasied and dreamed that his mother was in a plane crash in which she was killed. He would draw pictures of these preoccupations, and play them out with miniature toys. At the same time, he desired to have knives in his possession, which he polished and sharpened compulsively. He fantasied that he attacked his father with these knives. He slept with them under his pillow.[6]

---

[6] As he passed puberty, he became distressed by the obsessive compulsive force of these activities and their symbolic meaning. He never found it difficult to discuss them with his psychiatrist.

In early adolescence, he became interested in subway trains, the intricacy of the light signal systems, the schedule for the many subway trains, and the possibility of crashes. He would ride the subway for hours, get off at various major transfer stations, and watch the systems in action. He rapidly developed an interest in motors, in how they were made from magnets, and in electric batteries or other sources of electric current. He would make his own basic motor, and bought stronger and stronger magnets, carrying them about with him in his trousers pocket, sleeping with them under his pillow and always fingering one. He became concerned with the idea that this was a

There is not much doubt that we deal here with an extreme sadistic aggressiveness and anality. We did not attempt to exhaust the psychogenic problems. Billy's hate for his father was outspoken. For this reason, he denied the existence of his own penis, as well as his father's penis. One might be tempted to connect the whole problem with the congenital anal difficulty alone. However, the marital problem of the parents, rather than the problem of local organ inferiority and the sensations connected with it, was also of major importance. It is tempting to view Billy's primary impulsion with the "Stop" and "Go" signals, and the door checks, in relation to the partial obstruction of his anus. However, in this interpretation, one needs to remember that preoccupations in early life with the opening and closing of doors may also be present in children where there is no difficulty concerning the anus. Billy was fascinated with his impulsions and could hardly be induced to give up acting in this direction. As long as he performed the impulsion he was satisfied, although he sometimes remarked that he had to do so. The distress started when he was hindered, by outward circumstances, from following his impulses. The description makes it clear that Billy was a difficult child in other respects, full of sudden and destructive impulses. It is remarkable that these impulses changed from period to period. All of them seemed to have a symbolic character, although they were based on real interests such as doors, numbers, watches, knives, motors, light signals, and inhalant drugs.

---

masturbation substitute and a fetish, and developed absorbing sexual preoccupations. He thought a great deal about the functions and sensations of the woman and the various female organs, especially the breasts. He asked the woman psychiatrist many questions in regard to this.

He then became interested in ether, chloroform, and other volatile anesthetic drugs which would produce unconsciousness, and he began carrying about with him bottles of these substances, which he inhaled. He was concerned with death and various states of consciousness. As he felt unable to solve his problems, and was driven by his obsessive compulsive tendencies, he frequently thought of suicide as an easy solution. Three times he had to be revived by a physician from a state of coma, resulting from inhalation of volatile drugs.

In college, his problems apparently became overwhelming, and, after two more instances when physicians had to revive him after inhaling drugs, he was sent to a sanitarium. The frustration arising from isolation and lack of any opportunity to exercise his compulsions led to severe anxiety and hostility. This, in turn, led to further isolation. A transorbital lobectomy was performed when he was eighteen years old. For some time after this, he felt some relief from his tension states and compulsive obsessional activities. However, when they returned, he successfully ended his life with a soporific drug.

Larry was eleven at the time of his first admission to the children's ward. On the Stanford-Binet test his IQ was 131. In a retest a year later his IQ was 150. The family situation was desperate. The father had been a habitual criminal, who appeared at home only occasionally and was, at the time, serving a long term in prison because of a fur and jewelry robbery. His mother, a lawyer and a very intelligent person, suffered from paranoia and had been committed to a state hospital at the time that Larry first came for observation. She died there three years later. The family had always lived in extreme poverty. There was one brother, two years younger, who was also in the observation ward of the hospital, but merely as a neglected child. He was extremely well adapted, amiable, and considerate, and had an IQ of 150. He never showed any difficulties. Larry was brought to the hospital because he would not adapt himself, either in school or in camp. He ran away from home for hours at a time and came back exhausted. At camp he had sexual play with cats. He also tried to grab the genitals of other boys and put his hands under girls' skirts. His progress in school was poor, in spite of his brilliant gifts. When he came to the hospital, he was extremely indignant and abusive. He called the hospital a jail and the other children "jailbirds," and had fantasies of escaping or blowing the hospital into the air. He also had fantasies that a master criminal would come and throw a bomb at the hospital, so that he and other patients could escape through a hole in the wall. He threatened suicide and, indeed, made attempts in this direction. His preoccupation with the idea of leaving the hospital by far exceeded what one would expect under ordinary circumstances. Furthermore, he repeated the same motives and the same ideas again and again. It was as though he were compelled to do so, although he did not have the feeling of being compelled.

His attitude in many other respects was similar. He was extremely preoccupied with his possessions. He wanted to get as much as he could—pencils, toys, etc.—and he was continually afraid that somebody might take them away from him. He was particularly fascinated by the idea of money. He continually asked for money and tried to hoard it. He had an exaggerated opinion of the value of the things he owned. His attitude toward money was a compulsive one, but without the feeling of being compelled.

He had a similar relation to foodstuffs, especially candies, of which he favored specific types. He continually talked of how he could get them, and he devoured them with great pleasure. Irrespective of how much he received, he wanted to have more. On the occasion of ward parties, he made himself sick from eating. There was a continuous preoccupation with numbers. He calculated not only the exact number of days he was in the hospital, but also the exact number of minutes. Furthermore, he took an enormous pleasure in counting. For instance, one day he said that he had counted up to 7, 999. He bounced a ball and counted the impacts until the ball was taken from him. He counted his own respirations, and blew on a mouth organ with the same impulsion, to the exasperation of everyone else on the ward. He drew revolving curves and lines over sheets of paper and wrote numbers on the lines, so that finally the whole crisscross of lines and the sheet were covered with numbers. Later, he extended his interests to the fantastic numbers of astronomy.

He had a passion for walking the streets. He counted the numbers on the houses and wanted to see where the street ended. The longer the street, the better he liked it. Before he came to the hospital, he had walked for hours until exhausted. In the hospital he made maps of streets and houses, with the same end in view. After his discharge from the hospital for the first time, it was difficult to restrain him from doing this again. He used roller skates in order to extend his experiences. During his first stay in the hospital, he wanted to be a motorman in a subway train.

He produced all sorts of compulsive patterns with paper and pencil, most commonly village scenes, with elaborate details as to houses, streets, fences, streetcar tracks, labels, etc. His clay productions showed similar compulsive features.

He adjusted poorly to other children on the ward. He never tired of expressing his disgust, hate, and contempt for them. He called them criminals and guttersnipes. He wished that all of them would be bald. He did not form a real attachment to anyone. He made occasional attempts to pinch the genitals of other boys. He denied that there was any sexuality involved in this. He stated that he merely wanted to punish them and that this was, in his opinion, the best way. At the same time, he was extremely afraid of the children and continually complained that they were hitting and abusing him. He was cowardly in his reactions. His name was originally Howard, but he had changed it to Larry, since the children in school recited, "Howard is a coward." He liked persons as long as they yielded to him and gave him things. He reacted with enormous hate to the slightest deprivation imposed on him.

One might say that he considered other human beings merely from the point of view of what he could obtain from them. An attempt was made to psychoanalyze him. However, his associations remained mostly on the surface. Even his dreams dealt chiefly with his immediate wishes and preoccupations. On the whole, it appeared as if there had been a strong attachment to his mother, but he had felt that he was continually exposed to deprivation. This attachment, therefore, remained superficial, intermingled with hate and fear. A strong jealousy concerning his brother was always present. Fear dominated his relations with his father. He was not supposed to know about his father's criminality; however, it appeared that he knew all about it. There were numerous dreams of fears of being kidnapped and abducted by criminals.

After some months' stay in the hospital, various attempts were made to place him outside. With the help of an unusually tolerant foster mother, these attempts were successful for several months. However, he had difficulties in the public schools, because he could not tolerate other children, and assaulted a monitor. Finally, he had to come back to the school at the hospital. Further difficulties arose when he started to cover his face because he said he was ugly and people were looking at him—although he was quite attractive. This hiding of the face gave the impression that it was more a whim than a real paranoid idea. He was stopped in the subway by a policeman because it was thought he was going to jump in front of the trains, and he had to be admitted to the ward again. Psychotherapy was attempted, again without success. He had insulin treatment for two months, after which he was more adaptable for about two weeks. He did not cover his face so persistently, but his other behavior difficulties proved to be so severe that he was committed to a state hospital at the age of thirteen.[7]

[7] He remained in the state hospital for four years, with a diagnosis of hebephrenic schizophrenia. In the beginning he was withdrawn, held his hand over his face, and would not speak to anyone nor associate with other patients. He was untidy, said the whole world was against him, and masturbated excessively. He walked the floor, counting his steps and the number of times he turned. Later, he spoke of electricity in his body and of homosexual influences. He made several suicidal attempts. When he would discuss his problem, he spoke of being shy, introverted, and having an inferiority complex.

At seventeen, he was paroled to a social agency, but six months later was returned to the hospital because of another suicidal attempt. After another six months, he was again paroled, but was working as a messenger boy for the hospital where he had been a patient. Later, he moved into the city and had a very simple job. The next year he was found to have tuberculosis and was admitted to a sanitarium.

Larry was again examined in a psychiatric clinic when he was twenty-five. It was noted that in spite of spending most of his adolescence in a state mental hospital, where a diagnosis of schizophrenia was made, and a subsequent period in a sanitarium, he showed surprisingly good ego structure. He still functioned at a very superior intellectual level in a test situation (IQ 137, Bellevue-Wechsler Intelligence Test). However, his personality was immature, and his judgment poor. He showed schizoid features and obsessive trends in his overspecificity in approaching tasks. He was emotionally indifferent and somewhat paranoid. Renewed efforts were made to give him realistic vocational guidance. So far, he had been content with menial jobs, such as busboy in a restaurant or messenger boy.

In this boy we found not only overwhelming interests in numbers, streets, and houses, but also actions corresponding to them. His whole psychic life was so constructed that he had either no interest or an obsessive one, an impulsion. This picture was associated with obsessive greediness, pertaining not only to the oral sphere, but to everything in the nature of possessions. He had excessive hobbies, excessive likes and dislikes, and a tendency to collect what he liked. One may suspect that early deprivations and the wish to compensate for them may have had something to do with this picture. In spite of the unsatisfactory results of the intensive treatment, we did not feel that the diagnosis of schizophrenia should be made before he went to the state hospital. It was made at that time, although subsequent events led to the comment that the ego structure was surprisingly good. In spite of intellectual gifts, he functioned at a low level and was only interested in his impulsive and obsessional preoccupations.

Amelio, age twelve, was on the children's ward for two months. He was sent there by the school. The complaint against the child was that he was difficult to handle in the schoolroom because of his impulsive behavior, his emotional instability, and his maladjustment to educational routine. He had been classified, by the school psychologist, as a child of dull normal to borderline intelligence. There was apparently a suggestion of organic brain disturbance because of chorea-like motility and a doubtful family history of venereal disease. Examination and observation revealed that the child had an intellectual endowment above average, with special disabilities and special abilities, but with deep-seated psychoneurotic problems in reaction to a psychopathic father, an unstable home situation, and poor handling of his educational disability. Psychometric examinations, performed shortly after admission, revealed an IQ of 110. At that time, the psychologist expressed the opinion that the boy was still not functioning at his maximum level and noted a marked discrepancy between verbal and nonverbal performance, in that he showed an unusual capacity for handling verbal material. There were marked discrepancies here too, however, as he scored at an inferior level in social judgment and insight, and showed severe educational retardation in arithmetic, reading, and spelling; but he had an unusual fund of knowledge in geography, history, and astronomy. It was stated that the boy's intelligence was definitely above average and that he showed special facility in handling verbal material, but was handicapped in academic subjects, and

233

dealt poorly with performance material. He showed outstanding gifts in both graphic and plastic arts. There was, moreover, a reading disability, which he tended to compensate for by his ability in graphic art and by thorough development of verbal capacities based on information obtained by ear. His scoring on standard tests was obviously very much lowered by his emotional inhibition.

Observation on the ward showed that the child was exceedingly unstable and distraught, and that he was suffering from considerable tension. It was difficult for him to apply himself to the schoolroom routine, because of his inability to deal with tasks with any satisfaction to himself. There seemed to be constant impulses to draw, but even his drawings were incoherent and incomplete. During the second and third weeks of observation, when the boy was at his best, it was possible to motivate him to complete his drawings, at which time he produced some exceedingly interesting pictures, usually of wild animals attacking and killing men. These animals were mostly lions and tigers, but there were also dragons. They were usually in lively colors. Blood gushing from wounds in lively red was emphasized with particular gusto. The technical ability with which animals and persons were drawn was considerable. Of these series of pictures, there was only one in which a man killed another, with a sword. On this, he wrote the legend, "This man is just as small as the other man, but he put on big things to look strong so he can scare and kill this other man." When he was asked what he would do if he had the power to make the world over, he wrote "I would make the tiger and I would make the lion stronger than any men. I would make Africa and Australia stronger so they could conquer Great Britain, and would make it so that they could not die. But I would let the bad people die any time and I would be richer, better and make myself the strong man in the world."

On completion of the drawings, he often applied himself well to academic subjects. Otherwise, he was anxious to carry on group discussions about geography and present social events, especially in regard to Hitler and the Czechoslovakian situation. On the ward he was restless and frequently created difficulties with the other children, by whom he was not well liked.

In psychiatric interviews, the child gave evidence of being overeager; he made a good contact with the psychiatrist, showed marked capacity for verbalization and was anxious to discuss his difficulties. Briefly, his problems resolved themselves into a strong antipathy toward his father and an overwhelming feeling of being defeated and thwarted in any effort to obtain satisfaction. His hatred for his father often found concrete expression. He described his father as a slave driver of his mother, and a troublemaker, who made contacts with other persons in the neighborhood only to fight with them and make trouble for the family. He stated that his father pretended to be many things that he was not, and that he claimed to have been born in many countries other than the United States. He indicated that his father considered himself too good for his own family and made no effort to work, but that he often spoke of having superior positions and thus had thrown away many chances.

It was proved that the child's insight into his father's peculiarities was striking. It also appeared that the father would not allow the child any sort of satisfaction. The boy was not allowed to play on the streets, go to moving pictures, or listen to a radio in the house. The father attempted to drive the boy to do his homework, including reading and writing, of which the child was incapable and the boy was frequently beaten for failure. A final analysis of the child's impulsive and ticlike behavior indicated that it was an expression of the combined thwarting of his desire to express himself, and of his attempt to show his hatred for his father. His dream life, his pictures, his claywork, and even his dancing, all resolved themselves into some dramatic expression of an attempt to kill a man by a wild beast or by other means. We treated the boy with benzedrine, hydrotherapy, intensive tutoring, artistic expression, psychotherapy, and group activities, and he improved steadily for a few weeks. After that, he returned to most of his former behavior, although it was partially modified. For example, his drawings were less aggressive, but still compulsive.[8]

This boy had extremely strong aggressive impulses, chiefly directed against his father. He obviously identified himself with wild animals who kill men. He was completely preoccupied with this topic, and expressed it in fantasy, as well as in drawings. However, one had to keep in mind that the artistic ability which he had developed was closely connected with his reading disability; his pleasure in drawing and his capacity for it corresponded closely to what has been observed in children on other occasions. The special

[8] After he returned home, he continued to be a problem both at school and at home. Because his father was increasingly difficult, his mother separated from him and the family became dependent upon public welfare. Amelio stopped school as soon as he was permitted, but failed to keep any employment. He was abusive to his mother and stayed out late at night with bad companions. He was referred to a clinic for psychiatric treatment, but was not interested in cooperating. When he was nearly eighteen, he was charged with rape and imprisoned with a ten- to twenty-year sentence. It is of interest that an older brother, age twenty, was a problem because he was meticulous about his personal appearance, but unreliable in his work. A sister was attending art school on a scholarship because of exceptional artistic talent.

contents of these drawings, and the energy which he spent on them, were due not only to his reading disability, but also to his specific psychological conflicts.

We have described a group of cases in which preoccupations with specific ideas and fantasies, special interests in impulses, and the performance of specific actions with eagerness and satisfaction, dominated the picture. The ages of the children, when first observed, were between four and twelve. Marvin showed the transition from this picture to an obsession neurosis, when first observed on the threshold of puberty. We called this picture "impulsion." In their clear-cut form, impulsions have so far been observed only in children. There is, however, no question but that similar phenomena can be also observed in adults whose interests are more or less bound in one direction. Impulsions have close relations to hobbies, collecting, and overemphasis on a particular group of actions and occupations. We shall discuss this later in more detail, after having obtained insight into the range of the phenomena described.

In Billy, there was, at first, an overwhelming interest in door checks and doors in general. This preoccupation also expressed itself in actions repeated over and over again. Later, an interest in specific numbers and in dials was substituted. Here, too, the interest was not merely theoretical, but also expressed itself in actions. Both interests were also expressed in the contents of drawings. Billy had no particular tendency to resist his impulses, although he was in continual conflict with adults. He gave the excuse that he had to do it. Generally, he showed great stubbornness in following these impulsions, but it was remarkable that outside this particular field he was also obstinate and wanted to follow his own wishes only. He showed, furthermore, violent dislikes, especially for the male sex organ.

Larry showed a tendency to follow his impulsions, even to running and exploring the streets to the point of physical exhaustion. Furthermore, he generally did not want to stand for any interference with his wishes. He had the feeling that they must be satisfied. He expressed violent hatred against anyone who interfered with his impulsions and with his impulses. There was a particular preoccupation with counting, with numbers, and with space. All this was transformed as much as possible into action. Further, he was greedy, craving money and possessions, and he attempted to collect these things, all with the feeling that he was entitled to all he could get. He was self-righteous and self-satisfied. In his relations with others, he showed an enormous aggressiveness, in words and wishes. Physically, he was a coward and did not want to fight.

Stanley had a strong hate for his father and doubts concerning his own virility. He was preoccupied with drawing girls and he asserted that they too had a penis and testes. His father died when he was twelve, and, following that, he and his mother became more enrapt with each other. They could not be induced by social agencies to make a more normal relationship in any social situation or seek psychiatric help.

Amelio had strong aggressive tendencies against his father. He indulged in fantasies and drawings in which beasts killed men. That he chose this expression was partially due to the fact that the drawings compensated for his reading disability. In spite of help from schools and social agencies, he failed to make a good school, work, or social adjustment or to accept needed psychiatric care.

Finally, Marvin suffered when one of his strong wishes could not be fulfilled. In order to overcome his preoccupation with the wish, he threatened himself with death and then had to overcome his fear of death by special actions. This is a case in which the impulsion was clearly the nucleus of an obsession. However, besides the obsession, the boy retained the capacity for strong desires and wishes, and the necessity of having them fulfilled. There were aggressive actions in earlier childhood, followed by feelings of guilt. Since the boy felt that his wishes should be fulfilled, he demanded, and obtained, a bicycle from his family, a bayonet, admission to the naval reserve, and admission to and discharge from a public institution. He insisted, furthermore, that his wishes should be promptly fulfilled. His belief that he had a right to have his desires fulfilled led to illegal acts of fishing where prohibited, breaking open a parcel post package with friends, and hitching rides on trolley cars, although he realized the dangers involved. When he fell off a trolley car and broke his arm, he was preoccupied in a hypochondriacal way with the fracture, especially after it was cured.

Our observations show the wealth of symptoms in these cases: continuous looking at and handling of a specific object; drawing of this object; preoccupation with this object in fantasies or in thoughts; excessive walking; counting, and a preoccupation with numbers and space; strong desires, wishes, and demands for immediate satisfaction; resistance and hate directed against any interference; greed concerning food and money; collecting and hoarding; hypochondriacal preoccupation; stubbornness; and social actions which satisfy the strong desires.

This childhood picture of impulsions had not met with specific attention, as far as our knowledge goes. There exists a children's story, entitled *Susanna B. and William C.*, by Field (1934), in which impulsions are clearly described. Susanna has an overwhelming interest in shoes. She is magically punished by finding shoes which force her to dance forever. William is too curious about locks and keys. He is finally magically forced to wear a mailbag through life. Incidentally, such stories may have some value for students of psychopathology, but can only be harmful for children.

We might indicate that impulsions have a close relation to compulsions and obsessions. However, in the case of compulsions and obsessions, the subject protests against his impulses and thoughts. It is true that our patients also, from time to time, were bothered by their impulses. Their inner protest, however, was not as inherent a part of the picture as is the case with compulsions and obsessions. It is true that obsessions and compulsions are, at times, accepted or not protested by the patients, but this is the exception and not the rule. On the whole, one might characterize the difference by saying that, in the case of compulsions and obsessions, the patient protests with his ego and superego against his impulses, whereas, in the case of impulsion, this protest is weak or nonexistent. In this way, one may understand that impulsions are more characteristic of childhood, and compulsions and obsessions are more characteristic of adolescence and adult life. This statement should not be understood in a schematic way. Features of obsession neurosis have been repeatedly observed in early childhood and are also to be found in our material. Fenichel cited several cases of early obsessional neurosis. However, the question arises whether at least some of the so-called obsessions and compulsions in children are not impulsions in the sense described here.

In *The Psychoanalysis of Children* Klein (1932) expressed the opinion that obsession neurosis plays an important part in the neuroses of children. Obsessional neurotic trends serve, in her opinion that obsession neurosis plays an important part in the earliest levels of development. However, she stated that this early obsession neurosis is different from the later form. Indeed, she mentioned ceremonies, and exaggerated orderliness and cleanliness, as symptoms of the earlier neurosis. These, too, are symptoms which are generally accepted or are acceptable to the subject. On the other hand, the adult with an obsession neurosis, shows character changes which closely correspond to the impulsions we have described in children. They are tolerated by the ego, or even considered as a valuable part of the ego. Orderliness, cleanliness, parsimoniousness, collecting, and hobbies in general belong in this category. However, impulsions are compared with the obsession neuroses which may be present even without obsessions or compulsions. One immediately sees that while the impulsions are hardly socially acceptable, the obsession neurosis character trends are acknowledged by ego and society. Whereas, in the impulsions the ego is not concerned or is not considered as important, in the obsession neuroses the impulsions have been integrated, more or less perfectly, into the ego system. This is again understandable from the point of view of a difference between childhood and adulthood, in respect to the organization of the ego.

In spite of this, it would be wrong to believe that the impulsions, as described here, are the direct expression of primitive wishes. They have a complicated individual history and can be characterized as symbolic (as in Billy's case, in which the opening of the door pointed to his anal difficulties). The running, exploring, and counting, in Lawrence's case, have certainly not only a manifest content, but an unconscious meaning, and the same is true of the drawings of Stanley and Amelio. Complicated processes of interpretation are also necessary to understand the impulsions displayed by Marvin.

In this connection, it is worthwhile to point to the enormous aggressiveness which is represented in the impulsions and their allied phenomena. This is either direct aggression or curiosity, or

239

aggression hidden in counting. In the majority of cases, the impulsion often serves aggression in connection with the father problem. Only Stanley's problems were concerned with castration and femininity alone. It is perhaps worthwhile to mention that we have so far only observed impulsions in boys.

The aggression in these cases is by no means merely sadistic. In these impulsions, there is a great deal of curiosity, a wish to learn and handle, and a wish to experiment. This leads to the general problem of overwhelming interests in early childhood. We have observed, in very young children, that they have a close relation to the pillow. This may already be present in the second or third month. These children clutch their pillows, primarily in order to be more secure in their equilibrium. They want to have something to hold on to. Later, they retain the need for the pillow. It is gratuitous to say that the pillow serves the overcoming of anxiety and that this defense is retained. The anxiety has, in some way, to do with the maintenance of equilibrium. When children start to crawl, at the age of eight or nine months, they become deeply interested in doors. They play with doors and handle them well. This interest may last for several months, only to be replaced by another, such as wall plugs or light connections. We have observed these interests in children from twelve months to two years of age, when they shift to flags, boats, books, and other objects. It might be said that these overwhelming interests lead to a better acquaintance with the objects. They belong, therefore, to the ego functions. They may retain their importance when libidinous motives lead in a similar direction, as appears to have happened in our cases just discussed. This interest is transformed infantile curiosity and experimentation, and, also, a strong desire for satisfaction in the family circle.

In these cases, transformations and symbolizations, although they took place, did not go so far as in the character trends which appear in the adult. Such impulsive character trends can be found not only in the patient with an obsession neurosis, but also in the criminal who displays impulsions. One may suspect that deep, genuine interests, which lead to useful preoccupation in science and work, have a genesis comparable with that of impulsions.

It might be worthwhile to complement these observations from various angles. We might try to classify the possible impulses and impulsions of childhood. There are the impulses of sex, that emerge more or less directly in premature sex activities, which may be directed toward other children or may be autoerotic. One might, furthermore, find impulses concerned with motor activities in the narrower sense; for example, rocking, hitting the head against the wall, and manneristic and automatic movements. There might also be mentioned too much interest in motor play, and, finally, running away. As a third group, one might think of destruction and tearing, irrespective of the object. The fundamental change in the system of motor impulses, occurring in and after encephalitis, often induces pictures somewhat similar to impulsions. They differ in that, in the majority of cases of encephalitis, the impulses are less organized than in the impulsions. However, there are cases of postencephalitis, occurring in adults, in which the impulses are organized as impulsions, and one may also find instances in which impulsions, compulsions, and obsessions are present at the same time.

Most of these impulsions and impulses are not so much persistences of more primitive levels of expression as they are a return to these levels, when expression on a higher level is frustrated. These primitive actions and interests might be modified by the total situation and have, in addition to their direct meaning, a symbolic one. It is significant that most of the children, in this series, made poor adjustments at school and had various educational difficulties, in spite of good intelligence. This becomes more obvious if one considers their forms of impulsive eating (a particular emphasis on specific foodstuffs or eating rituals), and their impulsive fighting and hitting of other children. Habitual stealing and fire setting, as described by Yarnell (1940), have a still more symbolic structure, and many of the motor habits and ticlike mannerisms which the child cherishes are in no way a simple expression of primary impulses. Furthermore, one might draw attention to all so-called delinquent acts in children and adolescents. In many such patients, the constitutional motor and instinctual endowment plays an outstanding part. Some of the drives leading to impulses may be decidedly organic, although the group described here did not show such characteristics.

We have mentioned before that the so-called obsession neurosis of childhood might not really be that. Yaskin (1936) wrote, for instance, that he found neurotic trends existing from childhood in compulsive-obsessive reactions, "but [they] were thoroughly integrated in the personality makeup and did not produce disabling symptoms until somewhat later in life." Our own experiences, in analyses of adults suffering from obsession neuroses, did not disclose such trends, in the narrower sense, before prepuberty. However, there were many indications that impulsions were present. Moreover, we have observed children of about eleven or twelve years in whom the first symptoms of obsession neurosis had appeared at the age of seven. We are therefore inclined to believe that impulsions against which the ego and superego do not take a particularly strong stand are more characteristic of earlier childhood. They occur up to the age of ten or twelve years. Later, toward puberty, obsessions and compulsions make their appearance. In the impulsions, some transformations have taken place under the influence of the ego and superego system. At about the age of ten—sometimes earlier, sometimes later—the ego and superego take a definite stand, and the impulsions either become compulsions or are integrated into the total character as so-called obsession neurosis character trends. These character trends, as well as the impulsions, therefore express primitive impulses and are tolerated by the ego-superego system, but in accordance with the greater demands of the system in later years, the primitive desires have had to undergo more thorough transformation in order to be accepted as character trends.

## AGGRESSION[9]

Man, as a carnivorous animal, must kill in order to live. He is, at first, compelled to capture his prey, then overpower it, if he is to use it for the satisfaction of his needs. In this struggle for life, he is forced to defend himself against the aggression of the external world, which includes other human beings and animals. In such a pursuit of his needs, he must not only hurt animals, but probably human beings as well.

---

[9] From Bender and Schilder (1936a). This study has been condensed and partially reorganized because of its length. Brief footnotes, with follow-up data (1950-1951) from after Schilder's death, are added on ten cases which are given in some detail. For the more detailed case data on the remaining seventy-three children, see the original monograph.

In his relation to plants and the inanimate world, man makes use of his strength. He has to destroy structures and use materials without regard for their inner organization. A close relationship exists between such activities and aggressiveness toward animals and human beings. Thus, Freud has offered the theory that these "instincts of the ego," which serve self-preservation, are identical with the destructive tendencies, and that they are primarily directed toward one's self and only secondarily toward the outer world.

The studies discussed in this chapter are solely concerned with aggressiveness toward other human beings, and are not concerned with the general problems of the relationship between aggressiveness and human activities. Aggressiveness is here considered as violence against other persons, inflicted by physical means, and does not include psychic aggressiveness. We regard violence to be any action which damages the body of another person, or distorts the body image of another person by pain or discomfort.

Adler (1917) has always stressed the importance of aggressiveness in the fight for superiority. Klein (1932, p. 177) writes: "The idea of an infant from six to twelve months trying to destroy his mother by every method at the disposal of his sadistic tendencies—with his nails, teeth and excreta and with the whole of his body, transformed in imagination into all kinds of dangerous weapons—presents a horrifying, not to say unbelievable, picture to our minds. But the abundance, force and the multiplicity of the imaginary cruelties which accompany these cravings are displayed before our eyes in early analysis so clearly and forcibly that they leave no room for doubt."

She stated that the destructive impulses in the child culminate in his desire to suck and scoop out the breasts and later to do the same to the insides of the mother's body. Children also have the fantasy of destroying the inside of the body of the mother by poisonous urine and feces. The self-perception of these destructive impulses provokes anxiety in the child, by making him fearful of extermination by his own instinctive danger. This anxiety is increased by the external object against whom the sadistic feelings are directed. In addition, the combined image of father and mother, but particularly their poisonous excreta, is another source of fear of aggression against the child. Susan Isaacs pictures the child as defenseless

243

against untold dangers. In his superego, he suffers from frustration and punishment by the parents. He feels bad, since he is full of fear and rage and forbidden wishes.

Hostility is based on general feelings of anxiety and on the sense of possession of power and rivalry. For a child not to possess what others have is not only a denial of love from the parents, but also an aggression against the child, which provokes his counteraggression. Children feel that they should possess whatever they want. Ultimately, they want to possess everything, and will defend this attitude with hostility and aggression. The destruction of objects and the overpowering of others give the child a sense of power. Aggression is directed toward everybody who receives more attention than the child himself, and toward the beloved person who withholds attention. Children are also hostile to each other, as experimental play illustrates. They believe that when they become acquainted with other animals, it is well to assume that they are dangerous until proven otherwise. At least this is the attitude in the beginning of social behavior. Bridges (1931), asserts that fighting, punching, hugging, and touching are exploratory, and precede normal social behavior. Our study is not interested primarily in psychoanalytic interpretation, which Melanie Klein treats rather arbitrarily. We employed a definite method of another sort.

Since it is a general opinion that the degree of physical aggressiveness is a differential characteristic between the two sexes, our investigation included children of both sexes. The cases studied were children under observation in the children's service of the Psychiatric Division of Bellevue Hospital in 1934 and 1935. The majority of cases represented behavior problems of a more or less severe degree. The age range was from three to fifteen years, and there were 34 girls and 49 boys (which approximates the usual ratio of girls to boys on the children's ward). The IQ range was from 70 to 167. Thirty-three of the eighty-three children had IQ's between 90 and 110, while forty-three had IQ's below 90, and seven had IQ's above 110. The medium IQ was somewhat lower than that for the school populace.

It should be kept in mind that these children were referred to the hospital because they were problems in the community. Most of them came from underprivileged homes. Bilingual surroundings were responsible for limited language facilities in some cases, usually in Puerto Rican children.

The method of the study included an analysis of: (1) the case history; (2) psychiatric interview; (3) observation of behavior on the ward; (4) observation of specific play situations, especially with miniature toys; (5) the children's description of pictures with aggressive content; and (6) a questionnaire for the children who had sufficient verbal facility. They were often observed and interviewed in groups of two or more, as well as individually. Play with miniature toys was observed especially with the smaller children. They had the opportunity to play with a great number and variety of toys, but the following three situations were presented in a formal way, so as to constitute a test situation.

Doll Test: Examiner pushed over a small doll by touching its head. The same procedure was repeated three times, each time with the question, "What has happened to it?" If the child made no attempt to imitate, examiner said, "Would you like to play with it?" —then, "Knock it down."

Cowboy-Soldier Test: The examiner placed a small lead cowboy and Indian between two soldiers and said, "What are they doing?" If the child answered, "Fighting," etc., the examiner asked, "Why are they doing it?"—then, "Is it right to do it? Can you fight?" etc.

Automobile Test: The examiner placed a lead soldier between three toy automobiles, which were pointed toward the soldier. He then asked, "What is this? What will happen? Do you want to play with this? Do you want to play with them?"

The pictures[10] (see Figure 4) which the children were asked to describe or tell a story about, were of the following type:

(1)   A violent fight, with swords, between men of different colors and racial characteristics.

(2)   A parade of soldiers before going into battle.

(3)   A hippopotamus throwing a boy out of a canoe.

(4)   A half-clad woman defending herself, with a dagger, against a man.

(5)   A lioness taking a baby from the side of a sleeping mother, with the frightened father lying nearby, helpless.

[10] These are pictures 1, 2, 3, 8, and 10 of the fourteen pictures in the original monograph (Bender and Schilder, 1936a).

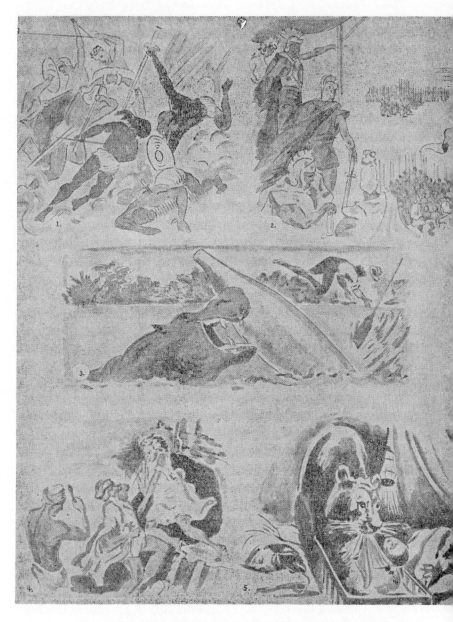

FIGURE 4. Sketches of Pictures Used in Studies on Children's Attitude
Toward Aggressiveness.

The questions asked them in the questionnaire[11] were:

(1)  What is courage (guts, nerve, bravery)?

(2)  What does it mean to be a coward (yellow)?

(3)  Why should one not be a coward?

(4)  Do you like to hit other children?

(5)  Is it right to hit someone who insults you?

(6)  What is a sissy? And what do you think of them?

(7)  Would you like to be a girl [to a boy] or a boy [to a girl]?

(8)  Should a girl fight? Should a girl hit a girl? Should a boy fight? Should a boy hit a girl?

(9)  Would you like to shoot somebody to kill them, or kill them with an ax?

(10)  How would you defend yourself against a stronger child?

We have divided the children we observed into two groups, those who were three to eight years old and those who were nine to fifteen years old. In the younger group, the questionnaire could be used only occasionally. The main emphasis was put on our observation of the play of these young children, and their description of the pictures. The three-year-old and four-year-old boys and girls showed the same characteristics in their play, irrespective of their sex. The following observation of play with toys is characteristic of this age. Nora (4-4) brought a small toy dog near the hand of the examiner and said "The dog is biting you." She arranged a number of toy soldiers in a line and pushed them down, saying, "Down! You got some more?" Rita (3-2) got particular pleasure out of pushing the toys over, and laughingly would say, "Play some more."

Both children very much enjoyed knocking over the toy men. They would say, "I fall that man down. I bite him." Both children would continue their aggressive play by beginning to bite the toys, but finally would bite themselves with great pleasure, and say, "Look!" When given a rubber doll, the older child, Nora, started to bite the doll and Rita immediately imitated. This is an instance of direct imitation. Nora said to Rita, "It's a bad doll baby. Don't take it." When the smaller child, Rita, started caressing the woman

---

[11] These are questions 1-4 and 15-21 of the original monograph (Bender and Schilder, 1936a). See also Schilder (1938c) for full questionnaire.

physician and the other child became obviously jealous, she continued to play with the rubber doll and ordered the smaller child not to take it. After the children had once established a pattern of knocking everything over, they continued, even with such objects as automobiles. It was only later that Rita started to push an automobile forward and backward.

Description of the pictures by children of this age was very incomplete. The following description by Nora was characteristic (see Figure 4):

(1)  "That man—laying down—oh look at the man laying down. He is - - - -. It is a picture—a man—they hurt each other." Why do they do that? "I'm mad on you—I'm going to smack you."

(2)  "We didn't look at that picture. The man is standing up. It is a dog." Knife? "Yes, they cut somebody." What is that? "Soldiers." That? "A flag." That? "A man."

(3)  That? "An airplane." Rhinoceros? "Man—he is laying down—another man."

One of our youngest hyperkinetic children, Joey (3-2), took the details of the picture very seriously. Joey hit the lion and the man in the picture with his fist, since he considered them to be bad. One must consider the play of children, as well as their spontaneous behavior. Three-, four-, and five-year-old children showed a distinct aggressiveness in play with toys, and in their tendency to knock them over and throw them from the table. When a toy fell down, they often considered it a sign of death. An early remembrance in an adult, psychoanalyzed by me, was of a servant maid stumbling and falling, whereupon the child exclaimed, "Julie's dead." The upright posture and the relation to gravity is not only fundamental from the physiological point of view, but also from the psychological point of view. In early play activity, children are also very anxious that the toys should remain upright. Nora's and Rita's play clearly revealed the primitive features in the organization of play and aggressiveness. Frequently, a doll is pushed over or a car is thrown away without any concern for their function. Our observation of the three-year-old Joey showed the formal features in his play. He first placed the soldiers in a row, then he put them near the border of the table; next he put a cluster of three men around a horse, and so on. This is mentioned merely to show that there are principles of organization, but they do not follow the concepts of the adult, and thus they lend themselves very easily to an aggressiveness directed against very simple units.

The tendency to bring the object to the mouth is present only in the very young children. When the children are older, the organization is often much closer to the patterns of adults. The soldiers are put into rows and groups, and placed along the borders of the table, or are otherwise arranged to conform to the background or field. Opposing groups are formed by placing those of different categories in different positions. A car knocks over a man. The wounded or the dead are carried away in a car. The character of the object becomes important for the type of aggressiveness expressed. The tendency for good and bad orientation comes out very clearly. The Indians are often "bad men" or the pirate is "bad" and it is quite justifiable for the others to shoot the "bad men."

Joey would let the Indians kill the soldiers and pirates, and then he changed the situation and said, "The Indian is running away because he is going to get killed by him [the pirate]." He then laid all the toys down and said "Look they are all dead." The car, by its suggested momentum, became a symbol for aggressiveness. The play tended to follow the course suggested by the nature of the objects.

In the development of play, motor impulses perform a very important part. Play implies the handling of an object. In the beginning, only the most primitive forms arise; in further development, more complicated structures form the basis for the action. Aggressiveness is based on this continuous interplay between form and motion. This has been shown in Bender's and my studies (1936) on the principle of form in the play of children (see Chapter I). Whenever the motor impulses are increased, their relation to the form is changed. There is a strong tendency to break up the form into smaller units and to destroy any form as soon as it has been created. For instance, the child will put up a row of soldiers and lay them down immediately or shift the row to a new formation. At first, the child may put soldiers into a car; then later he'll put one car into another. There is a strong tendency to repeat patterns of activity and, as these are increased, the single phase will be shortened. Joey gave short commands to the playthings. Not fully acquainted with the structure of things, he tried to make the soldiers stand in the air parallel to the wall. He ran the car around without any definite aim, making a sirenlike noise. Strong hyperkinetic factors made it necessary for him to form a quicker orientation concerning good and bad, and also regarding the physical qualities of the objects.

Nora, on admission (age 4-4), presented the picture of a small, emaciated child in a continuous state of fury. She would stamp her feet, spit, scratch, dash at things and destroy them if possible, grind her teeth, and fearlessly attack adults or other children. However, she was very responsive to affection and her behavior gradually changed. She proved to be very sensitive to the social environment and made herself the favorite in the group. She showed a great range of emotional responses and was dramatic in her expressions. She used her bodily motility and facial expression freely, with considerable histrionic ability. Her speech was no longer retarded and she showed a rich vocabulary. However, if she was thwarted or reprimanded she would still respond with exaggerated sullenness or dramatic temper outbursts, which, however, tended more and more to assume a playful air. She was usually the center of the play activities of a group, and played amiably as long as things satisfied her; but she became assaultive if anything went against her.

Hyperkinesis is a state in which the number of movements greatly exceeds the normal. It cannot usually be attributed to specific problems, but may be based on either constitutional factors or organic lesions of the brain, particularly of the midbrain region. It may occur in encephalitis or in reaction to other conditions, organic or psychological, which tend to disorganize the pattern of behavior.

But the aggressiveness of a child is not merely the expression of his motor constitution and constellation. It is also the expression of the child's total life history. Hyperkinesis can be a reaction to environmental psychic factors as, for instance, in the case of Nora. This case very clearly showed that hyperkinesis, coupled with aggressive activity of a very severe type, may be largely a reaction to unfavorable environmental factors. Although the child had been subject to neglect and abuse during the greater part of her life before she was four, and had suffered severe nutritional and developmental disturbances, her hyperkinesis and aggressiveness tended to disappear as soon as the environment and nutrition were improved.

The following is a protocol of one morning's activities with Nora. She started crying when the older children went to school and she was too young to accompany them. She threw a temper tantrum that lasted for ten minutes, during which time the examiner stood by her, but gave her no sympathy. Afterward, she was angry, but followed the examiner to the office. An effort was made to win her friendliness with toys, but she kicked them away, and then the examiner pushed them back until this became a game. Then the toy soldiers were put in a little wagon and first kicked back and forth and then pushed back and forth. She lined the soldiers up and counted them to three and, later, to five. She pushed one aside and said it had to be put there because it had been bad and had hit her. She admitted that she hit people too, but would not admit that she had been bad. She found a pencil and asked to draw a picture. She said it was "the boy friend" but it looked just like a scribble. She continued to be very friendly. She whirled on the top of the desk, humming, and said she was dancing. She whirled until she was dizzy and then whirled in the other direction. She continued this for a very long time. She asked the examiner to hold her hand and was very affectionate.

Joey was brought to us (at 3-2) by his mother, after his father had deserted the home. There was also a newborn brother at home. The home had always been inadequate because of the parents' marital difficulties, recurring separation, and immaturity. The mother felt unequal to caring for the children by herself. Joey was restless, untrained, and impulsive. It was suggested that he might have suffered from an encephalitis, following measles, but this was not confirmed. He spent some months under our care, partly because the mother could not decide what to do. Shortly after taking him home, she agreed to have him placed in a foster home. He was again seen by us when he was eight years old. Then he was dull, bewildered, and unhappy. He also had a reading disability and was an unsatisfactory student.[12]

[12] Later, the mother reunited the family, the father returning from time to time. Joey lived with his family, continuing as a poor student at school, but inconspicuous in his behavior through the age of sixteen, when the family was heard from because Joey's younger brother required some guidance service for aggressive behavior.

Rita was brought to our mental hygiene clinic when she was three and a half years old by her twenty-one-year-old mother. She had been an illegitimate baby, and had been raised by devoted foster parents. Meanwhile, her mother and father had married, and had two baby boys. After the father had been killed in a drunken brawl, welfare agencies attempted to set up a home for Rita's mother, with her two infant sons and Rita. Rita rebelled at being taken from her "Mother-dear," meaning her foster mother, and defiantly denied her mother and apparently deliberately regressed in habit training, wetting and soiling her clothes and bed, and indulging in crying tempers.

Against our advice, the mother insisted on taking Rita home from our ward, but soon openly neglected the three children, spending a great deal of time in bars. She also had another illegitimate baby. Rita and her two brothers were placed in foster homes, where they behaved in an infantile and undisciplined fashion. Rita was again seen by us when she was nine years old. She was alert and had a remarkable understanding of the family situation. She said her two brothers were "bad," but that they had not had a fair chance, either with their mother or in the foster home.[13]

*　　*　　*

Nora was the fifth child in a family of seven, that suffered many vicissitudes. The father of the first four children had died, and Nora was illegitimate. When she was six months old, the mother placed Nora, and the next oldest, Patricia, in an institution in another state, where they remained for two years. Meanwhile, the mother married Nora's father and the family was reunited. What the history of Nora and Patricia was, during their two years in the institution, can be only surmised from the description of their condition and behavior when they returned home. It was said that both were very much emaciated, and retarded in development.

Nora did not speak at all. She refused all food except milk from a bottle and dry bread. She wet and soiled herself. She did not respond to any human contact and would either sit or stand in the same position for hours, unless moved. At night she slept poorly, and tossed and moaned in bed. The behavior of the older child was similar, but she tended to re-

[13] The children were then all placed in a Catholic institution. For about a year, Rita showed signs of insecurity and hostility, by being frequently untruthful and aggressive. After that, she got along well, finishing high school, where she took a business course. She then attended a private residential business school, where she worked after school in return for her room, board, tuition, and spending money. Subsequently, she was happily employed and attempting to help her next youngest brother become independent.

turn to normal more readily. For six months, the mother attempted to care for Nora, but she did not respond and did not improve physically or mentally.

She was brought to the mental hygiene clinic in this condition, at the age of three and one half years. She was extremely emaciated, with a protuberant belly, and she was covered with scabs all over her body. She did not speak; she would stand or sit in fixed postures, and showed no facial expression. This was looked upon as an extreme regression due to institutional deprivation. Convalescent care was recommended to build up her physical condition. She was sent to a convalescent home for three months and gained some weight, but then showed a different type of behavior difficulty. She was negativistic, irritable, defiant, and disobedient. She could speak by then and expressed an open hatred for everyone. The mother cared for her at home, again, for a few months, until the father was sentenced to jail. The child was then placed with a pediatric service for further care (and study) for her nutritional deficiency and developmental retardation, but she responded slowly. When taken home again, her defiant and antagonistic attitude had increased. She was subject to temper tantrums, and still openly expressed her hatred for everyone. On one occasion, she turned on the gas and said she wanted everybody in the family, but herself, to die.

Meanwhile, the father had been released from prison, but had died of pneumonia, and the family situation was again in a turmoil. Social agencies were making investigations to determine who should support this mother and her seven small children. In one of Nora's severe temper tantrums, she presented a picture which suggested a convulsion and was taken to another hospital, which recommended observation by our service. Then she was on the Bellevue children's ward for about two months.

She improved physically, although, in two months, the actual gain in weight was less than two pounds; there was a redistribution of body weight with flattening of the abdomen, straightening of the back, an increase in height, and a filling out of the limbs and face. Her IQ was 91 at this time, although she had been previously considered defective. She was well adjusted to our group, except that she often wet the bed. She was always domineering, when possible with sweetness and charm, but when this failed, with open aggression. She rebelled at going home, when her mother called for her, and left the hospital crying.

Subsequently, we learned that Nora was like a new person at home, pleasant, no problem to her mother, healthy, and gaining weight. Within two months, however, there was a report that her sister, Patricia, had attacked her in bed with a saw, and that Nora was just intercepted from

253

throwing a knife at her brother. When a social agency entered the home to investigate, they found that she had regressed in her behavior, was not eating, was undersized, would not play with the other children, and was again negativistic and defiant to adults.

When she was six years old, she was again admitted to our service, where we found that she was again underweight, with a protuberant belly and a toneless posture, and she contacted both adults and children poorly, was sullen and antagonistic, and given to severe temper tantrums and long heartbreaking crying spells. She improved, both physically and emotionally, more slowly on this occasion. A psychometric examination gave her IQ as 76. We recommended that she be placed away from home in a normal environment.[14]

* * *

While Clare (4-11) was less than five years of age, she was bright and consequently could give some description of the pictures and some answers to the questionnaire, although her verbal connotations were incomplete. [The attitude of these young children toward the pictures was very objective. There was a tendency to react with a simple moral orientation.] The child was primarily interested in whether a person was good or bad, without obvious justification, but she retained a completely objective attitude toward many of the violent acts depicted. When asked why the violent deed had been committed, she frequently answered "Because he likes to do it."

Clare's history showed that she had fed leaves and dirt to her younger sister. She would pick up her little sister and drop her with a thud. It was said that she would undress herself, her sister, and her playmates in the open yard; and that she broke all her toys and those of her playmates. When scolded, she laughed, screamed or kicked. Her IQ of 116 was in keeping with her alert behavior. Observation showed her to be an extremely hyperkinetic child and her mother claimed that she had been so from birth. There was no historical or clinical evidence of encephalitis or other organic condition. She showed no sense of danger with her

[14] However, she was returned to her home again, as we got an inquiry concerning her from one of the public schools, about three years later. We learned that, in 1944, at fourteen years of age, she was admitted to a state school for mental defectives and, after a period at home, was returned again in 1947, to remain until 1950, when she was nineteen years of age. When she was in the institution her IQ was 66. It was reported that she was a quiet, steady girl, who gained steadily, but slowly, in all school work and who made a satisfactory institutional adjustment, although she occasionally got into minor difficulties with other girls. After this, she remained at home under the supervision of the institution. It appears that this girl's normal maturation had been sacrificed by the early period of gross deprivation, and that the early aggression had given way to a final emotional flattening and intellectual retardation.

hyperkinesis. She would jump on the running boards of passing cars, etc. She described the pictures as follows (see Figure 4):

(1) "Cowboys. They are cutting him up because he is chasing him because he is going to cut him. He has one fellow dead." Why? "He sticks that down into him." Why? "Because they are bad. He is chasing them." How can you tell they are bad? "They are bad."

(3) "The alligator pushed the boat up and threw the man down in the water. He is going to bite him all up."

(4) "He is going to take that lady away because he is going to take her away." What is he going to do? "If he stabs her, then he will be deader."

(5) "This man is sleeping and he waked up and the bear is looking at him. He woke up and saw him and then the baby was sleeping and he bite the blanket." Why? "Because."

She answered the questionnaire as follows:

(1) What is brave? "I don't know."

(2) What is a coward? "I don't know."

(4) Do you like to hit other kids? "Yes." Why? "Because." Is it nice? "No, but I like to hit people." Which would you rather hit, a boy or a girl? "A boy because he is bad." Aren't girls bad? "No." Should you hit a kid who is bigger? "No because I want to be a little girl." Are you bad? "No." Why are boys bad? "Because they throw things." What would you do if a small boy hit you? "I would smack him." If a small girl hit you? "I would smack her too." One your size? "Smack him too." A bigger one? "I would smack him." Suppose he smacked back? "I would get a piece of wood and throw it at his head." Suppose he threw it back? "I would run in to my mother." Is it right to hit someone who hits you first? "No." Why do you hit them? "Because I like to hit everybody."

(9) Would you rather kill with a gun or an ax? "Shoot him." Why? "Because he is bad. I like to hit him."

(7) Would you rather be a boy than a girl? "No, I rather be a girl." Man or lady? "A girl." Why? "Because."

(6) What is a sissy? "A lady." Like them? "No." Like to be a girl? "No. I want to be a boy." Why? "I like to be a boy. I like to smack." Should girls smack? "No. I like to. I like to hear other people cry. I want to smack my little sister." Doesn't it hurt her? "No. If she smacks me I will smack her back."

She started to play with miniature soldiers and talked while she played. "He is going to fall down too. He is going to go in the truck. He is going to shoot him and he is going to shoot the arrow. He is going to turn around so he can't see him and he will shoot him in the back." Why? "Because he likes to. He is going to throw him right down. This car will smack into this one and he will move this car away and go in. This one will back right into the Indian's leg and the Indian will go over it. He will come up here. If he stands in the sidewalk, he will get run over. The horse is going out in the middle of the gutter. They are all standing there. These are on the bicycle."

It is remarkable how freely this child expressed her tendency to aggression. This girl has already accepted the symbolism that men and boys are aggressive, and said, on one occasion, that she wanted to be a boy. "I want to be a boy. I like to smack." She was also not averse to killing.[15]

* * *

James was a seven-year-old white boy of Catholic parentage. He was brought to the clinic by his mother, because of stealing, setting fires, misbehaving in school, fighting with other children, and disobedience. Psychological tests revealed that he had an IQ of 93, and a reading disability. He was an extremely aggressive child, who freely expressed this quality both verbally and in play. He too showed a tendency toward simple moral orientation into good and bad with the toys, by creating hostile and good groups, such as Indians and cowboys. On the ward, he made a good adjustment at all times and was well liked. Behavior difficulties occurred only occasionally. He was cleverer than other children in covering up his behavior, and would usually behave well under supervision.

In play, James was paired with nine-year-old Dorothy who, though actually older, had approximately the same mental age, with an IQ of 75. She was not an aggressive child in the usual sense, but showed aggressive tendencies in order to bring punishment upon herself. She was aggressive when the formal character of the toys would naturally give a pretext for this type of play.

In an interview with James, he was asked why he had been brought to the hospital. He answered, "Because I am crazy for fighting. As soon as my mother gets a house she is going to take me home. She is going to be dispossessed. Sometimes you are put out in the street. I know one woman downstairs from where we live got put out in the street. Because you don't pay your rent. Because we didn't have no money." Why fight? "Be-

---

[15] Clare returned to her family after leaving Bellevue. In the ensuing years, the family suffered many vicissitudes and frequently solicited help from various welfare agencies. One brother was before the children's and adolescents' court because of delinquency. However, Clare finished her schooling without further difficulties and, in 1950, at the age of twenty, was living at home and working regularly as a soda fountain clerk in the drug store.

cause I like it. You have a lot of fights and you have a black eye. Once they get me going, then it's too bad. Then there's black eyes, two or three, not one. Once they get me going—I like it more than anything." Like to get hit yourself? "I like to get hit from my mama when I am bad." Bad purposely so you will get hit? "Yes." What do you do? "Run out in the street and when my mother calls me up I come up and I get a whipping. I could be hit with an iron and I could never cry." Fight big or small boys? "Bigger ones because it's better. The smaller ones can't fight and the big ones can. I jump at their feet. Next thing, I like to get hit. The big boys can fight with me and I can be tripped." Always like to be hit? "Yes." Like to get black eyes? "One. I would like to have two."

He stated that he liked being hit and punched in the stomach, but not to the extent of being knocked out or made black and blue. "I get my feet tight around her and sock her and yell at the top of my voice. It's more fun than anything. Then you have rags and wipe up the floor." Why? "From the sink water—I turn it on." What do you think of Dillinger? "I think he is the same as me. I am glad I ain't big. I'm afraid I might be Dillinger. I would be in jail. He is in jail. He is going to the electric chair." Think he should be? "Yes. He held up a lot of people." Right to kill? "No."

What are you going to be? "An aeroplane detective. They have guns to shoot people, gangsters." Like to go to war? "Sure." With toy figures, the boy again expressed unrestrained aggressiveness. The figure with a knife is a "bad guy." Indians are also "bad." "They shoot arrows." He did not like to be pinched or to see blood come. He said his mother whipped him "in the can." Do you like to make fires? "I am crazy for fires. You can cook mickies [potatoes]. The lot was on fire." Did you light it? "No. Some woman said I did it. The night before I came here and I stayed out so late until I got off every gate and rang their bells. Then I run. We put the gates back loose how they were and when the people come out they open the gate and the gate comes off." Fun? "Sure." Fun to start fires? "No. Sure, in case they said I could, it's fun." How many have you lit? "Ten. I had an ax so I chopped some trees. It's really my father's. Then I chopped it in little pieces and brought it in the lots and lit it. We put mickies in it and when we went away put it out." When? "Saturday." How did the one start on Sunday? "A big boy. He had a pack of matches. One didn't light, the other one lit and then he smoked." You? "One. I lit that one and it didn't light, then I went looking for some more and lit them and then I lit the fire. What the heck day was it? I got a little mixed up."

Do you swear? "Since my father went away I don't do that no more. He used to swear at me and I would curse right after him. I thought it was fun. The state hospital came out after him. He got gassed from the war." Do you lose your temper? "Yes, my mother can't move."

In an interview, Dorothy was timid and shy; she spoke in a low, inaudible voice, appeared disinterested, and walked away during questioning. Why are you in the hospital? "Because I fight myself." Scratch yourself? "Yes." Don't you like yourself? "Yes." Nice girl? "No. I fight, I get bad. The teacher tells me to sit down, then I fight." Brother and sister? "Yes, I fight the little one, Barbara. Because I want to." Don't you like her? "Yes." Then why fight her? "Because I want to. I push her down. Then she cries." Fun? "No." Why do it? "I don't know." Hit others in school? "Yes, they bother me. They scratch me." Who made that scratch? "A girl." You said you did it. "I did." Then why hit the girl? "I don't know." Do you like your teacher? "Yes." What do you do? "I sew and write." Make the teacher mad? "Yes, I fight with her. I don't fight with the teacher. I put my feet on the table when she goes out of the room." Like to make her mad? "No."

Tell about the toys. "Soldier; no, a cowboy, Indian. The cowboy is going to shoot the Indian." Right? "No. The soldier is going to shoot him [farmer]. The Indian is going to shoot him." All right? "No." Who is best? "This one [peasant]. That man [in car] is running over that one [horse and rider]. He won't get out of the way. The horse will get smashed too. You get killed." Nice? "No. You are buried. You get some flowers." Nice? "Yes. They put them over the coffin."

Afraid of something at home? "My father. He hits me because I talk back to him. My mother don't like him." Like it here? "Yes, better. I get pretty books." How often get hit? "A lot. Because I hit them." Who starts? "My sister." Should you hit? "No." Most scared of? "My father. He took all the clothes and my mother told him to get out. He is too mean. I like him now. He brings me fruit." Ever hurt mother? "Yes, he fought my mother. He threw her in bed. He shakes the bed." Where do you sleep? "In the next room. She screamed. She said bad words. I wouldn't say them." Mother bad? "No."

Toys were arranged before Dorothy and James, so that a pirate and a soldier were shooting and stabbing an unarmed man.

Dorothy said, "This one is shooting this one. This one stabs him." Why? "I don't know." She brought the unarmed man closer to the pirate. "This man [pirate] is going to stab this one."

They were presented with two soldiers shooting two Indians.

James said, "They are shooting each other. Indians don't like soldiers and soldiers don't like Indians." Why shoot them? "I don't know."

258

Dorothy was asked, Think he should shoot? "No." Why? "I don't know."

James was asked, What do you think? "That guy [soldier] and this guy [pirate] is a bad guy. He got a knife." Isn't it also wrong to have a gun? "A knife you can throw and a gun you can shoot." Better to have knife or gun? "Because the bullet goes farther than a knife." Why is this man bad and this one good? "Because he has a gun."

In the discussion, James used the word "good" in two different ways. Once he used it in a moral sense, and once to describe a more effective weapon of aggression. He apparently felt that the aggressivity of the dagger was greater than the aggressivity of the rifle, and the hand-to-hand fight was more cruel than fighting with bullets.

Why is it better? "Because a bullet can go further than a knife." Which is the bad guy? "This one. He has a knife and this one has a gun. A knife is bad and a bullet comes out of you. A bullet you got a little hope, but if you are stabbed you are dead."

Dorothy grabbed one of the toys. "I don't want to get stabbed."

James was shown two Indians shooting at each other. "Two are fighting." Would you like to be with them? "Sure. Because Indians are Indians. They fight much better with bow and arrows." Like to be there? "I would. I would like to see how far the arrows go from the knife." Indians shooting cowboy with gun. "It's two men against one man." Fair? "No. If you put one out then it would be fair." Fair now? "Yes." Like to be in such a fight? "No." Why? "Because it ain't right."

To Dorothy: Would you like to kill somebody? "No." Like to shoot any Indians? "Yes. They are bad." Dorothy took the cowboys from in front of the Indians. "I took them away. I don't want them to get hurt." Would you like to be very strong? "Yes—so I could fight." Want to fight? "These [toys] hit them, scratch them. They would shoot me." She said this with an angelic expression on her face.

Both children were continually changing the order of the toys. Dorothy finally put them together, and said, "I am going to put them away. I want to play with the doll."

To James: Would you like to be strong? "Yes. So I can fight." Like to hit other children? "No." Why not? "I don't know." You really like to, don't you? "Not so much." What would you do if a stronger boy hit you? "Fight back." Smaller boy? "Just let him." If he hurts you? "Just let him." Right to hit a girl? "No."

To Dorothy: Like to hit somebody? "No." Why not? "They would hit me back." This girl had a continual fear of retaliation if she became aggressive. She was always trying to hide and take away one of the tin soldiers.

They were presented with a man surrounded by three cars. Dorothy started rolling a car. James ran a man down with a car and put him into another car.

To James: What did you do? "I knocked him down. He was run over. The guy was carrying him." Why stand him up like that? "He will be run over again."

Dorothy: "The car will run over him and he will be dead." Bad to be dead? "No." Good? "No." Like to be? "No."

To James: Would you? "No. It's bad. When God comes he wakes you up." For what? "To take you to Heaven." What is Heaven? "I don't know. It's better to go to Heaven than anything when you die."

Dorothy kissed the car. Why? "Because it's little." She put it in another car. "I don't want it to get knocked over."

It appeared as though there were a pattern of aggressivity which had to be followed. The objects implied a tendency that expressed motor activity in connection with momentum. Momentum led immediately to aggression.

James put two men in a truck. He said that he put them in so the other car would not run over them. Should girls be strong? "No." Why not? "I don't know." Should a man? "Yes." What are you doing? "I am making a war."

To Dorothy: Should one hit other people? "No." Why not? "You get hit back."

To James: Should one? "No. It ain't right. When you do that you go to jail." Suppose you get away with it? "Anyhow I wouldn't do it. One day they will find you." He showed a marked tendency to play with things on the edge of the table.

Dorothy had a reading, writing, and spelling disability, and was left-handed. She was the oldest of six children, in a Negro family. She had been a disturbing element in her class in public school, interfering in the activities of other children, and showing little ability to play with them. On one occasion, it was reported that she tore up the papers of other children and threatened to punch them in the back; she threw everything, within reach, to the floor, such as pencils, paper, scissors, etc. When she picked up other pencils and scissors, she buried the scissors in the sand and put the pencils down an iron drain in the floor. She then tore up more papers, banged herself with her fists, and scratched her arms.

A social investigation revealed that the mother was subject to severe temper outbursts that terrorized the children, and that the father also showed temper outbursts at times, especially when he was drunk. His outbursts were probably secondary to those of the mother.[16]

The play method and picture descriptions were less fertile study methods with older children; but in children from nine to eleven, interesting reactions could be observed.

Nine-year-old Marshall came to us because his father had asked for temporary placement, following the birth of the second sibling. Marshall's mother was an inadequate woman, who had trained Marshall poorly. Up to this time, he was the only child and, as a result of his insecure relationship with his mother, had shown poorly organized and aggressive behavior, which was too much for the family, following the birth of his sister. In the hospital, his behavior was infantile, attention-seeking, and impulsive, with his striking out at any child who thwarted his impulses. However, he had good intelligence (IQ 104) and respond-

[16] Dorothy returned home, and to the public schools. Within a year, she had a grand mal convulsion, her first. Her IQ was found to be 62 then. She was placed in a state school for mental defectives, where she stayed for two and a half years, having occasional convulsions. She returned home at thirteen and was cared for by a private physician. Although quarrelsome and excessively religious, she was managed at school and at home until twenty-one, in 1946, when she had a series of severe convulsions followed by confusion and excitement. She was placed in a hospital for the mentally sick for one year, and then cared for at home under convalescent supervision from the state hospital. Her convulsions were controlled by Dilantin and behavior became subdued.

James's father had been sent to a state mental hospital before James came to us. He was diagnosed as psychotic, with meningovascular syphilis, for which he was treated. He was in the hospital from 1934 to 1943, and subsequently took care of himself in the community, but took no responsibility for James. James did not have syphilis. Meanwhile, however, the mother felt inadequate to care for James, and he was placed in boarding homes through a Catholic agency. The mother died in 1941, when James was fourteen. In the boarding homes, James at first seemed to do well, as he was a likeable, intelligent child. But he was soon found to have a bad temper, was a frequent truant from school (probably on account of his reading disability), and was addicted to lying and stealing. He did not complete the eighth grade until he was sixteen. After holding a job for a year, he enlisted in the Navy, during World War II, before he was eighteen. He was discharged after a year because of two threats to shoot a superior officer. He claimed he had no grudge against them, but did not wish to take orders from them. He had been drinking, but had not been intoxicated. He was discharged with the diagnosis of schizoid personality. He took a job in a railroad freight yard and burned down a storage building "on an impulse." He was held for arson, but was committed to a state hospital, where he was diagnosed as psychotic with a psychopathic personality. He received insulin shock treatment, and was said to have improved. Although his behavior in the institution was generally amenable, he was held, because of the seriousness of his antisocial behavior before admission. One can speculate that the inadequate home and parental relationships throughout his life, and his reading disability (which was never overcome) led to his antisocial personality development, for he was an otherwise intelligent and promising child.

261

ed to the security and training offered through the ward routine and his relationships with the adults. In addition, he accepted his role as one of a group of children. Consequently, the father gave up the idea of any further placement and took the child back into the family group. We had no further contact with this family.

Marshall described the pictures as follows (see Figure 4):

(1) "A man, they are fighting for their country." Is it right? "So you can live. They have a war." Is it right? "No, because most of the people get killed. It is better not to fight. If somebody hit me, I wouldn't fight; I wouldn't start the fight."

(4) "I won't tell you that one. This girl must have got sore at him. And there is a man who tries to get his knife out and there is a black man. That man wants to blackjack him over the nut." What do you think of girls who stab men? "She would go to prison and get the chair, or get a rope around her neck, or prison for life."

In play with the tin soldiers and Indians, he said, "The Indians hit white people because Indians has red skin. And these people have white skins and these people are their enemies." Confronted with another group of playthings, he actively enriched the play with his fantasy and said, "These three guys are looking for a treasure and they want to kill these people so they don't get the treasure. One guy gets behind him and this guy calls him and he goes all around and goes over here. Then he pushes them. They shoot down the enemies." He took particular pleasure in having the toys fall over. When the physician pushed the doll over, the boy said, "That is no way to do it. I'll show you how to tip a girl over."

In play with the toy soldiers, as well as in the interpretation of pictures, Marshall showed aggressiveness. He felt that any slight difference was justification for group hostilities. It was also enough reason for hostility that "one gets sore on somebody." Furthermore, he approved strict and thorough punishment. The psychological features of the earlier stages of development, as seen in the younger children, were preserved in this hyperkinetic boy of good intelligence.

No fundamental difference was observed between the younger boys and girls in their reaction to the pictures.

When nine-year-old Vivian was shown picture 4, she said: "A lady; she is going to kill a man. Maybe he did something to her." In play with the tin soldiers, she said, "This is a soldier. He is going to shoot Indians." Why? "Because they are having a war. They are fighting because it comes to the end of the world and everybody dies." Who makes the end of the world? "God. Sometimes it is rainy and stormy; everybody dies." Two Indians were placed so that they faced the soldiers. "They are going to jump on the two Indians." Why? "They don't like them. They shoot with bows and arrows." Which ones are right? "The Indians because they did not hit anybody." Which ones would you rather be? "The Indians because they don't hit people first."

Vivian was sent to us from her public school because of her antagonistic behavior. Since she was seven years old in the second grade, she had been subject to temper outbursts and periods of sullen, stubborn resistance. Her intelligence was average. She lived with a married brother and his wife, as her mother had died when she was an infant and her father had deserted her. About herself she said, "I'm bad. I fight in school. I don't know why. One boy is worse than I am but I whip him. I like all my work in school." She responded to the warmth and socializing activities of the hospital and returned to her brother's home and school.[17]

This nine-year-old Negro girl clearly identified herself with the Indians. Her play with dolls was not merely determined by form elements such as are seen in the younger children. Still, even the china dolls were paired off by her, and she arranged them in different symmetrical forms, moving them from one form to the next, sometimes by means of the cars. One gets the impression that, in the play of older children, the objects and figures are used much more in accordance with imagined situations than according to the formal laws which determine the play of younger children.

These nine-year-old children faced the death of others with an astonishingly cool objectivity. It seems to be sufficient reason for killing that "one is sore on somebody," or just that one does not like him. But even at the age of eleven, similar features may be observed.

Charles (11-4) was sent to our children's ward, by a children's court, as a delinquent child. His mother stated that she could not handle him.

[17] She was next traced to an institution, in a southern state, where she had been sent at fourteen because of temper tantrums, stubbornness, and being without a guardian. She remained there until she was nearly eighteen, escaping several times and returning of her own free will. Vivian's problems were essentially related to insecurity, deprivation, and neglect.

He threw things about the house, used vile and indecent language, and ran away from home many times. On several occasions, he and his siblings were in court as neglected children, because they were in the habit of street begging while in a filthy condition. The boy was asked what he would like to be when he grew up and he said, "A cop. You have a uniform and you will be able to kill somebody. You get some crooks and lock them up." Why do you want to kill people? "I want to save people. I could kill crooks because they kill everybody else." Whom do you want to save? "People who are being killed."

He was given a group of soldiers, carts, and automobiles to play with. He said, "They had a war, the Americans and Indians. I am on the side of the Americans because that is my nationality." What is the matter with Indians? "They can't fight so good. I am only playing with them. Here is the battlefield." He put all the soldiers in the cart and moved them to another position. "Bang-bang, that guy is dead." The soldiers killed four Indians. One Indian knocked down an American. Why does he do that? "I don't know. These are Americans. They are having a war because they don't like Indians because they fight too much. They are just having a little war. That [the automobile] is the place where you carry things because they can't carry them in their hands; they are too big." He put all the vehicles in a line, and all the soldiers along the edge of the table. "I am going to line some over here too. These are going to be the guards around the blockade. These are near the gate so the people don't come in and rob things. They have to have a place for the car to go through." He laid them down to put them to sleep. "The other men may come after them, the men who try to make war with them. They think they are bad. They kill everybody." Why? "I don't know." He put the vehicles, which were parallel before, in a series and imitated the sound of blowing taps. "Now you have to get up. They have to get up at six o'clock in the morning to get dressed. They go two by two. This is the rear guard." He divided the men into two groups. "These are all his men and these are his."

Children have a tendency to make form and structure an important part of their play. Army maneuvers seem to have a similar origin. Charles responded to the questionnaire in the following way:

(1) What is courage? "I don't know. Courage is brave. You are not scared of anything. Like when a soldier is against anybody they have to be courageous; they have to be brave because maybe the people might kill them." Is that good? "Yes." Won't you get killed then? "No. Your mother tells you not to fight and not to go to war and then you wouldn't

be killed." Would you be brave then? "I would say I want to go but my mother won't let me." Suppose you don't have a mother? "I would go to war and be killed."

(2) What does it mean to be a coward? "You are scared of everything. When you are afraid of anything you are a coward." Is it good? "No, because everybody thinks you are scared, because they all make fun of you and then you don't like it." What is best? "It is best to be brave and don't get killed. You just go to war." Suppose you get killed? "That is all right." What is it like? "You get shot. Then he is buried." Is that good? "No, ma'am, because then you don't go no place; then you get no candy and you go to heaven." Is it nice there? "Yes, it is all right to be dead." What does one do in Heaven? "You get shelter there. God is up there. He helps you. I know He is there because my house mother told me that."

(4) Do you like to hit other kids? "No, because then you get hurt yourself." Is it right to hit other kids? "No, because then you get hurt yourself."

(5) Is it right to hit someone when they insult you? "No, you will walk away from them. You don't like them no more." Don't you hit people you don't like? "Yes I guess you do hit them when they insult you." Suppose they are bigger? "Then you don't do nothing." Smaller? "Then you do."

(6) What do you think of sissies? "Sissies are people who are afraid to fight. They don't know how to fight so good. They are girls; they don't know how to fight." Don't you like boys who don't fight? "Sure I like them. I like girls, too. Sissies don't know how to fight and it makes me sore."

(7) Would you like to be a girl? "No. They can't fight and they wear dresses. A dress goes up and everybody looks underneath. That is being sloppy. You are being a slob. A slob is a person who don't know any manners." Is a slob a person who eats with his fingers? "Yes, I mean you make a lot of mess. You are eating and the stuff spills."

(8) Should a girl fight? "They can't fight. I put on one of the boxing gloves upstairs and tried to hit Mr. D." Why is it important to be strong? "Then you can beat everybody up." Is that good? "No, ma'am. You have to win everything. Then you have some victory. You get prizes."

(9) Would you like to shoot somebody? "No, then you are killing them and then you get the electric chair." Cop? "Oh that's all right. Then you kill gangsters instead of a good person." Why would you like it? "Because they kill somebody else. They always kill somebody else." Would you rather kill them yourself? "Yes, then you are saving people." When is it right to hit somebody? "When they are sore at you. Even if they have a right."

265

(10) How should you defend yourself against a stronger boy? "You go like this—bang. If he is much stronger, I would tell my mother. That would be a coward." Would you do it anyway? "No, I would tell somebody else."

He described the pictures as follows:

(1) "That is a war. This is Flash Gordon and he is fighting with all the men. He is a man on the funny sheet. He is all right because he is an American and these are from other countries. He can fight them if they are bad. These are bad because they kill everybody." Which one would you like to be? "This one because he is strong. We take the swords and stab them. I would stab with the sword because they shouldn't kill anybody. It would not be so good because then you are killing everybody else."

(2) "I don't know what that is. Some soldiers marching, going into the country." What is going to happen? "I don't know." Is it nice? "Yes, because they are people there and swords here. They are going to have a war because they don't like them."

(3) "This is Tim Tyler. The hippopotamus turned over his boat and he lost the oar. He going to drown." Is that nice? "No, maybe he can't swim."

(4) "He is going to kill the man." What for? "I don't know." Why? "Because she doesn't like him because maybe they are bad and she is good. They might kill somebody." Is it better for her to kill them? "Yes, because they are bad and she is good." Is he good if she kills them? "No, maybe they are in another country."

(5) "This is a bear taking a baby out of a cradle. These are good men. These men are going to kill the bear with a gun or with fists." What will happen to the baby? "It is going to die. The bear will bite it."

Our examination of Charles had shown that he was undersized, had a mild congenital heart lesion, and small genitals with undescended testicles. His intelligence was not good. His IQ was 81, and he had a reading disability. His home was inadequate to care for him.[18]

The case of John, a twelve-year-old boy, shows that the infantile trends, which we saw in the younger children, were no longer effective in him. We give a short report, on this extremely aggressive boy, in order to show that, at this age, the aggressive tendencies do

---

[18] He was sent from us to a cottage type of boys' institution. He did well there, and after three years returned home under the supervision of an agency, and did not get in trouble again.

not express themselves in the questionnaire and in the interpretation of the pictures, although his behavior was dangerously aggressive and asocial. We know very little, in this case, about the psychogenesis of the aggressiveness.

John was a Negro boy, who had been referred by school because he had been subject to very peculiar behavior, with moods of deep depression, during which he suddenly assaulted other children. It was also said that he would hold and beat a child until the child was rescued. He nearly tore the ear off one boy. He was subject to bad temper tantrums followed by stubbornness, and this, in turn, was followed by the so-called depressive period. This boy was in a class with retarded children, although our psychometric examinations showed an IQ of 84, and he should have been able to make advancement in regular grades. However, he was a chronic truant and, at one time, he was placed in a correctional school. When first admitted to the ward, he was cooperative and communicative. He admitted his bad behavior and said it was due to poor associates. He showed a strong sense of guilt. From his descriptions, it became apparent that the periods of so-called depression were sullenness, with feelings of guilt following bad behavior. He stated at once that he had been told that he had come to the hospital just to be examined, and that under no conditions would he remain in the hospital. John immediately became sullen and uncommunicative for a day or so, but this was followed by a period in which he seemed to be making some sort of adjustment to the activities of the other children. It was noted that he was becoming a ring leader to a group of adolescent boys, and he would bully the other children into accepting his leadership. It was finally revealed by the other children that John was organizing a well-calculated plot to escape. He had, hidden under his mattress, an iron bar from a bed and a rope which painters had left in the ward. He also stole a crank used to open the windows from a nurse's desk. His plans were to knock a nurse unconscious at night, take her keys, and open the door; but to make his plans doubly sure, he calculated that, if necessary, he could open windows and escape from the eighth floor by means of the rope.

His description of the pictures was as follows:

(1) "Flash Gordon is fighting. They are fighting for their country." Why? "They don't want anybody to take it away." Is that right? "Maybe they are trying to take his country." Is it right? "If they haven't got any." Who would you like to be? "I wouldn't like to be anybody." What would you do in the war? "I would have to fight." Would you like it? "No."

(2) "They are Flash Gordon's men. They are standing still. They are going to fight." Why? "For their country." Do you like Flash Gordon? "I don't know." Would you like to be him? "No." Good or bad? "Good." What makes him a good person? "Don't know."

(3) "A rhinoceros is turning over the boat to get the people and eat them." Why? "He likes it." Why? "I don't know." What will happen to the man? "He will get killed." What does that mean? "He will die." What does that mean? "You can't talk, you can't do anything." Is it good? "No." Why not? "I don't know."

(4) "The girl is going to stab the man." Why? "I don't know." Is it right? "If he did anything wrong. If he killed somebody."

(5) "It looks like a tiger. He is taking a baby out of the crib. The mother is sleeping and the father is waking." What is to happen? "He is going to kill the baby. He is hungry."

His answers to the questionnaire were as follows:

(3) Why shouldn't one be a coward? "I don't know." Should one be a coward? "If they want to. If you don't want to be a coward you don't have to."

(2) What is a coward? "Some people are afraid. A coward is afraid of animals, afraid to do things." Is it good? "No, if you are a coward they will pick on you and you are afraid to hit them back." Is it good to be a hero? "Yes." What is a hero? "You fight for your country and win." Can you be a hero without war? "Yes. You can stop bad people like gangsters." How? "You can shoot it out." Suppose you get shot? "You can be a hero anyway." Which would you rather be, a live coward or a dead hero? "A dead hero."

(4) Do you like to hit other kids? "If they hit me first." Is it right? "No." Is it ever right to hit somebody else? "If they ever do anything to you." What? "Telling lies."

(7) Would you like to be a girl? "No, there is too much housework." If the men were doing the housework and the women were working, would you like to be a woman? "No."

(8) Should a girl fight? "If they want to." Do you think it is right? "Yes and no."

(9) Would you like to shoot somebody? "If they shot at me first." Suppose it is too late? "They may miss you." Would you like to shoot a gangster? "If they shot first." How about a German? "I would shoot them."[19, 20]

[19] We recommended John be sent to a correctional institution. He stayed there for two years. During this period, his abusive, alcoholic father died. His inadequate and

Of the thirty children, three to eight years of age, thirteen responded, at least in part, to the questionnaire. Each question was often answered with an "I don't know." The following is a summary of the remaining responses:

(1) What is courage? What does it mean to be brave?—Although most of the children up to the eighth year did not exactly understand the meaning of the word "courage," their answers showed that they reacted to the word in a general way. Such answers, by girls of three to eight, were, "When you are strong," "Somebody who fights," and "You are big." Boys, three to eight, said "You are big," "You don't let nobody do nothing to you," and "It means you grow up, you can take it, you don't cry or anything." Girls of nine to fifteen years said, "Strong and not afraid of anything," "You can take it," and "You are not scared."

(2) What is a coward—yellow?—Besides the "I don't know" answers, several young children, three to eight, said "It is a cow, it gives milk," and "A cowboy." Others answered, "When you fight," "It means you are afraid," "It is bad, very bad, you holler at everybody and everything," and "You are afraid to hit anybody."

---

sickly mother did not give him much support nor did he give her any support when he got his working papers and quit school; he spent his earnings on a "girl." He was rejected for military service when he became of draft age, during World War II, but he was employed through the United States Employment Service, in a Navy Yard in California, as a general helper.

[20] A summary of the outcomes of the children whom we followed into adulthood showed the following: Joey was a failing student in school, apathetic and unhappy in his home, where he remained. Nora, who, at the age of four, had scored an average IQ after a period of intensive physical and socializing care, entered a state school for mental defectives at fourteen, her IQ dropping through 76 to 66. She returned to the community from time to time, but remained dependent on the institution. Rita had done well with the aid of social agencies and foster homes. She became independent and tried to help her brothers. Clare has also done well in her own home, in spite of many unfavorable circumstances. These girls both had good intelligence. James was in constant trouble in schools, in foster homes, in the Navy in World War II, and on jobs. He was sent to a state hospital for the mentally sick and held there because of his record of asocial behavior. Dorothy developed epilepsy, which was controlled with medication. Her intelligence dropped from an IQ of 75 to 62. She spent most of her time in an institution for defectives. Marshall, as far as we could learn, got along all right after his period of observation in our hospital. Vivian was placed in a state mental hospital in a southern state at fourteen, apparently because there was no place else she could go. She escaped from this place several times, and voluntarily returned whenever she needed a refuge. Charles was sent to a correctional institution for boys and was not heard from again. John also went to a correctional institution and, later, made an asocial adjustment.

Girls, of nine to fifteen, said, "You are afraid to hit back," "You are scared," "When you run away," "When you can't fight," and "When you kick, scratch and bite." Boys, from nine to fifteen, said, "You are scared of everything," "Scared to fight," and "You run away."

(3)   Why shouldn't one be a coward?—The answers from boys, three to eight, were, "I like to be a cowboy," "I don't want to be a coward," "Because you are called a coward," "It means they are fresh," and "Nobody will like you." Girls, from nine to fifteen, said, "Everyone will pick on you," and "You get hurt." Boys, from nine to fifteen, said, "They kick you and make fun of you," "You can't hit back," and "A coward might cause death."

Although children from nine to fifteen still had no clear conception of what a coward was, they had a good understanding of the negative value expressed in the term. They crammed into the word everything of a negative value connected with fighting, wrong methods of fighting, running away, etc.

(4)   Do you like to hit other children?—The responses were varied. Girls, three to eight, said, "Yes, because I like to hit people," "No, some are good," and "No, because they will hit me." The younger boys said "When they are bad because they hit you back," and "No, I am afraid of their mothers and fathers and brothers and sisters. They will tell them and they will hit me and make me cry." The children considered this problem from a practical point of view. They were afraid of the consequences and tried to avoid them. Their connotations of bad and good were purely practical and facilitated their orientation in a dangerous world. Girls from nine to fifteen answered "No, because they might hit you," "No, you will have no friends," and "No, unless they hit you first." Older boys said, "Not unless they hit me first," "No, you might get hurt," "If they start," and "Only in order to hit back."

The answer to this question, in the group of older children, was clearly formulated and reflected the morality imposed by adults, in a more or less schematic way. But the child's fear of getting hurt was still clearly expressed, although in a more objective form.

(5)   Is it right to hit somebody who insults you?—The little girls said "Yes, because they call me bad names," and "No, you should call them back." The little boys said "No, call a nurse," "Little ones, no; big ones, yes," "If I touch something of his he has

a right; if he has no right, I hit him back," and "Of course it is right." The girls, from nine to fifteen, said, "No, but I did it," and "No, call them back." Most of the rest simply said "No." Boys of this age said "You tell them not to," "No, I would tell the nurse," "Bigger boys, no; smaller boys, yes," "Sometimes no and sometimes yes," and "No, ask for an apology."

Among the younger children, cursing was often considered a worse offense than hitting. Older children did not see the absolute necessity for retaliating to insults by hitting, nor did the younger children. But observations not included in this study have shown that curses against the mother, especially of a sexual nature, always justified an aggressive counterattack.

(6)    What is a sissy and what do you think of a sissy?—The girls, from three to eight, said, "A lady, I don't like them," "When you are bad, when you go with boys," "A boy who plays with girls," and "A sissy is a girl, I don't like them." The boys, of this age, said, "A girl, I like them," "If a boy goes with a girl it is not allowed, the teacher hits them," and "Pussy cats, I like cats." Is a boy ever a sissy? "If the boy is like a cat. A boy that fights girls, I don't like them." "A boy that plays with girls and other boys that play with sissies; I don't like them."

The older girls, from nine to fifteen, said, "Boys who fight with girls and can't fight," "Boys who play with girls," "Boys who dress like girls," and "They are not nice, they are all like girls." The boys, from nine to fifteen, said, "A sissy is a show-off. He is no good," "Anybody who can't fight," "He is fighting with girls, he is a coward," "When they play with girls," and "They act like girls."

The older children express a definite dislike for sissies, although they hardly know what the word means. For them, it is a boy who does not live up to some of their social expectations. It is interesting that their social code forbids boys to play with girls.

(7)    To girls: Would you like to be a boy?—The girls, three to eight, answered "Better to be a girl, don't know why," "I like to be a boy, cause I like to smack," "I don't like to be a boy," and "No, because I don't like to be rough." Girls, nine to fifteen, said, "No, girls have more hair," "You can be smarter as a girl, boys can't sew," "No, because I don't like boys, when you are older you can go out with boys," "No, they are fresh," "No, they go to war," "No, boys

271

are fighting, girls can wear rings and bracelets," and "I would rather wear dresses than pants."

To boys: Would you like to be a girl?—"Yes, because nobody can touch them. They can go to war too, I saw a picture of it," "No, boys have more fun," "Boys have more toys and wear pants. You can pull up a girl's dress any day, but if a girl wants a boy's pants off she couldn't do it," "I wouldn't like to be a girl because I like to be a boy," and "No, because a girl is weak." Boys, from nine to fifteen, said, "No, bad boys hit you and a lot of things," "No, they can't fight, they wear dresses," "I would like to be a girl in wartime. I like to use a gun but I don't like to get shot," "No, a girl can't play baseball," "No, girls have too much housework to do," and "No, boys are stronger and girls wear dresses."

The paucity of responses to this question, in younger children, was partially balanced by the study of play material, in which comparable responses were obtained. There was evidence, in any case, of pride in masculinity and femininity, which increases with age, and which is at least partially due to social influences.

It is remarkable that only the younger, and physically small, children accepted the idea of a change in their sex rather readily. Seemingly, the difference between boy and girl did not mean very much to them. They saw only the superficial characteristics. The superficiality of the answers of the older children was astounding. By merely studying these answers, one would come to the conclusion that many of the so-called sexual differences are more or less a matter of habit. But the pride in masculinity in boys, and femininity in girls, was so outstanding that it is probable that there are much deeper motives responsible for the unwillingness to consider being changed into the other sex. The only one of the older children who expressed a desire to be changed into the opposite sex was one boy, and it was questionable whether his wish to be a girl in time of war expressed a real wish for a change in sex.

(8) Should a girl fight? Should a girl hit a girl?—Three- to eight-year-old girls answered, "No, but I like to. I like to smack my little sister. I like to hear her cry," "No, because it isn't nice to fight and hit," and "No, because you get hurt and a cop may chase you." The younger boys said, "No, they will hit me back," "No, they are not ladies," "Sure if they want to," and "No, never." If a boy hits

her? "She should sock him back," and "Yes, if another girl hits her she should sock her back."

But when the younger children were asked if a boy should fight, all of the girls said only "No," while the boys said "No, because they will hit you back," "Yes, because they are boys," and "No, unless the other one hits him first."

It appears to be the general opinion that girls should fight less than boys. When the older girls were asked if girls should fight, they answered "No, then you get in trouble," and "No, then you are a tomboy and the boys hurt you." All of the rest simply said, "No." The older boys said "No, she shouldn't start up either. Girl to girl is all right. If one starts it, the other should hit her back," "A girl should not fight with boys but with girls," "No, they can't fight," and "No, they pull hair and scratch, but they do it." In answer to the question whether a boy should fight, most of the older girls said "No." One girl said "Yes," and one said "No, it hurts." The older boys said "Yes, when they hit you," and "Yes, when somebody starts up with them it is O.K. If they don't it's out." The rest said "No."

The older children, as well as the younger ones, denied the advisability of fighting. This was probably partially due to the way in which the question was put to them. The answers show that some amount of fighting is expected from both boys and girls. The younger children usually gave utilitarian reasons why one should not fight, while the older children felt more strongly that fighting was wrong in itself.

(9) Would you like to shoot someone to kill them?—The younger girls said "Yes, because he is bad, I like to hit him," "Yes, my real daddy," and "No." Gangsters? "Yes, because they shoot me," and "Yes, if somebody is bad." The smaller boys said "Yes, Jimmie K," "Yes, if they shoot me," "I would love to for hitting people too much," and "No." Gangsters? "Yes, because they want to shoot the man on the other side," and "No, if there was a war you could kill them but I wouldn't like to, they might blame me."

Would you rather kill somebody with an ax?—The younger girls said "I'd like to shoot him or hit him," "No, the gun would kill you really," and "The gun is better because it has bullets." The younger boys said "Yes, Jimmie K," "If somebody shoots me, I'd rather shoot them, but if I only had an ax, I would throw it," "I'd rather have a gun," "No, I would like to chop wood but not people. You would be in jail. But if you shoot them they can't catch you," "Yes, because they throw it on your back and kill you that way," and "No, I would rather shoot with a gun, it has bullets and an ax takes too long."

Even small children who showed their aggressiveness so clearly in play did not freely profess their murderous wishes, unless there was a specific reason; for example, Gertrude, who said she would like to shoot "my real daddy." In this girl, the aggressiveness against the father had been stimulated by the mother, who was divorced from the father and had taught the child (who had never seen the father) to express herself in this way. In other cases, the children said that it was all right to kill gangsters. The preference for the gun as an instrument of killing was already present at these early ages. This was due, in part, to the recognition of this weapon's greater effectiveness, and, in part, to the recognition of the danger and unpleasantness involved in direct physical violence. Although these motives were present in the smaller children, they found a much clearer expression in the older children.

When the nine- to fifteen-year-old children were asked if they would like to shoot somebody, the girls answered "No, only the man who steals," and "No, you get hung." The boys said, "No, only in war you have to or they will destroy the country," "No, they put you in jail," and "Only in self-defense." With increasing age, the expression of aggressiveness became diminished. The utilitarian point of view of the younger child was supplanted by more general ideas of right and wrong. War and justice seemed to allow some outlets for aggressive tendencies (as we found in our later studies on the aggressive ideologies expressed by children during World War II). When asked if the older girls would prefer an ax, they said "An ax is better than a gun, a gun is more dangerous." Boys, nine to fifteen, said "It would be worse than a gun, there would be more blood," "The ax hurts worse than a bullet. I would like a bullet better," and "If I have no gun."

Children of this age, more than the younger ones, seemed to shy from the violence of an ax, and preferred the gun to the ax as an instrument of murder; but they were still willing to consider using the ax.

274

(10)   How would you defend yourself against a stronger child?
—The small girls said, "I would get a piece of wood and throw it
against his head," and "I'd hit him back." The boys said, "I would
give him a bloody nose," "I'd hit them back just the same," "I
would run," "I would hit them back or tell a nurse," and "I would
hide somewhere."

The tendency to reactive aggression is obvious in these answers.
A smaller child must either hit back himself or get someone stronger
to hit back for him. Revenge by some other method, such as hiding
the possessions of the stronger child, is not accepted as morally
correct.

When the older children were asked how they would defend
themselves against a stronger child, the girls answered, "Hit him,"
"I would be afraid," and "Hit him back." The boys said, "Hit him
and run away," "I don't know, I would try to hit him back but he
would hit me harder," and "I would try to get somebody to fight
him." In these few instances the tendencies for counteraggression
are also obvious.

Aggressiveness, as the tendency to use violence against the bodies
of other human beings, is undoubtedly one of the characteristic
trends of human psychology. It becomes manifest in the attitude
and behavior of the younger children. The destructive tendencies
are directed against animate, as well as inanimate, objects. The
destruction consists of tearing the objects to pieces, either by hand
or by mouth, or the object may be put into the mouth and devoured.
Mild destructive tendencies may be expressed through pushing the
object away, throwing it away, or by inflicting pain on an animate
object.

Aggression results from experimentation with objects in the
external world. In order to explore an object, it is not enough to
touch it; to learn its texture and consistency one must literally tear
it to pieces. The resistance of an object to this procedure is one of
its characteristics. In this respect, the reaction of animate objects is
particularly interesting to the experimenting child. The search for
the physical qualities of an object tends to become a hard test for
that object's endurance.

Of course, the child necessarily gains a sense of power by this
aggression. He becomes the master of the object. In trying to in-

vestigate the bodies of others, through more-or-less destructive methods, he also becomes better aware of his own body. In wrestling, he discovers how far a body can be compressed, and in scratching, biting, hitting, wounding, and pushing, other important qualities reveal themselves. The child learns how much he can do with objects and how far he can master them. Our protocols corroborate the contention of Isaacs that children are never contented with what they have. They want all the playthings and toys available. A possessive greed, with strong oral tendencies, is a characteristic feature of childhood activity. This greed is liable to interfere with the rights of others. The satisfaction of the child's greed is possible only by aggressive behavior.

There exists an immediate pleasure in the destruction of objects, just as there is also a pleasure in reconstructing them. In order to build, however, it is first necessary to destroy. Destruction might be a direct aim, although not a final one.

The case history of Nora illustrates an aggression which was immediately directed against the integrity of the other person's body. She tended to inflict pain and discomfort as the first step on the way to more complete destruction. It may be that she inflicted pain in order to have a sense of power, but she was unmistakably delighted when she succeeded.

It is very probable that, in the world of the child, the obvious destructive tendencies directed against others are not the final aim. Children expect that the destroyed object will be restored. In our studies on children's attitudes toward death, we have found that, for them, even death is not final, but appears to be reversible. The child chiefly considers death as a deprivation due to violence. Since he knows deprivation primarily as a consequence of the ill will and hostilities of others, he does not hesitate, when ambitious to punish others, to entertain violent ideas of their death. Since the child needs other persons, he has a decided wish that the integrity of the other person should be restored. There is a real bond of sympathy, which urges the child to seek and favor reconstruction of the other person's body.

In the play of children, especially those under nine years of age, the dead soldiers arise again. The suffering of another human being is, in a deeper sense, also present in the aggressor. From this point

276

of view, the child wants to restore the other person and to relieve his pain.

The child very early experiences punishment as a result of his own aggression. The child fears to be deprived of food. He requires continuous support and help, since his muscular coordination is imperfect and he is uncertain in his struggle for equilibrium. If he loses the adult's love, he may also lose his help. He also fears pain and dismembering, or encroachment on his body image. He soon learns that he has to check many of his aggressive acts, in order to escape punishment. The child feels continually threatened. Of course, children tend to disregard the dangers to which they are exposed, especially when they have seen that deprivations imposed by adults are not final.

When children are deprived of parents' love, their support, and food, they experience this deprivation as a direct aggressive attack with destructive tendencies. To this, they answer with an unbridled aggressiveness as a reaction to the withdrawing of love, as demonstrated in the case of Nora. It was as if this child felt that the deprivation could not become worse, even if she became extremely aggressive. A similar reaction was also present in the case of Rita; but her aggressiveness was specifically directed against a mother who not only had not given her sufficient love herself, but also interfered when Rita *was* able to get love from a foster mother.

In general, it seems that the withdrawal of love increases aggressive tendencies in children. Psychoanalysis would speak about the diffusion of instincts, with destructive tendencies coming into the foreground. It is preferable to remain closer to the described facts. The child who is deprived of love tries to get satisfaction from other sources, and starts with his destructive search. He has learned, in addition, that the deprivation which he may receive as punishment is not so severe as he had feared. He not only receives satisfaction by embarrassing the adult, but may also receive more attention.

Withdrawal of food may have a similar effect. Nora was decidedly undernourished and retarded in her growth. She was a nutritional problem, due to early deprivation of food. In two other cases, severe nutritional problems, with retardation in growth, were factors in increasing the aggressiveness in children. Dissatisfaction with food leads to destructive tendencies. In the case of Johnny, a five-year-old

277

boy, dissatisfaction was partially in the form of jealousy directed against a brother, eighteen months younger. There was a well-directed tendency to kill and destroy him, as well as two other siblings who came later. This boy was not only undernourished, but dwarfed. One wonders if it were possible that he knew, at eighteen months, at the time when the younger brother was born and the aggressiveness started, that his body was going to be too small, and that he reacted to this as a serious deprivation. We know that his parents considered him retarded in growth and undernourished. He must have felt this double deprivation.[21]

At any rate, aggressiveness appears as a reaction to deprivation, which is understandable, since the child always feels that deprivation is inflicted through ill will. In this sense, aggressiveness is reactive and an answer to the aggression of others. In this respect, the results of this study closely tally with the results obtained by Keiser and myself (Keiser and Schilder, 1936) in a study of aggressive criminals.

Aggressiveness in children is, from the beginning, checked by the forceful counteraggression of the adult. Even if the adult is not completely successful in suppressing the aggressive actions of the child, the child soon learns that there is good and bad behavior. The bad behavior is that for which one gets punished. This simple moral orientation thus becomes the pillar of the social psychology of the child. Many of the decisions of adults appear completely arbitrary to the child. Good and bad are merely actions which the adult, with authoritative power, likes or dislikes. The child decides to be good in order not to be exposed to any deprivation. The child is therefore utilitarian in his attitude. When children provoke punishment by their aggressiveness, they merely react to a deprivation which is unbearable. Even when children act contrary to the order of the adult, they have a strong feeling of guilt and consider themselves to be bad.

They accept the morality of adults, at least verbally. At any rate, they need a simple system of moral orientation. It is due to Freud that we understand this process. The outward force becomes incorporated in the ego, by identification, and the superego condemns the actions which previously have been punished by the adult.

[21] This case was reported as one of masked hypothyroidism by Dorff (1935, 1939).

In order to understand the morality of children, one must try to understand their attitude toward the world. Their world is a narrow one. They live in the immediate present, and do not coordinate a great number of facts. It is difficult for them to determine what is good and what is bad in the adult sense. Guided by immediate impressions, they often change their moral orientation. Actions which are alike for the child may be different for the adult, and vice versa. The world of the child consists of the arbitrary actions of human beings who do something because they like to. The child does not understand his own or others' aggressiveness. Human beings are bad because they like to be bad. The child wants certainties. One should be punished and should be severely punished. As Piaget (1932) has indicated, the punishment is expected to be proportionate to the actual damage caused by the wrongdoing. The motive is less important from the point of view of the child, or he feels rather sure that any damage wrought is intentional. Every deprivation is felt with equal severity. Death is a deprivation like any other. The child, therefore, does not think that the death penalty is a particularly severe punishment.

These general principles are derived from our clinical observation, as well as from the children's descriptions of pictures and answers to the questionnaire. It is worthwhile, however, to discuss the material offered in the questionnaire in more detail.

The questions which required answers in terms of basic connotations called forth responses from the children which showed that their thinking did not concern itself with the abstract structure of things. For instance, courage meant to them, "Somebody who fights," or "You are big." A coward meant "When you don't fight," or "If a boy is fighting he takes a rock and throws it." Some children believed that a coward, a cow, and a cowboy were more or less synonymous. The partial identity of sounds (signs) is sufficient to make children believe that they mean the same object. Children do not differentiate between strength and health. They use these connotations more or less at random. The child tends to understand the emotional implication of a word, rather than the cognitive implication. The child feels these uncertainties of his intellectual orientation, and he tries to escape from them by going back to the single experience.

The same difficulties are observed in their perception of pictures. Younger children do not correlate the various details. Partial similarities, for instance (as Piaget has shown), often stand for complete identity. Young children do not make a differentiation between the question "Do you like to hit other children?" and the question "Is it right to hit other children?" Children are generally taught not to hurt smaller children. They themselves are afraid to be hit by bigger ones. They come, therefore, to the obvious conclusion that it is probably all right for them to fight with somebody of equal strength. It is very interesting that this attitude also persists in adults. Hitting of a girl by a boy, or hitting of a smaller child, is similarly rejected, since girls are better protected by the rules laid down by adults. But the aggressiveness of a smaller child, insults by a smaller child, especially if directed against parents, and, finally, the greater strength of an aggressive girl, justify counteraggression even against a smaller child or girl.

To strike back, on attack, is generally considered as correct—also true in adults. Even small children, who show their aggressiveness plainly in play, do not freely profess their murderous wishes unless there is a specific reason. Preference for the gun as an instrument of killing is already present in the smaller children. This is partially due to the generally acknowledged greater effectiveness of this instrument, and partly due to the feeling that killing with an ax is more bloody and violent. Even smaller children justify aggression against gangsters.

It seems to be the general trend of development that aggressiveness is very soon covered up, and only dares to show itself as reactive aggressiveness—as when one is first attacked—or as aggressiveness against those who have sinned, or those who belong to another social group (Indians, Germans). Aggressiveness thus becomes organized into the general social structure. The comparison between the answers of the younger age group and the older age group gives a rather clear insight into this process of organization of aggressiveness, which perhaps more readily takes place in words than deeds. A great amount of aggressiveness finds its expression in play, when a child has already obtained a higher degree of morality, at least in words.

Popular psychology considers boys more aggressive than girls.

Passivity has even been considered a feminine characteristic, and it has been said that masochistic trends are the basic ingredients of female psychology. Only small children readily accept the idea of change to the opposite sex. Seemingly, the difference between girl and boy does not mean very much to them. But that there is some deeper meaning, in their unwillingness to change their sex, was evident from the case of Milton, in whom passive and masochistic elements were outstanding, as a result of his relationship to his mother. She developed a bone cancer during her pregnancy with him, from which she knew that she must die, and she could not help from feeling that he was to blame; she rejected him accordingly. Around the fifth year, all children develop a great pride in their respective sexes; this increases with age. In both sexes, the reasons which they give for their preference are very superficial. One girl wants to be a girl because a girl has more hair; another one because a boy can't sew; another one doesn't want to be a boy because boys are fresh; another one because the boys go to war; and still another one prefers to wear dresses instead of pants. Boys want to be boys because they want to play baseball and football; because the girls have too much housework to do; because boys don't have to wear dresses; and because they have more fun. In our material, there was only one boy of the older group who said he would prefer to be a girl in wartime. Our material does not offer any evidence that girls would prefer to be boys. One may have doubts as to whether the questionnaire method is sufficient to exclude a deep-lying penis envy as one of the roots of female psychology. But our cases were also individually studied, although over a comparatively short time. We do indeed think that the classical Freudian teaching of the castration complex in girls is not justified, and that our questionnaire study comes closer to the deep-lying facts.

It is true that girls are considered, by boys as well as by girls, to be weaker and should, therefore, have the protection otherwise given to the smaller child. For both the younger and older children, a sissy is a boy who goes with girls; a boy that is like a cat; a boy that fights girls and is a "show off"; a boy who can't fight; a boy who dresses like girls; boys who "play around" with girls; and anybody who can't fight or who is afraid to fight. With the exception of five-year-old Milton, all the children expressed a definite dislike for sissies.

The general definition of a sissy, for children, would be a boy who, in his relations to girls and fighting, does not live up to the social standards. These answers of the children show clearly how so-called secondary and tertiary sex characteristics are arbitrarily attributed to one sex or the other. The answers of children show the strength of the social conventions, and point to the importance of convention for the determination of masculinity and femininity.

If one considers the differences between the younger and older children, in the problem of aggressiveness, one sees that the chief difference is in the older children's better coordination of the different parts of the problem. The younger children want immediate satisfaction, and are in immediate fear of punishment and retaliation. In the older children, the idea of right and wrong gradually emerges and is independent of their idea of immediate advantage and disadvantage. The youngest age groups must resort to play, to reactive aggressiveness, and to the idea of punishment of others for sinning. Only particularly gifted children, of the oldest age group, had doubts as to whether aggressiveness was justified under any circumstance, as in the case of Max, nine years of age, who had a mental age of sixteen. We did not have the impression that we dealt with abrupt changes, in the psychology of the different age levels, and we separated the groups between the ages of eight and nine in a rather arbitrary way. We had the impression that we dealt with a process of gradual organization, in which the attitude of the surroundings was of paramount importance. Nature is continually modified by nurture.

The case histories showed the influences of the home situation and the psychological problems of the child on the final crystallization of his aggressive attitudes. It should be emphasized that we did not merely put the questionnaire before a group of children and supplement it by play and picture interpretations; every child of the group was studied individually, concerning his aggressiveness. It was astonishing that, in a great number of cases, the actual behavior of the children did not particularly differ from what they expressed in reply to the questionnaire. In the very young children, there was an almost complete coincidence; in the older group, the verbal morality was often higher, but still, in the aggressive children, the aggressiveness was often expressed rather clearly.

Perhaps the term "aggressive child" is an unjustified generalization. Children were often aggressive at home and not aggressive in the hospital. In other words, we should not speak too readily about the general quality of aggressiveness. Aggressiveness occurs in specific situations. It is true that there is a general drive, a general activity in handling objects, which we tried to characterize in the beginning of the discussion. It is difficult to distinguish between activity, which is a general characteristic of life, and aggressiveness. Generally we speak of aggressiveness when the activity leads to an encroachment of the physical integrity of others. This aggressiveness is mostly combined with destructive actions concerning other animate and inanimate objects.

This activity in aggressiveness has a close relation to motor drives and to instincts in general. It doubtless has its foundation in the organic structure, and its variations are in close relation to the child's constitution. Organic processes may influence the general output of energy. The hyperkinetic child shows a great increase, not only in activity, but also in aggressiveness. His hyperkinesis can be due to constitutional factors, encephalitis, birth injuries, or head traumas of all kinds. Two instructive cases were the M. brothers, where constitutional components played a great part. The older brother was the more inferior and a head injury at birth may have played an additional part. But even in their cases, psychological factors played some part, as a reaction to neglect by an unstable mother. It seems that with constitutional predisposition, psychic traumas can lead to a general increase in activity and hyperkinesis. It is characteristic that this hyperkinesis leads to a rather diffuse aggressiveness and destructiveness. In the majority of cases, psychic traumas lead to a direct aggression, which expresses itself in a specific situation (for instance, at home or against a younger sibling only).

The criticism might be made that we have studied abnormal children. We cannot deny that our material is not as homogeneous as could be obtained from so-called normal children. On the other hand, the majority of our children were not more abnormal than many children who attend the public schools, and they showed the same problems as many normal children. The particularly difficult circumstances under which many of them had lived tended to focus attention on many specific trends more clearly than would be the case in a so-called normal group; but they were not qualitatively different. Even an organic brain lesion does not create fundamentally new trends; it merely underscores specific psychological problems. We believe that the conclusions which we have derived, from this so-called pathological material, are valid for children in general.[22]

The psychology of physical aggressiveness in children, based on the clinical observation of eighty-three children, between the ages of three and fifteen, was studied. Violence was considered to be any action which damaged the body of another person, or distorted his body image by pain or discomfort. The children were not only clinically observed, but were subjected to a definite play situation, to series of pictures depicting aggressive situations, and to a questionnaire on aggression. Ten of the children were followed for fifteen years.

Aggressiveness finds expression more directly in younger children, in actions as well as in play, in words, and in the description of pictures. Young children seek immediate satisfaction, and are in immediate fear of punishment and retaliation. The narrowness of their world does not allow the coordination of a great number of facts. Good and bad, in the adult sense, is more or less an abitrary decision of the adult. Deprivation of love or food increases the aggressive tendencies of children.

In all the children, there gradually emerged the idea of right and wrong, dependent on immediate advantages and disadvantages. The youngest children expressed their aggressiveness freely, both verbally and in play. The older children were inclined to be inhibited,

[22] Of the ten children that we followed into adulthood, two bright girls did very well; two boys remained in their own homes (one, at least, failing in school and dependent); two other boys were in correctional institutions (one, again, was a social failure); three girls were dependent on state institutions and showed dropping IQ's; and the remaining boy has been held in a state hospital, because of his serious asocial behavior.

The final effect on the adult, who has suffered from early childhood deprivation and reacting aggression, has, with some favorable exceptions, been a retardation in affect, in the social aspects of the personality, and even in intelligence. As adults, they have tended to escape from the conflicts of life and to settle into or become dependent on asylums or refuges, in the form of state institutions for the mentally defective or mentally sick, or correctional institutions, where they either deteriorated or became dependent on the institutional regime for discipline and control of their aggressive impulses.

284

and often needed a play situation, or other indirect method, by which they could express their aggressiveness unconsciously. Aggressiveness against a group was expressed more freely than aggressiveness against single individuals.

There was an apparent process of gradual organization of aggressive tendencies into a socially accepted concept, in which the attitude of the environment was of paramount importance. The psychological situation of the child leads to the final crystallization of his aggressive attitudes.

In the youngest children, there were no discrepancies between their actual behavior and their answers to questions. In the older group, however, the verbal morality was usually higher, while aggressiveness found expression in play and tended to become more or less unconscious and repressed.

Aggressiveness has close relations to motor drives and to instincts in general. It undoubtedly has foundations in the organic structure, and its variations may be constitutional. Organic processes influence the general output of energy. The hyperkinetic child shows increased aggressiveness. The aggressiveness on an organic basis is mostly more diffuse, whereas psychic traumas lead to an aggressiveness in relation to specific situations.

# VII

# Clinical Considerations

## ANXIETY NEUROSIS[1]

It was a great contribution when Freud (1926) stated that anxiety is a reaction to danger.[2] This danger may be external or internal. According to Freud, anxiety is a danger signal on the part of the ego, which initiates repression. The internal danger, according to him, is the perception of the rising sexual tendency in connection with the Oedipus complex. If the individual gives in to his sexual urge, he becomes in danger of being punished; the love of either parent may be withdrawn from him. Furthermore, the boy may think he will suffer castration, mutilation, and dismemberment. The girl might be torn by her father's penis, or robbed of the inside of her body, and she might face mutilation and dismemberment. These formulations go beyond the Freudian formulations, insofar as Freud considered merely castration as the final threat. He considered castration fear of the body as the model, and the structure of the girl's castration fear equivalent to that of the boy. I have repeatedly stated that I consider the castration complex of the girl to be fundamentally different from the castration fear of the boy. The girl is afraid that her sex organ might be torn by a disproportionately large male organ or she is afraid that her sex organ might be occluded. There is also the fear that she might lose the receptacles within her body and would not have any organs in which

---

[1] From Schilder (1941).
[2] Compare Schilder's *Medical Psychology* (1924), which precedes Freud's contribution.

she could take and carry either the male sex organ or the child.

The external danger is, for the most part, incompletely described in the pyschoanalytic literature. If the child loses the love of its parents, it is threatened not only with the lack of love, but also with the lack of food, and the loss of help with its equilibrium. There is, furthermore, the danger of mutilation and dismemberment. The final fear of death summarizes all the dangers mentioned and contains, furthermore, the fear of being deprived of the power of movement.

Klein (1932) has justly pointed to another fundamental fear. This is the fear of being deprived of the inside of the body. I have mentioned that the girl may be afraid of losing the receptacles for the genitals. There is also, however, the fear of being deprived of the gastrointestinal tract, and of the whole inside of the body. This fear is, of course, common to both boys and girls. Experiences with schizophrenics have shown me that the individual may, finally, be afraid of being deprived of the ingested food and the feces. This fear is linked with the fear of being deprived of food, since, in the unconscious, the infantile idea prevails that the inside of the body consists largely of the food which has been eaten, as D. Wechsler and I have shown. Bromberg and I (1933a) have shown that castration and dismemberment fears form the main contents of the picture of alcoholic hallucinosis. I have seen these fears reach a peak in a case of alcoholic hallucinosis who was threatened by voices telling him that everything would be taken out of his body, so that he would merely consist of bones and skin, until he actually felt that this had happened to his body.

Klein is correct when she states that the child considers that his weapons of aggression are not only his striped muscles in action, but also his feces and urine, which might burn and eat away parts of the body.

It is to be expected that an individual threatened with the dangers just described, will not, and cannot, react to these dangers merely by giving in and suffering terrible punishment. Furthermore, the more aggression there is in himself, the more he will experience aggression in others. In other words, the fear of aggressiveness by others is, in part, the projection of one's own aggression. The sexual urge is, in itself, combined with aggressiveness, and an

287

overwhelming sex tendency will be experienced as colossal aggressiveness. We may also expect that the individual will be more afraid
of the consequences of his sex urge, the more this urge is coupled
with aggressive tendencies. Fear of punishment may be followed by
a feeling of guilt and a tendency to self-punishment. Deutsch (1932)
has shown that, in a case of anxiety neurosis with agoraphobia, there
were hostile tendencies against incestuous love objects. At the same
time, the patient identifies himself with his love object.

Anxiety is a phenomenon which may originate from experiences
of very different types. In the earliest stages of development, the
child is particularly threatened by the loss of equilibrium, and by
the physical forces of gravitation. Only gradually does he learn to
orient himself in space and to appreciate the definite importance
of the vertical and horizontal direction. In this stage of development, it is very probable that the love object also represents an
insurance against the danger of falling. In this respect I have called
the love object a supportive figure. However, the child also reacts
with anxiety when the supply of food is not assured. Furthermore,
food means, for the child, the inside of his body, since, according
to the connotations of the young child, the inside of the body consists of the food which has been ingested. Direct threats against the
integrity of the body are probably experienced only at a later stage.
They are closely connected with aggressive tendencies of the child
which are directed against the bodies of others. At this level, fear of
dismemberment in general will become of importance, and later
on, with the awakening of the genitality, will culminate in castration motif. During this whole development, the love object will
offer protection against deprivations, on the one hand, and will, on
the other hand, be feared as a possible aggressor. Fear of losing the
love object will come into the foreground when the sexual development has reached a higher level. When there are hostile tendencies
against the love object they will be reacted to with feelings of guilt.
At the earlier levels, there will be fears of the counteraggression of
the love object. At the higher levels, there will be identification
with the love object, who is also hated, and the insecurity connected
with the dreaded loss of the love object will be increased by the
guilty feeling, which increases the identification with the person
who has been killed in fantasy.

If one considers the variety of situations which provoke anxieties in the course of development, one will not be astonished to see great variety in the types of anxiety neuroses which revive the various types of developmental anxieties. Any anxiety state may contain all the possible anxiety situations, but in various degrees and proportions. One should further keep in mind that, in spite of deep regressions which have been described, the typical case with neurotic anxiety has usually reached levels of heterosexual adjustment, in terms of the Oedipus complex, and illustrates one point of fixation in genital relation to parents. This separates these cases, from a clinical point of view, from cases with obsession neuroses, although the anxiety cases with space distortions often show obsessional trends. It is the characteristic of neurotic anxiety, in contrast to psychotic anxiety, that there is always some appreciation of the love object.

## Concept of Hysteria[3]

The hysterical character is characterized by the tendency to build up a strong attachment to both parents. The attachment to the parent of the other sex prevails (Fenichel, 1934). This attachment is connected with decided genital sensations or genital activity. In many of our cases, more-or-less close actual contact of the girl with the father has been reported, and, in one instance, there is a report of early sex relations with the father. The actual conflict obviously provokes the previous attitudes, which later on are transferred into the symptom by the mechanism of conversion. The conversion is either based on an actual scene experienced in childhood, a disease observed in another, or a previous organic disease. There is always a real event at the basis of conversion. In this event, the body image or a somatic experience always plays the most important part. The conversion is based on childhood experiences, but the later organic trauma may be the nucleus and pattern for the final formation of the symptoms. For instance, amnesia and memory disturbances often occur in patients who have suffered from an organic unconsciousness due to trauma or carbon monoxide poisoning. Erickson (1937) even reports that he has revoked such a preceding organic unconsciousness, by hypnosis.

[3] From Schilder (1939c).

The psychogenic problem remains paramount in all cases of true hysteria. However, there are all kinds of gradations, of interaction between psychological attitudes as described, to pictures in which the organic problem is in the foreground, and the particular hysterical attitude becomes more and more unimportant. However, hysterical attitudes may prevail when the organic disease is either not so severe, in its beginning, or at its decline. If the organic disease is severe, attitudes appear which try to neglect the organic disease. One may define this tendency to devaluate the organic disease as akin to hysteria. At any rate, the indifference which one has so often observed in the hysterical patient, concerning his or her symptoms, has a close relation to the attitude of the organic case.

Hysterical phenomena in children show, with marked clarity, the continuous interaction between the attitudes of the patient and the parents. In the case of Jenny, all the fears of her childhood were in close relation to the attitude of the beloved mother. I now report an instructive observation which Bender has made, on the children's ward of the Bellevue Psychiatric Hospital.

Jenny, who was thirteen years old, closely resembled her mother. The mother had limited intelligence, and some dramatic hysterical phenomena, which Jenny's behavior closely resembled. The older sister, Salvina, born of a former marriage of the mother, was sixteen years old, and had spent a period in a psychiatric hospital, as a child, for "seeing things." The family history was filled with sickness and operations. The mother and three children had all received antiluetic treatment. The infection had probably come from her first husband. The present husband was said to be an alcoholic.

Jenny was a colicky baby and, at the age of three, after a slight cold, the mother noticed a slight strabismus, which she felt had developed at that time. She claimed that Jenny had been nervous ever since then. At the age of ten, she had an operation for the strabismus and since then she had been more or less hysterical. She also had measles, whooping cough, chicken pox, and mumps.

Jenny's hysterical phenomena all related to body sensations. She had periods when she felt as if she were shrinking; other times when she was dizzy and going around, and sometimes she felt hot all over, and got pins and needles and pains all over her. She was sometimes afraid of death and stated that she was dead. Other times, she had optic phenomena with blurring, seeing double, or blindness. On other occasions, she could not hear well. Almost all these phenomena had, in one way or another, been suggested by the mother. We had observed them on the ward, especially after visiting hours by the mother. She also had periods when she was suspicious of the environment. She refused to eat for two days, because she was afraid the nurses would poison her. This was the outgrowth of a hysterical excitement which the mother demonstrated on the ward, stating that she was afraid the nurses would get even by poisoning the child. These phenomena were all very superficial, and the child could be quickly relieved of them, settling down to a fairly normal adjustment until she was again disturbed by her mother.

The child was poorly developed and, although of good height, was of asthenic build; there was no evidence of approaching puberty. Blood Wassermann was negative, and complete serological examination of the spinal fluid was also negative. There was a refractive error of vision, as well as an alternating convergent strabismus. Hearing tests showed a hearing loss of 22 per cent in the right ear and 19 per cent in the left ear. Neurological examination was otherwise negative.

The following is a summary of the psychometric test: Stanford-Binet, IQ 68; Bellevue Adult Test, IQ 63; Otis Classification, Pt. 2, IQ 85; Pt. I school placement, 4B; Woody-McCall arithmetic, 5A; Monroe spelling written, 3B; Monroe silent reading, 3A; and comprehension, 3B. We classified her as a high grade moron mental defective. The higher results obtained on the Otis Classification were attributed to her having pushed herself beyond her actual capacity.

In this case the low IQ facilitated the hysterical fixation. However, since the conflict in such cases more easily provokes the hysterical symptomatology, it is also easier to bring the individuals to insight. In children, an accident may play an important part in the genesis of the neurosis, as in the case of ten-year-old Oliver, who showed a similar symptomatology.[4] In such cases, one can easily show that the car or truck which caused the accident symbolizes the forceful father who pushes the child into an infantile, masochistic, and dependent position.

Early disappointment in the relationship with the parents plays a leading part in the structure of hysteria. Later traumas bring this early disappointment again into the foreground. In the early relations to parents, organic disease plays a very important part. It

4 See p. 330.

291

makes the individual still more dependent on the parent. It also concentrates the love of the parent on the child. Organic ailment is, therefore, of fundamental importance for the whole psychology of hysteria. It reinforces the masochistic attitude in the afflicted person. The affinity of the hysterical patient to organic disease and trauma has to be considered from this angle. Hysteria thus becomes the expression of suffering, by disease, in its human and social aspects. It stresses the helplessness and dependence of the child on the love of the parents. From this angle, it is understandable that the actual cause of the hysterical difficulties in women is often to be found in erotic disappointments, whereas, in men, social conflicts and accidents play the most important part. At any rate, the person afflicted with hysteria addresses himself to a highly organized social structure. The hysterical patient acknowledges reality, but he cannot get a definite hold on it. Therefore, he is curious, eager, and full of interest in human beings.

The passing hysterical symptom is thus based on the same mechanism as the lasting hysterical symptom and the hysterical personality. However, even the passing hysterical symptom is only possible when the individual has reached the level of the Oedipus complex, and also the level of a lively interest in the outer world. When the erotic or social situation becomes too prohibitive, the individual takes refuge in the symptom.

On the basis of this discussion, it becomes obvious that attitudes which lead to hysterical symptoms are facilitated by organic disease. However, it is of fundamental importance to note that people with such attitudes, asking for erotic and social help, are only those with organic diseases which are not too severe. In general, it will be found in chronic diseases, or the beginning or decline of an acute disease. If the organic disease is at its height or completely incapacitating, the individual will get the full social recognition for it, without hysterical symptoms.

Our material accordingly contains a great number of cases of organic disease with hysterical symptoms. However, one should not speak of hysteria when the patient merely has an attitude of neglect toward organic symptoms, as is true in very many organic cases, or when the individual does not put up a particular fight in the face of organic disease. One should stick to the definition that hysterical symptoms are the expression of the attitude of love toward the parents, in a symbolic form. As in all products of unconscious thinking, many tendencies are condensed in hysterical symptoms. However, whatever the share of pregenital and destructive tendencies in the hysterical symptom may be, it is less than the share of tendencies in immediate connection with the Oedipus complex. This is, after all, the definition of hysteria.

It is difficult to decide when the Oedipus complex makes its appearance. Many analysts believe that genitality and the Oedipus complex make their appearance before the third year, and my own observations point in the same direction. Hysteriform phenomena have been observed in children at the age of one and a half years. However, it seems to me that the structure of these cases is not identical with the structure of cases of hysteria. They probably represent comparatively simple emotional outbursts, in which aggressive and destructive impulses prevail. The conversion connected with these outbursts is different in its mechanism from one of a strictly hysterical type (see Friedjung, 1925).

We speak of the hysterical character in individuals who easily develop hysterical attitudes or retain such symptoms through a longer span of their lives. I have also observed hysterical symptoms in schizophrenias; however, they were merely in connection with those parts of the personality which obtained a fuller adaptation to reality. One finds, accordingly, hysterical phenomena in almost every type of neurosis and psychosis.

## CHILDREN'S ATTITUDE TOWARD DEATH[5]

Death is a frequently recurring theme in human psychology. It is indeed surprising how often thoughts of death creep into the consciousness of the average person, during the course of his everyday activity. But ideas concerning death are especially prominent in psychopathology. Thoughts of death and dying occur as everyday symptoms among psychoneurotics of the anxiety, hysterical, and obsessive types, and in depressions, melancholias, schizophrenias, epileptic psychoses, panic reactions, etc.

Death attitudes are apparently formed chiefly by experiences

---

[5] From Bromberg and Schilder (1936).

derived from the early life of the individual. The early "natural-istic" attitudes of childhood toward death and dying (mainly an open expression of sadistic, destructive tendencies of infancy) are modified, during early life, by experiences with funeral situations and the adult conventions of bereavement. Later, during the course of the years, repressions, rationalizations, and religious acceptances further modify the instinctive unconscious attitudes toward killing and death. Thus, in our case material (Bromberg and Schilder, 1933), sadomasochistic trends, expressed by suicide fantasies aimed at injuring society, a wife, husband or other loved ones, etc., were clearly unconscious death thoughts against the parents, borrowed from infantile situations. Other death fantasies may show a desire for increased love or for punishment of persons in the environment. The commonly expressed horror of violent, gory death, and the wish to die calmly and serenely, represent a repressed interest in pain, and mangled and destroyed bodies. At the same time, the overtones of serenity and pureness, that color the tradition of the funeral ceremony, are based on the idea of narcissistic perfection in death. As is commonly seen in childhood, anal influences (interest in ani-mal corpses, decayed objects) form an active part in the death fantasies and ideas of adults. In many fantasies of our subjects, death meant the perfect sexual union, a union with an ideal, not to be found in life. This desire for such an unattainable love object was, in unconscious terms, the incest wish.

By the genetic method adopted, we came to the conclusion that death has several meanings in psychological experience: (1) An escape from an unbearable situation—one lives, in death, a new life without any of the difficulties of the present life; (2) a method to force others to give more love than they are willing to grant in life; (3) an equivalent for the final sexual union with the ideal mate; (4) the final narcissistic perfection, which grants eternal and unchallenged importance to the individual; and (5) the gratifica-tion of masochistic tendencies, since death perpetuates forever the suffering inflicted by self-punishment (the eternity of the hell-fire reflects this psychological attitude).

Human individuals apparently do not have a primary tendency to die, but they may have a primary wish for their own destruction, which is an expression of sadomasochistic trends against those in their environment. It was evident that the idea of death serves the libidinous tendencies of the individual; hence we may say, the idea of death psychologically serves in the interests of the life instincts. Baudouin (1933) says, "Death is . . . an instinct of retreat . . . death may be interpreted as the supreme refuge." Fear of death is the fear of a loss of something positive and is, therefore, closely interrelated with the castration complex in its widest sense. Psychologically, we never die, and the belief in immortality is but the expression of this inherent tendency in our psychic life.

A case is presented in which the pleasantness of death expresses the sadomasochistic trends of the patient.

Arthur F., a sixteen-year-old boy of superior intelligence, was admitted to the hospital with a history of numerous delinquency difficulties, psychopathic behavior, and disobedience. He had frequently been in children's court. He was bright in school. Trouble consisted of impulsive behavior, hypochondriacal symptoms, and sexual conflicts. He had shown behavior disturbances for years. His father was a psychopathic type, alcoholic, excitable, and unfaithful; he often talked to the boy about his sexual life. Masturbation was reported at the age of nine or ten years, and Arthur started having sexual relations early, about the age of thirteen.

The patient had obsessional symptoms. He frequently thought of death, had dreams of coffins, and frequent thoughts of death that were pleasurable. He saw naked, unmutilated dead people, who looked peaceful and were mostly men; he fantasied himself in a silk-lined coffin surrounded by a sorrowing family. He wanted to die by hanging. He said he had often imagined having sex relations with dead people. At times of intercourse, he thought of dying. He wanted to be an undertaker. He said "Dead people look beautiful." He felt angry, and wanted to beat persons with whom he had intercourse to death. He had vivid pictures of heaven, with people without clothes and indistinct features. He liked to handle dead bodies. He never thought of suffering in connection with dying. He often thought of killing his father. He said he would like to kill someone and hear him scream as he died. Two years ago, he had the flu and was delirious. "I got funny feelings in my head. In the last six months I heard a voice which must be mine, telling me things about myself and about dead people. I am sort of able to look at myself, can imagine I see through myself, my intestines. I see a lot of veins, just red streams of blood. I see a big long tube more like a bone."

In this situation, the dead person is the love object to whom the patient is attracted. The sadistic elements in the love relationship are expressed in the aggressive fantasies about a dead person. The masochism is reflected in the desire for submission to the father. For Arthur, death means final sadomasochistic gratification in a homosexual reunion with the father. It is true that the presence of strong sadomasochistic tendencies brings this case very close to the obsessional group which we shall discuss later. It is quoted here in order to show the erotic symbolism that death has for some types of psychoneurotics, notably the hysteric and anxiety groups.

## DEATH FEARS IN NEUROTIC CHILDREN[6]

We present here two cases of neuroses in children in which death ideas play a prominent part.

Nathan I., a Jewish boy of nine, was admitted to the children's ward for observation because of difficulty at school, inattention, restlessness, talkativeness, and a preoccupation with fantastic ideas. He constantly talked about death, religion, etc., and would not interest himself in school subjects. He was unwilling to play aggressive games or adjust to the conventional school or play life of the average boy his age. Physically, he was hyperkinetic, and showed a tendency toward choreic movements which gave him an effeminate appearance.

Observation showed he was a boy with dull normal mentality, who was able to attract attention because of his high verbalization ability and consequent tendency toward fantastic inventions. He was particularly low in practical and manual ability, and was content to withdraw into his fantasy world, without displaying any aggression, but at the same time being able to attract the attention he desired. His productions concerned themselves chiefly with religious, ethical, aggressive fantasies.

For him, death was an agent of his sadism. He brought death into his fantastic stories easily, but it was not so easy for him to imagine his own death: "I want to live forever because I don't want to be eaten by magic . . . I don't want to be no devil." However, he could easily put himself into death situations. For example, when asked, Do you ever think of being buried alive? he replied, "No, I'd start kicking with my feet and I'd holler 'help' and then they'd take me to the hospital. God came early by magic." Magic? "When you want to change something into something else. If you want to change things upside down you can do it by magic."

[6] See footnote 5, p. 293.

Can one die? "Maybe by sickness, heart attack or shot. God can kill you by a touch or magic word. After death you come to life again and maybe He makes you an angel. He is invisible and goes up to heaven."

"God can kill you with magic. The devil can kill you with his nails. He sticks you with hooks when he gets mad." How does God do it? "When you are good He gives you presents and likes you but when you are bad He tells you you will not be a good man when you grow up. He says a few words. God watches so that the devil will not hurt you. God is good and the devil is bad. The devil might touch you with his hand, then you are killed. When he touches you you get frightened. He sticks his nail into your body." Poison under the nail? "Yes, when you die you are carried up to heaven. When a person dies his body is eaten by flies." What does he look like? "When you are dead God brings you up to heaven and brings your own flesh back. When you are in the grave you look like a devil."

What would you rather see, a skeleton or a dead man? "A dead man. A skeleton gets you scared but the dead man doesn't." How does he scare you? "His eyes, he is only made of bones, he hasn't any eyes." If you should see a dead man now what would you do? "I would test him. I would say, 'put your hand on this card.' " Ever think of dead people? "I am thinking about it now." Do you think you could die? "I don't know. I am scared to die." How would you look if you die? "Look nice. If people die, other people look at them and be afraid, they would have to close their eyes; they look fierce if they were shot." Grimaces to illustrate. What diseases have you heard of? "Heart attack." What would a man look like if he died of a heart attack? "Maybe he would look bad." Patient insists upon dramatizing dying situation by assuming various grotesque postures.

"I want to be a Catholic. Jesus makes people well. He is an old man. God is a good man too. God is older than Jesus. Moses is good too. He was a good man; he was old. He is 300 years old."

What pictures do you have when you think of death? "They're killing, smacking bones on death's back . . . the cruel, mean, no good people are going to be like dead . . . there's no death in this world. Death is a man who has eyes—like [skeleton]. If someone could invent life, he could kill death. When life comes, death dies."

Nathan showed an obsessional interest in punishment, and devised many ways of punishment. He talked of being a "cop, detective, soldier, cowboy" in order to punish people who do wrong. He was very graphic in his imagination and portrayed the struggle between good and evil. His devil is bad, poisonous, and kills. God is good and kills only by magic if He must kill at all. God is right, the father, the judge, and executor. He expresses fear and antagonism of the father, and unconscious sadomasochism, in a way that is closely related to religious (theological) cosmology.

Death is here closely connected with the fear that violence will be inflicted on him by the stronger and unrelenting force. The greatest punishment is mutilation. It is part of the inherent psychology of childhood that the child cannot conceive of a lasting deprivation. Wechsler and I (Schilder and Wechsler, 1934), in studying the attitudes of children toward death, found that children are ready to believe in the death of others, since death is merely deprivation. They do not tolerate the idea that deprivation is the nature or structure of life and reality. They view deprivation merely as the result of the ill will and hostility of others, and hence death seldom has the character of something definite and final. A child's own deprivations are usually not of a permanent or lasting kind, and it is therefore easy for the child to wish the death of others and to speak of killing people, without any conscious feeling.

In the neurotic cases described here, the general attitudes of children toward death are clearly expressed. Another important attitude that is expressed is the child's feeling that torture and punishment seem to be everlasting. In other words, the idea of death is closely connected with the idea of a continuous, eternal torture. The following case has a similar psychologic structure.

Leonard S., a Jewish boy, ten years and eleven months old, was admitted to a mental hygiene clinic because the mother stated the boy was nervous, afraid to stay home alone, afraid if someone knocked at the door, and afraid to go out alone. "About four weeks ago a woman in the house died. He saw the coffin and since then is badly frightened."

The patient was alert, frank, friendly, and tractable. He had a good fund of information, good scholastic attainments, good reasoning, insight, and judgment, but he was apprehensive and fearful.

The patient described his feelings by saying, "I got scared when I saw the lady come down in the coffin. After the funeral I walked upstairs. Saw a door open and close three times. Thought her ghost was doing it or maybe a spirit. You can't see spirits. Nobody was there to do it so it must be spirits. On the fifth floor a kid died too, he got a scratch, blood poison and died. A lot of people go upstairs. I imagine the boy's and lady's spirits are in the house and go around to hurt somebody who done them wrong. They put spells on them because they have magic. I am more afraid of lady ghosts. I went downstairs by myself and heard the lady ghosts whispering and talking, they got a hideout in the halls.

"Everybody is spirit when he dies. They stay in the hall, the spirit stays down and the soul goes to heaven. It represents you over there. The heaven is in the sky. The soul talks for the lady who dies. Hell is down there. A ghost kills somebody, it chokes you because it don't like you, the ghost chokes you by magic.

"If a man dies in a hospital his ghost stays around his bed. If you want to get rid of ghost from hospital take the body home. Ghosts see each other, can get angry if the people they came from fight. They could fight by saying words to each other, but nobody could hear. They have their own language in whispers. Sometimes when they talk I could overhear them. Ghosts change themselves to shelly bones, then they could eat and drink. They can fly around the world in no time."

What is a sin? "If you light the gas on Sabbath. If you tear things on Sabbath. Telling lies is a sin too, saying bad words. I can't say it but I can spell. As long as I don't say it it's all right. Saying it is bad. If a person gets me mad, I get mad but say nothing. All the bad boys say the word. I figured it out like that myself, that it's worse to say them than to spell. The chief word is f - - -. S.o.b. is not so bad, it's weak. Another bad word is p - - - but I can't say it. If I say 'ball' I mean a ball that you throw. If the boys say 'ball' with an 's' that means something bad."

The patient says he is mostly afraid of women, that they will attack him, but he adds that that is because so many women have died in his house.

This was a neurotic boy with definite obsessional tendencies. He was afraid to say obscene words out loud, but would spell them out. He seemed much impressed by the idea that dirty work (housework) leads to sickness in women. His equivalence of women, dirt, death, and evil seemed to represent strong repression of anal tendencies that, in his early life, may have had a relationship to the cloaca theory of birth. His preoccupation with being "good" represented a struggle against the possibility of eternal punishment, which, as we have seen, is the meaning of death for children. The whole structure of the neurosis seemed to be built around women, a substitute for the mother. He was afraid that they would kill him—an expression of guilt feeling. For him, death meant to be killed by the mother (women), especially the ghosts of women. His fear of women represented punishment of some kind for his "bad" ideas (obscenity), and his hypermoralistic attitude is an anxiety reaction arising from his perception of his own guilt feelings. In his sadistic fantasies centering around ghosts, he allowed expression of his sadomasochistic tendencies.

In these two neuroses in children, the fear of death is the fear of being killed, mutilated, or choked. A dead person or ghost of God kills. But, as is commonly seen in the psychology of childhood, death is nothing final. After a person is killed, he starts killing himself. These ideas of children unmistakably have a close relation to the concepts of primitive peoples; destructive tendencies seemingly do not know the limit of time. There is a distinct difference in the internal structure of children's anxiety neuroses as compared with that of adults. In the hysteriform group, the idea of death brings up the libidinous relationship of the total personality of the individual to the object person, whereas, in the neuroses of children, death ideas are related to aggression of the child against the object person. In children, this aggression is expressed by the fear of death through mutilation and dismembering motives. In this way, the cases in childhood approach the structure of an obsessional neurosis.

The conception of death, in anxiety and hysteria cases, is dominated by the idea that death is separation from a love object. The beloved person is an unconscious incestuous object. The separation is a separation in space, which may be expressed symbolically. Death is feared as a sudden removal. Basically, death may mean reunion with the love object of incestuous character. The anxiety is partially a defense against the incestuous danger, and partially due to the libidinous conflict. Cases of this type may also show obsessional features, where death may give sadomasochistic satisfaction by punishing others and oneself. The fundamental psychopathological formulation of the hysteriform group, as regards death, is that of struggle against libidinous tendencies which are interfered with by spacial separation.

In summary, two cases of neurosis in children were studied. Cruel and sadistic attitudes expressed themselves in connection with the fear of death. Death was connected with the fear that violence would be inflicted by a strong and unrelenting force. But death was not conceived as a lasting deprivation.

## SUICIDAL PREOCCUPATIONS[7]

According to Hall (1905), suicide in children was not rare. In Italy, in the years 1885 to 1896, there were 222 boys and 80 girls who committed suicide, out of a total of 3763 suicides. However, according to the statistics of Corré (1891), in France, of 514 suicides below the age of sixteen years, only 34 were below the age of twelve. Cavan (1928) considered suicide below the age of twenty as rare. She even said that "children are non-suicidal." She quoted figures showing that in Chicago, 1919-1921, the incidence of suicide for 100,000 for the ten-to-fourteen age group was 0.27, and for the fifteen-to-nineteen age group was 4.12. She further stated that, in London, in 1922, there were no suicides reported under fifteen years of age, and that from fifteen to twenty-five there were 4.0 per 100,000; while in 1910, in Denmark, France, and Germany, there was a rate of 2.0 to 5.0 per 100,000. And in Austria, the suicide rate for children was the highest in Europe, being 0.5 per 100,000, under fifteen, and 18.3 per 100,000 from fifteen to nineteen. United States mortality statistics, from the Bureau of Census, show that 30 to 55 children, ten to fourteen years of age, annually lose their lives by self-inflicted death (quoted by Leo Kanner). However, these do not appear to represent suicidal deaths alone, but, rather, accidental ones for the most part. It was shown that the most common methods were by firearms, hanging or strangulation, corrosive substances (such as lye), other forms of poison, and drowning.

The following study deals with children who expressed suicidal preoccupations. The material was taken from children observed on the children's ward of the Psychiatric Division of Bellevue Hospital, between 1933 and 1937, with follow-up reports thirteen and seventeen years later, in 1950-1951.

The youngest boy was Edward, age six, IQ 120. Both of his parents had died within a very short time, the father of pneumonia, and the mother during antiluetic treatment. Edward also had to have antiluetic treat-

---

[7] From Bender and Schilder (1937).

ment, which very much depressed him. His suicidal ideas were a protest against his various unhappy experiences. He was afraid of being injured, physically and mentally. At times, when his feelings of deprivation became intolerable, he would threaten to kill himself, usually offering some incidental and even inconsequential reason. For example, he once said, "If I were a court case I would kill myself" (meaning if he were like one of the children who came to the hospital with a children's court charge of neglect or delinquency). The term "court case," as it is used here, is an empty word shell. At another time, he said, "A kid told me about devils. I don't know if it is true. How should I know if my mother and father are in heaven? I am not a fortuneteller. I heard somebody say the angels take the soul. But I am not sure about it. They read about it in the Bible. I did not see it myself but I am sure they are lying under the ground. I saw it."

Three boys, seven years of age, with suicidal preoccupations were observed.

Joe[8] was an illegitimate boy, who spent his early years in institutions, later in foster homes. He tried to drown himself in a puddle. He often stated that he did not want to live. He wanted to go to heaven and be good. He had a number of obvious sadistic and masochistic tendencies. He tortured animals and had astonishingly rich fantasies. His activities prevented his free association with other children. He was cruel with animals and children, and told fantastic stories about death, killing and torture.

In the hospital, he was threatening and assaultive to other children, impulsive, and overactive. He spontaneously spoke of his fantasies of death. He seemed to have no feelings of remorse for his asocial behavior, and frequently attempted to impose sexual activities on other children. An example of his productions follows: "When I am hungry my mother lets me starve. If she does not give me what I want, I knock her down. My teacher has a spanking machine, he spanks the children and it hurts . . . He jumped from his chair and jumped in a lot of blood that came from his nose and died. A kid threw a knife at my feet and all my toes fell off. Then the ambulance came and took me to the hospital where they were going to give me two new legs . . . I had my eyes pulled out seven months ago. It didn't hurt. I couldn't sleep. I had my eyes pulled out again. The kids were killing me . . . I took ether to die. I don't want to live. I want to go to heaven and be good . . . They are going to

[8] From Bromberg and Schilder (1933).

take out my teeth and eyes but I told them they better not . . . The children cry and the teacher bangs them on the floor . . . My mother cried till her bones cracked."

\* \* \*

Armand had refused to go to school when he was seven and when efforts were made to force him, he demonstrated severe temper tantrums with acute anxiety, and threatened and attempted to throw himself out of a window to kill himself. He became increasingly unmanageable at home, having temper tantrums and nightmares, quarreling with his brothers, stuttering, and defiant to his mother, and enuretic. His mother told him that his behavior was making her more nervous and might kill her. Armand answered defiantly that he would like to see if he could make her go crazy and if she would die then.

On our wards, he showed acute anxiety; he could not take part in the activities of other children, but clung to adults. He was enuretic, chewed his fingernails, and stuttered. His intelligence was average and he could do good schoolwork, if he had the undivided attention of a teacher. He had temper tantrums when pushed into activities, and threatened and attempted to squeeze himself out of a sixth floor window of the hospital, in order to kill himself. He abused his parents at visiting hours, insisting that they take him home, and promising to go to school and "be good." They finally acquiesced and, in the following three days, took him to several different schools, in each of which he became acutely disturbed and ran away screaming. They brought him back to the hospital; all three in a hysterical state. The mother had a fainting spell on the hospital steps and subsequently reported that this brought on a miscarriage.

Armand was the oldest of three boys of very disturbed and inadequate parents. The father had been a sailor at fifteen. When he was drafted in World War I, he was said to have feigned illness, been put in a straitjacket, and developed a severe stuttering which has persisted. He was a longshoreman, but because of a strained back did not work; he was on public welfare relief.

The mother had always been very nervous. She believed that the landlord had put a curse on her family, as a result of which she had insisted on moving three times within the year. It was when Armand was entered in the third school that he refused to attend, although he had done well in the other two schools. He said that the school was "funny" and had a "curse" on it. He said his teacher was ugly, crippled, and used a cane. He was afraid that she would hit him or put him in a closet.

The mother was said to have pampered Armand to a fantastic degree, as she believed he was something special because he was so beautiful and had been "born circumcised" (subsequent physical examination suggested a mild grade of hypospadia). He had been accident prone; at four years he tripped, fell, and cut his lip, which necessitated five stitches; at six years he fell against a wall and bruised his head.

On his second admission, Armand was even more anxious, withdrawn, and disturbed. Arrangements were made to send him to the children's service of another psychiatric hospital, where he stayed nearly two years. There, he responded well to psychotherapy and seemed well enough to return home. But when this was arranged, the mother had a fainting spell and broke her leg. Even so, he was doing well at home until she returned from the hospital, when he again became anxious, would not attend school, expressed death wishes against the father, said he was to blame for his mother's conditions, and said he would kill himself.[9]

Armand's suicidal preoccupations, which recurred throughout his childhood, were clearly both a reflection of, and reaction to, his mother and his inadequate relationship with his disturbed parents.

The third seven-year-old boy was Joseph:

Joseph's mother reported that he had started showing suicidal tendencies, at the age of three, by throwing himself from beds, chairs, and shelves. At five, he ran out into the traffic in the street, and "escaped being run over 25 or 26 times." However, there had been no accidents, although his mother said she had "saved his life a hundred times." He did not verbally express any suicidal intentions. He did show open anxiety in the hospital because of separation from his mother, which, in turn, brought out some anxiety and guilt on the part of the mother, who told us that although she had wanted her first three children, when she

---

[9] Armand and his two brothers were sent to an institution for normal boys. His mother's mental condition became more unstable and she was finally diagnosed as a severe idiopathic epileptic with epileptic equivalents. On one occasion, she wrote a letter to the clinic physician saying she would kill her sons if they were left at home with her.

All three of the boys got along quite well in the institution, but when Armand was twelve and a half years old, he refused to return to the institution after a home visit; he then ran away from the institution, to his home, a half dozen times. At home, he would not attend school and had temper tantrums, threatening to kill himself if he was not given what he asked for, especially money to go to the movies. After seeing mystery stories at the movies, he would come home in a panic and try to smother himself in his bedclothes. He would not go on the street without a weapon, such as a stick, knife or toy gun. He set fires and fought with other boys. He knew of his mother's threats and said that he was to blame for her nervousness and that she had a miscarriage although he wanted her to have another baby. However, he said he did not really believe that she was very sick. He was committed to a correctional institution and got along well, remaining there until he was sixteen. He then went to live with an aunt in a distant state. He was rejected for military service in World War II.

became pregnant the fourth time, with this child, she attempted to abort herself with lots of pills and foot baths. She had also tried to get rid of the fifth pregnancy, and said the fifth child, a little girl, was also nervous.

On the ward Joseph was shy, anxious, and tense, often crying. His intelligence was dull normal, IQ 83. He said he was bad and therefore his mother and father did not like him or his small sister; but they liked his older sisters because they were good. He cried to go home, until his mother took him. But she returned him in a few days, saying that he had run in front of a bus and might have been killed, that he fell off a chair and hit his head, and that he fought with his siblings. When he was readmitted, he clung to his mother so that he had to be forcibly separated. He threw himself on the floor in a panic of anxiety, screaming, "All right, I'll be good, mother, I'll be good." The mother admitted that for more than a year she had been threatening to send him away if he were not good. After a second period in the hospital, with some satisfying socializing experiences, Joseph returned home, where he remained.[10]

Although his mother had claimed that she wanted her first three children and that therefore they did not present any problems to her, three years after Joseph first came to us his next oldest sister, Lucy, then eleven, came to the hospital in a similar anxiety state. She had been refusing to eat because she did not want to get fat like her mother. The mother was obese. Lucy said that the mother thought of nothing but eating. She called her mother "a fat slob," and "a balloon." The mother said Lucy wanted to spend all her time in movies, and that she would not eat because she wanted to look like a movie star. She said she had lost 25 pounds.

Lucy spoke of dreams in which her mother was dead, and she was afraid her father would fall off a ladder and get killed. Her intelligence was dull normal, IQ 84, but her schoolwork was as good as could be expected for her intelligence. She quickly fell into the ward routine, and ate her meals like the other children. She was sent to a convalescent home for two months, and gained 19 pounds. When she returned home her mother received her halfheartedly, saying that she could stay home as

[10] He was never a satisfactory schoolboy and the schools complained about him and, especially, the home, from time to time. We attempted to do some guidance and other agencies attempted to help in the home, but none of us was ever able to penetrate the mother's dullness and self-satisfaction. In junior high school, Joseph was still presenting problems relative to his dull intelligence. He was a poor student, a flat indifferent personality, and a frequent truant. In 1944, at sixteen, while still in junior high school, he received his working papers and left school. This boy seems to have become submerged by his anxiety and the limitations of the facilities to give him relief.

long as she behaved herself, but if she lost as much as one pound she would send her to a worse place than the convalescent home.[11]

Both Joseph and his sister, Lucy, suffered because of the inadequacy of their mother. It seems probable that when the mother interpreted their behavior as suicidal, she was projecting her own guilt feelings, as well as recognizing their feelings of being hopelessly overwhelmed.

Eight-year-old Frank came to us because of his excessive preoccupations with death. He expressed suicidal intent, and thought continuously of the death of members of his family. He dreamed of death, and was preoccupied with death fantasies most of the day. He was the second of three boys in a substandard Sicilian family which was on welfare relief most of the time. He was born by a breech delivery, and was said to have been black. His development was reported as normal, but his "bad" behavior started when he was four years old. He cried at night and seemed to have frightening dreams. He cried all day and hit his head with his hands, and bit his hands. He quarreled with his siblings, especially his younger brother. He did not want to play with other children.

When he was six years old, he did not want to go to school. His father carried him to school forcibly and slapped him into submission. He refused to enter into the school activities and upset the classroom routine. He started talking about killing himself and others. He tried to cut himself with a knife, and ripped his clothes to pieces. He threatened his brothers, especially the little one, with a knife, but never actually touched them with it.

In the hospital, he was acutely anxious, crying most of the day and crying out in his sleep at night. He said he was bad. "I jump about the house all the time, I scream and kick. I go in the streets and hit kids. My brothers and the other kids bother me. They hit me and I can't fight back. I want to kill myself. I want to kill the kids with a machine gun." Do you have one? "Yes, a BB gun. My father has it to shoot birds. I don't like my mother and father. They don't treat me right. They don't give me supper sometimes. Nobody likes me and I don't like nobody else." What do you want to do when you grow up? "I want to die now and grow up in heaven. I want to be an animal man and kill people." What is an animal man? "A man who lives in the woods like an animal and kills people. I'll starve myself for one hundred days and then I'll be that."

---

[11] Subsequently, complaints came from school of behavior antagonistic to authority, and stubbornness. Arrangements were made to send her to a girls' home, where she was contented and did well.

Dream? "I dream of a red thing with horns, claws and pitchforks. I can't say the name. It's a d - - - . If you touch it, it burns you because you are bad."

He was poorly developed, and undernourished, with an umbilical hernia, refractive error of vision, and a conjunctivitis associated with his continuous crying. No specific neurological deviations were noted. His intelligence was dull normal, IQ 83. He had numerous excoriations on his body which were evidently self-inflicted. Other children reported that he scratched himself with objects, especially on his left arm. The nurses reported seeing him pull a piece of skin from his eyelid. There were fresh abrasions daily. When asked if he still wanted to kill himself, he said, "So I said. I do it to make my father mad. Not exactly that but I don't want to eat and they yell at me and say that I want to kill my brothers."

He was transferred from our service to the children's service of another psychiatric hospital, where he stayed two months. He got along well there, and was reported to show no suicidal preoccupations or tendencies, but when he was returned home he again became disturbed, refused to go to school, fought with his brothers, and started to talk about dying. He was returned to us, and said that, in school, the other kids called him "crazy" because he had been in the hospital, made faces at him, and hit him and pushed him around. He had similar trouble with his brothers at home. He said "I felt like killing them again. I said before, I wanted to die. I wanted to go off to a quiet place and be by myself. My father and mother don't like me, they bring me here."

On this admission, he improved very rapidly, entered into the activities of the other children, and could talk about his previous preoccupations quite objectively. He said that he had felt before that he was so bad that it was hopeless, and he wanted to die, and he wanted his parents to die. Everyone was always hitting him and he felt like hitting anyone near him. It was difficult to understand the dynamics of such a severe reaction.

It was felt that a diagnosis of schizophrenia could not be maintained. Although the marked anxiety and guilt in this boy seemed to be in reaction to the poor and inadequate relationship with the parents, the full implications were not understood at that time.[12]

[12] He returned home, but within a year was having trouble in school, became a truant, was involved in gang activities, stealing, etc., and was sent to a correctional institution. There he had an attack of pneumonia and, while under medical care, it was discovered that he had a muscular weakness. He was referred to a neurological hospital, where a diagnosis was made of progressive muscular atrophy, the fascioscapular form of Landouzy-Dejerine. It was of interest that he said that he had felt weaker than other boys since the age of six, and realized that he could not whistle or blow up a balloon.

Frank's feeling of inadequacy and weakness obviously stemmed from the heredo-degenerative disease, even before the muscular atrophy was evident. In addition, he felt threatened, overwhelmed, and inadequately supported by his parents.

Nine-year-old Peter was preoccupied with death, in all its manifestations. He had threatened suicide since the age of seven, and he expressed the fear that other people would kill him, and the wish that other members of his family would die. He had dreams which included suicide, murder, graveyards, funerals, and various forms of death by violence. He also had waking fantasies on the same subject, and would confabulate freely. At the age of twelve, he was observed again, and showed the same preoccupations. He would get up at night and walk in his sleep. When awakened, he would claim that he was being led by skeletons or Frankensteins who wanted him to follow them "into death" and be their companion. He also expressed open suicidal desires, while under observation. The boy was mentally defective, with an IQ between 60 and 70. He was deeply attached to his father, who had similar preoccupations. On one occasion, the father removed Peter from the hospital because he said that he had heard that we might throw the child out of the window into the river.[13]

\* \* \*

Howard, a ten-year-old boy, had outbursts of violence against others. He expressed the desire to die, and threatened to kill himself. His family

---

At the age of fifteen, while he was home, he stole several hundred dollars that his mother had in the house and spent it on himself and companions. He was returned to the adolescent service of our hospital. His muscular atrophy had progressed considerably, so that his face was atrophied, he was weak, and he limped badly. His intelligence was very dull, IQ 79. He no longer was anxious, depressed or preoccupied with his own death or that of others. He said he had a frequent impulse to have money, and stole it when he could get it, without compunction. He felt that his parents had never cared for him much. A year later we received a communication that his younger brother also had progressive muscular atrophy of the same type as Frank.

[13] Peter was later transferred to a state training school for mental defectives. That institution informed us that he remained there for two years, receiving formal class instruction, and that he did fairly well, although he was neurotic, emotionally unstable, manneristic, and prone to tell fantastic tales. His IQ was 59. At fourteen he was paroled to his parents, remaining under the supervision of this institution for one more year, when he got along fairly well in a public school class for retarded children. In 1942, when he was sixteen, he was taken to an adolescent court on a charge of sexually molesting little girls. He was then referred to a mental hygiene clinic for evaluation, where it was found that his IQ was 55, and that he showed some psychoneurotic and depressive features reactive to his inadequacies and adaptive failures. The court charge against him was not pressed and was, therefore, dismissed.

life was characterized by great violence, due to epileptic furors exaggerated by heavy drinking in the father and hysterical outbursts in the mother. The boy identified himself with the father, for whom he expressed a great hatred and fear. He continually felt threatened and would respond by violence, using such weapons as chairs or window poles. When restrained from injuring others, he would express the desire to die himself. While Howard was in our hospital under observation, his thirteen-year-old brother, who was said to have shown similar behavior, died by hanging himself from a tree in the backyard—although the mother maintained that it was an accidental hanging.

Howard was violently disturbed on our ward, threatening injury to himself, the other children, and the personnel, whenever he was frustrated or even expected to comply with the activities of the other children. His intelligence was good, IQ 96 to 120.[14]

\* \* \*

Ten-year-old Alice, a case of arrested congenital syphilis of the central nervous system without intellectual deterioration, wanted to kill herself when asked to stop a game in order to go home to dinner. She was found in a window with a string about her neck, in an attempt to hang herself. It was a passing episode. The child had suffered enormous psychic traumas throughout her life, at the hands of a mother who was a drug addict and prostitute, who had psychotic episodes, and often used the child to serve her convenience, even to soliciting or obtaining drugs for her. Alice had been in several foster homes and institutions, and had had antiluetic treatment of all forms. Her intelligence was good (IQ 100 to 116).[15]

[14] He was transferred to a children's service of a state hospital. At first, he was violently disturbed there, to the point of requiring restraint. But he soon benefited very much from the program of activities, and had several visits home. Howard remained in the hospital for three and a half years, returning home when he was ready for high school. Although the home situation was unfavorable, as his father was abusive and fed and clothed him inadequately, Howard, while under parole supervision, did well in school and kept out of trouble for a while. Later, however, he was charged with an auto theft and possession of a gun. In 1952, when he was twenty-six, his father died. His two brothers returned home (one from an army camp); the three brothers became intoxicated and desecrated a synagogue, for which they were charged with vandalism.

[15] From our ward, she was sent to the children's service of a state hospital, where she presented a rather erratic picture. At times she was very active, happy, cooperative, and functioned at her highest intelligence (IQ 116). Intermittently, she was acutely disturbed, meddlesome, and seemed dull and deteriorating (IQ 89). On one occasion, when she was twelve, she made suicidal threats and an attempt (by swallowing pins), but this also seemed like a passing occurrence. Her mother died and parole to an aunt was tried, but was unsuccessful. When she was fifteen, she was paroled to a second aunt, had some trade training, and finally secured a simple job placement without further turmoil. This girl was certainly reacting to a completely overwhelming situation, in which she had totally inadequate support from parental figures.

John, a ten-year-old Negro boy, was mentally defective. He had been placed in a pediatric hospital because of an attack of acute rheumatic fever. He had previously been antagonistic and unruly in school. He resisted hospitalization. When forcibly admitted, he threatened to throw himself out of bed and out of a window. He was aggressive to the other children, and threatened to kill them if they came near him.[16]

\* \* \*

Ruth, eleven years old, had been reared in institutions. Meanwhile, her mother remarried and had another family. Ruth resented this deeply. She wanted the attention of her mother. When at home, she wanted her mother's constant expression of affection. She once told her mother that her baby brother had thrown himself out of the window and had been killed. For this story, she was severely reprimanded by her mother, whereupon she threatened suicide by throwing herself out of the window. In the hospital, she accepted the charge nurse as a mother substitute and was contented as long as she had the attention of this nurse. When the nurse was off the ward, she repeatedly attempted to kill herself. She would hide, try to choke herself with her hands, and try to climb on the roof to jump off. She would talk to the other children of her desire to die, and encouraged them to join her. She threatened to cut her throat.[17]

\* \* \*

Paul, an eleven-year-old boy, was brought to us because of persistent truancy and stubborn antagonistic behavior in the home when he was disciplined. In the hospital he threatened to kill himself and said he would be taken out of the hospital in a coffin if he were not allowed to go home. He escaped and returned to his home, but willingly permitted his parents to bring him back for more help. His intelligence was average

---

[16] When he recovered from his acute illness, he was transferred to a training school for defective children, where he remained until he was sixteen years old. His IQ was 73. He received schooling through fourth grade and then trained in the work groups of the institution. He was paroled to his home at sixteen, and, for a year, was reported to be steadily employed and behaving well at home.

[17] She was transferred to the children's service of a state hospital, but was kept there only a few months. At home, she again ran away and was sent to a girls' training school. She ran away from there to get home. When she was paroled home, she ran away from home to get back to the training school. She was returned to the training school, where she remained until she was sixteen. She ran away, traveled through several states, but kept her mother, or the social worker of the agency that was interested in her, posted as to her whereabouts. When last heard from, she was with a small western traveling carnival, where she did various jobs, from being the lady that was sawed in half to ticket taker. Ruth's suicidal tendencies, and confabulations of death of a sibling, were clearly a reaction against her deprived childhood, separation from, and rejection by, the mother, and, in part, a spite reaction against this mother.

and he was capable of average schoolwork. He had defective vision and infected tonsils. Glasses were fitted, his tonsils removed, and, with some guidance, he later did well in school, except for one period when he was again truant for a short time.[18]

\* \* \*

Anthony, an eleven-year-old Italian Catholic boy, developed acute anxiety, with feelings of guilt, in connection with an episode in which he confessed he had played sexually with little girls. He wanted to kill himself by jumping from a window. For that reason, he was brought to the children's service at Bellevue Hospital. He said that he had played "doctor" with a six-year-old girl. He confessed it, and felt that all the neighbors knew about it. He was also hypochondriacal. Subsequently, there was doubt as to whether the episode was real or fantasied.[19]

\* \* \*

Gilbert was first known to our mental hygiene clinic when he was eight years of age. He was the only child of a psychopathic mother and had been deserted by his father. He was a forceps delivery, and had a swelling over the anterior fontanelle for six weeks after birth. At four months, he had a severe convulsion. The mother had always rather openly expressed her rejection of him, and he spent most of his early childhood in two different institutions and several boarding homes. He had broken his wrist, at seven years, and had several minor head injuries. He had average intelligence.

At eight years, when he came to our clinic, he was preoccupied with his own death, his mother's, and that of anyone else who played any role in his life. He threatened to kill himself by drinking various fluids, and threatened and attempted to stab and choke his mother. To the clinic physician, he said, "I really mean to kill myself. I'll drink ink. I'll be in the papers tomorrow."

[18] He joined the army in 1941 and served in Army Occupation in Germany until 1947. He married and had a child. In this case, the suicidal threat seemed to have been rather casual and not a serious preoccupation.

[19] At fifteen, he came back to the hospital because of an acute anxiety episode, in which he was preoccupied with masturbation guilt and had hypochondriasis. This time, it was learned that his father was a seriously disturbed person, who made sexual advances to his daughters; and he had many serious hypochondriacal complaints, which resembled Anthony's. The mother, and the rest of the family, as well as Anthony, were all reacting to this disturbed father, with various anxiety responses. Anthony was considered schizophrenic by some of the physicians who saw him, at this time, but others thought that he showed a mixed psychoneurosis. He was discharged and referred to a neighborhood clinic for psychotherapy, but he reported there only once, in 1940. After finishing school, he stayed home unemployed, while the family was on public relief, and was classified as unacceptable (4F) for World War II military service.

At eleven, he received antuitrin-S for several weeks, for an undescended testicle—unsuccessfully. Afterward he was brought to the children's ward. His mother related that for two years he had been increasingly impulsive. For a year, he had been having convulsions. She said, "He tried to choke me. Maybe I got mad and choked him. Maybe he saw it in the movies. He bit me and I told him to bite himself and he has done it ever since. 'Kill' is his first, last and every word, 'kill' and 'murder.' He talks a lot about Dick Tracy. He got nothing but hatred from his father. He was always looking for him just the same." In the interval, he had been in several other psychiatric and neurological hospitals and clinics, and had been variously diagnosed as epileptic, psychoneurotic, and psychopathic. It was our impression that he had an organic brain disorder related to anoxia at birth, with an impulse disorder, an increased anxiety, and a need for much more emotional support than his rejecting mother gave him. He also tended to mirror, or overreact to his mother's instabilities and inadequacies.[20]

This boy, like several of the others described in this section, showed the development of increased impulses on an organic basis. At the same time, he was deprived of the needed support and love of his parents, and reacted with strong anxiety and aggression. As a young adult, he adjusted at a retarded or deteriorated level, with emotional flatness. He found refuge in an institution, and no longer showed either anxiety or aggression. It is true that he also had convulsions, and, as an adult, was obviously organically inferior. Most of his irritability was turned against his mother, while, according to her, he constantly sought for the absent and disinterested father.

Edward, a Negro boy of eleven, had suicidal dreams. He was a high

[20] He went to a private school for problem children for several years. In 1941 at the age of fifteen, an air encephalogram showed a left cerebral cortical atrophy. The next year, he was sent to a state hospital, because of increasing aggressiveness, which was described as vicious. He was diagnosed as psychotic, with epilepsy with deterioration. A year later, he was paroled to his mother. In 1950 at twenty-five years of age, he was returned to a state hospital, because of his excessive irritability and assaultiveness to his mother. He was described as disproportionately developed, with a large head, small scrawny limbs, and a dwarflike body. He had a bilateral nystagmus. Intellectually, he appeared immature and showed organic deterioration, with repetitiveness, misuse of words, and impairment in general knowledge, calculation, and insight. He was emotionally flat, seemed contented to be in the institution, expressed no resentment against his mother, showed no interest in his future, and continued to be amiable and undisturbed in the institution. The general impression was that of an epileptic deterioration.

grade defective with an IQ of 63, who was placed in the ungraded classes at school. He was referred to us by the school, because of excited outbursts—usually rages in which he menaced the other children. He admitted this difficulty and said his worst trouble was his temper. He said he couldn't learn in school and felt bad about it. The other children called him dumb and this angered him. The same thing happened at home with his brothers and sisters. He said he dreamed that he killed himself because the children called him dumb. In his dream, he jumped out of the window and crushed his skull. When he woke up, he didn't know what had happened. He said he once threatened to jump from a window, in school, when he had been taken to the principal's office for one of his temper outbursts. When the principal expressed his disbelief, he actually attempted it, but was caught on the window sill. He also said that he dreamed he was a lonely boy, without a home or place to go, with nothing to eat, and no one to care for him, so he killed himself by leaping from a window. He reported that when he was a baby, he actually did jump from the window of a fourth-floor room. He heard his brother calling him from the yard, and, on finding the door locked, he jumped out of the window because he didn't know better. He fell four floors but his fall was broken by a clothesline and he was not injured.

This boy told us that he had a religious problem. His father was a deacon in the neighboring Baptist church, which all of the family attended, all being devoted to their religion. For two years, however, Edward had found himself unable to attend this church, but attended a neighboring Catholic church, instead. Something inside of him made him do this. He felt that it was a real problem, but his father did not blame him and let him attend the church of his choice. He seemed very devoted to his father, and often expressed his love for him. He carried a little wallet with a picture of his father. He said that his father gave him the rosary, but later explained that he meant the Catholic father or priest of his church. He had another dream in which he was down South. Someone had committed a murder and he was accused, tried, found guilty, and had the rope around his neck to be hung, when they brought up a man who said he was the guilty one. This man looked just like his father so Edward decided to take the blame and was hanged. Subsequently, he remarked that this man could not have been his father.

This was a mentally inferior boy, inadequate himself and inadequately cared for, or emotionally supported, according to his need. He identified himself with his father. He had an accident, falling out of a window, at four, when he was nearly killed. He

313

seemed compulsively to re-enact this episode throughout his life, in dreams and fantasies, threats and attempts. He had remarkably good insight. The dynamics were remarkably clear, as they may be in the dull child or high grade mental defective.[21]

Two boys of twelve considered and threatened suicide because of epileptic convulsions which made it impossible for them to live normal lives or plan on the future as other boys could.

Harris was the only child of a psychotic mother who suffered from a manic depressive psychosis which led to repeated hospitalization most of her adult life. She had been in a hospital continuously since Harris was one year old. The father had taken a widow into the home; a woman with two children of her own to care for. He believed, or he stated, that Harris thought this was his mother, though everyone knew differently. There were no problems until Harris was eleven, when he began to run away from home and claim he had no parents. He seemed to be in doubt as to his identity. He was sent to a camp, where it was first noticed that he frequently dropped things in what seemed to be slight spells. On our ward, he said, "I'm here because it goes like that— (snapping his fingers). I am doing something and it goes like that—. I used to steal before I was ten or eleven, everything I could get my hands on. I'd steal perfume from the dime stores and give it away. My mother is dead. This one is an aunt, sometimes she is too severe with me. She tells on me to my father and she exaggerates, and then he hits me."

He had many types of twitches, tremors, tics, and, also, frequent petit mal absences, when he would lift his right hand and turn his head to the side and drop whatever was in his hand. He also had one grand mal convulsion in the hospital. He was impulsively domineering and righteously indignant at the misbehavior of other children, but stubborn in insisting that his own behavior should not be criticized. The father would not consider institutionalization because of the mother's history.

He was taken home, but his condition got rapidly worse. He was irritable, stubborn, and unadaptable. He was apparently interested in self-

[21] Edward was transferred to a state school for mental defectives, where he remained for two years. It was reported that he did not adjust very satisfactorily, and had to be continually watched. After a visit at home on vacation, the father asked to have him stay, which he did on a parole basis. It was again reported that the adjustment was not satisfactory, and he was followed in a mental hygiene clinic, where he had been referred from a school because of rages. The school considered him dangerous, but there was no serious difficulty. His parents refused to let him return to the institution. He applied at the hospital, where the clinic was located, for a job in 1943 when he was seventeen, but this was not given to him. In 1945 he stated that he had been in the Navy and had been discharged. He refused specific information or authorization to obtain data. In 1949, he was at home in a dependent position.

314

injury. He would insist on long baths, where he would duck his head under the water and hold his breath. His foster mother was in terror lest he drown himself. When he was readmitted, he was having pyknoleptic seizures ten to fifteen times an hour. He was tense, irritable, and assaultive, and could not get along with the other children. He admitted he wanted to drown himself.[22]

Edward, a twelve-year-old epileptic boy, was living in a Catholic institution. His father was a barge captain and his mother worked as a maid in a hospital. He had been a chronic truant, a runaway, and begged on the street, telling tall tales of his lack of home and parents, etc. He had "spells" two to three times a month, in which he described prickly sensations in the chest, extending down the left arm, when his left hand became numb and was clenched, and he started to feel faint. He felt that he had to grasp out for something to keep from falling. He did fall, if he did not catch on to something, although he never became completely unconscious. He frequently became very depressed, in the institution, and once cut himself with a razor. He said he would do away with himself, and, on another occasion, was found in the bathroom with the window screen out, obviously intending to jump. On our children's ward, he was impulsive, irritable, and moody. He said he would rather die than have these spells. He was afraid he would clutch at someone when he was having the spell and choke them or tear their windpipe out. Since the convulsions were focal, it was thought possible to operate. He begged for this operation, but his parents would not consent.[23]

The suicidal trends of these two epileptic boys were of interest, because of the general belief that epileptics do not commit suicide. Charles Prudhomme, however, found from questionnaires to private physicians and institutions who cared for epileptics, and surveys of incidence of suicide in epileptics, that this was not true. He found

[22] He was transferred to a state hospital, where it was subsequently reported that his condition continued to deteriorate, and he was not able to be cared for on the wards with other children for some months, but after that his convulsive phenomena subsided, and he spent two years on the children's ward, before he was discharged. He attended a vocational high school, where his work was satisfactory and he was active in student activities. However, he became increasingly irritable and, after a series of convulsions, was sent to the state epileptic colony, in 1941. He was said to have been a difficult patient there, getting into disputes with other patients, until he escaped three years later, in 1944.

[23] He was transferred to the state epileptic colony, where his behavior was reported as unsatisfactory. He frequently ran away, and disobeyed all reasonable rules. He had two grand mal convulsions while there. He finally escaped, in 1939, and was kept home by his parents.

that the suicidal incidence in epileptics was about three times as great as that of the general population.

Jean was a thirteen-year-old girl who had attained puberty. Her mother died when she was three years old. Because she was a bed wetter, and not an attractive child, none of her relatives felt that they cared to take her, and she was reared in a Catholic institution. She was visited by her father and always looked forward to the time when she would leave the institution. Her father died when she was twelve years old and at the age of puberty. She became depressed and moody, and withdrew from the other children. They called her "crazy," and she said she tried to live up to this role. She devoted herself to religious ceremonies, sometimes deliberately acted as though she were in a dazed state, would eat ants, and attempted to kill herself by scratching her wrists, which would become infected because she continued to pick at them.

In the hospital, she continually protested that no one loved her and that she might as well be dead. She was an unattractive, fat, pudgy child, with hypertrophied breasts. She admitted to one of the doctors that she would rather be a boy than have such breasts and that they were her chief grounds for distress. After this confidence, she was badly upset and said she wanted to die. She wandered from window to window, either trying to get out or trying to find a chance to break a piece of glass and cut her wrists. Later, she improved, with weight reduction, and returned to the convent, but, in a few months, she was brought back because she would not allow anyone to approach her when she was undressed. In the course of routine admission care, it was found that she had a large breast abscess, which she admitted was the result of a self-inflicted wound. This healed slowly because she would probe the area with pencils or hairpins, when not observed. Subsequently, she again improved, especially as she developed an interest in some of the boys on the ward. But on one occasion, when one of the boys refused to answer a note, in which she asked if he would be her boy friend, she again scratched her wrists and said she wanted to die.[24]

Jean had been badly traumatized by the death of both parents, and deprivation throughout childhood. Her physical deviation,

[24] She was sent to the children's service of a state hospital, where she remained for seven years. At first, she was inclined to be seclusive and emotionally unstable, unable to relate to other people. She had frequent temper outbursts. A diagnosis of schizophrenia was entertained, but as the behavior disorder seemed to subside, leaving a mildly withdrawn, socially cold, and slightly unstable personality, it was thought that she showed the dynamics of psychopathic personality development. Her intelligence remained about average. After leaving the hospital, she entered domestic employment and was getting along without difficulty when last heard from.

316

especially her large breasts, further made it difficult for her to relate to other people. Her serious personality deviation may have been primary or secondary.

Tony was a fourteen-year-old boy, constitutionally inferior, from a family with poor social standards. The father had been in a state hospital for a year. Tony was a borderline defective, and had a congenital or rachitic deformity of the back and chest, which dwarfed his height and distorted his posture. He had been in children's court several times, for serious charges, including entering a store with a loaded gun, the source of which he would not explain, and threatening another boy with a knife. His family always protected him. Both he and his family were openly antagonistic to hospitalization, and resented any efforts to examine the boy in any way. For example, they opposed every effort to examine his deformity or correct it. When he was not discharged at the time he wanted to be, he burst into an unreasoning emotional frenzy. He threatened and attempted to kill the nurses and doctors about him by throwing chairs and every object he could get. When thwarted in this, he screamed that he would kill himself, and attempted to bang his head against the walls and choke himself with his hands.[25]

This boy had a deforming and disabling organic disorder, inferior intelligence, and an inferior family, who did not give him adequate social concepts or protection. The whole family was characterized by antisocial, explosive, and aggressive behavior. Interestingly, this boy, as he passed through adolescence, tended to become compliant and conciliatory, although he engaged in antisocial acts when he could.

[25] He was sent to a state hospital, but was paroled in a few months on the insistence of his family. He threatened to shoot his mother with another gun that he had gotten, if she did not give him money for the movies. He was returned to the state hospital, but subsequently escaped with the help of a brother. He was next heard from five years later, when he was twenty. He received a reformatory sentence for petit larceny, having snatched a woman's pocketbook because, as he said, "I needed money." While in the institution, he confessed to setting a fire in some papers under a bench, but later insisted that he was forced into the confession by other inmates, who would otherwise have beaten him. He claimed that because he was small, weak, and couldn't protect himself from the other inmates, he was forced to do their bidding, give them cigarettes weekly, etc. He was transferred to the penitentiary, because of the fire. His earlier history was apparently not known in either of these institutions, at that time. He was described as a docile, infantile, immature, small man, with a rachitic deformity of the chest. He was always afraid of being abused by others. His family insisted that there was no history of difficulties, and that the boy was slow because he had been kept back in school. Several psychometric examinations gave him an IQ of 55 to 66. The family again wanted him home, but he was sent to an institution for the criminally defective.

Emily was a fourteen-year-old girl who was unusually mature for her age. Her mother had died, and her father was an abusive, alcoholic individual, who expected this child to keep house for him and accept his abusive, alcoholic behavior. She took iodine as her only way out of an impossible situation, but gladly accepted the help we were able to give her.[26]

\* \* \*

Helen was a fifteen-year-old girl who was brought to us from a child placement agency, because of recurring episodes of hysterical behavior, in which she would attempt or threaten suicide. These episodes seemed to coincide, to some extent, with her menstrual periods, which had begun at the age of thirteen. She was the child of a psychotic mother, had been born in a state hospital and had been reared in her early years by one or another relative, much of the time by her inadequate grandmother and indifferent father. She began running away from home at the age of eight, when her mother was home on parole for a period. She was deeply sensitive concerning her mother's condition, and felt that if she were properly understood and cared for, she could be at home and the family reunited. She wrote to her mother regularly and fantasied the ideal home life, which she expressed in the stories, plays, and poems that she wrote and the pictures she painted. She had been living in boarding homes for years, but repeatedly ran away in order to get to her own home. She made dramatic scenes, apparently to gain attention in the schools and homes. Her suicidal efforts included tying jumping ropes around her neck until forcibly removed, swallowing pen points, running into the road in the path of automobiles, swallowing ink, slashing her arms and legs with long scratches and smearing the slashes with ink, trying to choke herself with her hands, and scratching her neck with her fingernails. Similar episodes were observed in the hospital, together with silly, annoying behavior, which always brought disapproval and punishment from the other children and nurses—which seemed to please her. She considered herself very dumb, unattractive, and unlovable, and seemed to do what she could to act out this role.[27]

---

[26] She was sent to a Catholic home for girls where it was reported that she needed a good deal of training. The father subsequently remarried and Emily went home to him and the new stepmother. Apparently things did not go very well as she was subsequently sent to a Catholic correctional institution.

[27] She was sent to a children's institution, where she remained until she was eighteen years old. At the age of twenty-one, in 1941, she was admitted to a state mental hospital for chronic patients, where she remained. She has had to be catered to and has acted in a childish, dull, almost defective manner, although her IQ was 83, as late as 1947, when she was twenty-seven. She has had periods of excitement, when she has made suicidal gestures or attempts at self-injury, usually by swallowing small objects.

This girl had a deprived and traumatic childhood. She had a psychotic mother with whom she tried to identify. Finally, she herself was psychotic.

Frank, fifteen years old, turned on the gas when his mother married a young man. He said that his mother was not happy and he wanted them both to die. Lily, fifteen years old, took Mercurochrome, because of the home situation. The father had deserted and Lily saw her beautiful mother exhausting herself trying to do laundry work to support the family, while Lily was expected to prepare the family meals. The situation seemed equally hopeless to both child and mother. Lily had threatened suicide three times, before actually trying it. She would not accept the offer to go to camp, but insisted on returning home to continue aiding her mother. Louis, age fifteen, took iodine, because of school troubles. He wanted to change a program which he found too difficult, but the whole family argued against him and he found himself in an untenable position. Lucy, age fifteen, threatened to kill herself and her father, because of her inability to dissuade her father from his old-world ideas of how a girl should act. She wanted the freedom and independence of a young American girl. When she came in after eight o'clock, and her father attempted to beat her, she responded with threats of death against him and herself.

These adolescents are referred to rather briefly, because they did not stay in the hospital long enough to permit the intensive studies that are usually possible on the children under observation for more general behavior disorders, in which the suicidal preoccupations were incidental. The adolescents were frequently admitted to the hospital because of the suicidal episode, and then discharged in a few days. It will be noted, however, that, in the case of most of these adolescents, the situation that precipitated the suicidal attempt was an incident in family living, in which the girl or boy felt that his position was untenable, often because of the relationship with an unsympathetic or asocial father, and sometimes because of sexual problems of the parents. G. Schmidt reported a number of attempts at suicide in adolescents, and discussed the mechanisms involved in terms of the psychology of adolescence. He claimed that suicide, at this age, could not be explained by the interplay of character abnormalities and traumatic events alone, nor by the

319

adult mechanism of escape, but, rather, it was more closely related to real inner difficulties and the emotional lability that characterizes this age period, combined with the conflicts arising from the outside.

As Zilboorg (1936, 1937) pointed out, psychiatric studies, concerning suicides in children, are lacking in the literature. Our material is too small for statistical conclusions. Our cases were observed between 1933 and 1936, when about 2000 children were admitted on the children's service of the Psychiatric Division of Bellevue Hospital. Our reports are complete only concerning the children under the age of thirteen, as adolescents were usually cared for by services other than the children's service. There were eighteen children, under the age of thirteen, who showed preoccupations or tendencies to suicide. In this age group, the preponderance of boys is obvious, even considering that, on the average, there are twice as many boys as girls admitted to our children's service. In the other statistics quoted, suicide in childhood is two to three times as common in boys, as in girls. Dublin and Bunzel (1933) found only a small prevalence of suicide in boys below the age of fifteen. According to Zilboorg, Argentine statistics point in the opposite direction. In the majority of our cases, we found obvious conscious motives for the suicidal preoccupations in the situation of the child. The child seemed to want to escape a situation which appeared unbearable to him. The only six-year-old boy feared being committed as a "court case," after both parents had died. Others felt unhappy in foster homes, resented the separation from parents, or felt inadequate and insufficiently protected and supported by the situation, because of constitutional weaknesses, epileptic convulsions, or intellectual inferiority. In puberty, preoccupations about ugliness and deformity played a part and worries about the family situation, especially in connection with the sex problems of the parents, played an outstanding part. Some cases included school troubles and parental interference with desired activities. In several instances, psychotic or psychopathic parents were openly aggressive, sometimes against others, in defense of the child or themselves; but, often, their aggression was also directed against the child. In some instances, there did not seem to be an obvious motive at the time, as in seven-year-old Joseph, who continuously exposed himself to dangers. But later, when his sister came with the same problem, it was more evident that the mother was insufficient and, at times, aggressively hostile. In two cases, children with suicidal tendencies came from aggressive families. One child had a father who was pre-occupied with problems of death, and one boy had suicidal dreams, which originated in connection with impulses which remained unconscious, of hate for the father.

Unwillingness to stand a difficult situation can be the motive for suicidal threats and attempts in some children. It was remarkable that two of these children were decidedly inferior, from an organic point of view, and a third one proved to have a progressive muscular atrophy. However, suicidal reactions may also be found in children without organic damage to the central nervous system.

Hall (1905) mentioned that suicide may be committed by children for trivial causes, and often from blind and sudden impulses. No psychological reaction, however, can be completely isolated from a specific background. In all these children, the immediate situation was important in that it was overwhelming. In all the preadolescent children in this study, with the possible exception of Paul, the situation seemed genuinely serious enough, and even more so after our follow-up studies indicated that serious degenerative diseases or psychoses followed in the family pattern, in nearly half of the group.

On closer scrutiny, it appeared that, even in acute reactions, escape was not the only motive. The suicidal threat asserts the independence of the child and punishes those who have interfered or proved inadequate. There is hardly any suicidal case in which the motive of spite does not play an important part. This was not so obvious in the two epileptic cases, but, in both of these cases, resentment against parents was also present, and it might be expected that the general aggressiveness found in epileptics played some part.

It is doubtful whether children expect to actually succeed in committing suicide, or even realize what suicide or death implies. It may be that they hope to be thwarted, and thus be reassured of love and care. These motives are not fully conscious, even in the children who react to an immediate situation. One cannot understand the unconscious motives for suicide, in children, unless one gives careful consideration to their family situation. The child needs the parents and their love, both biologically and psychologically. Death of the parents, especially when it occurs suddenly and mysteriously (as in the case of our six-year-old), must necessarily make the psychological situation so unbearable that even a small deprivation can lead to the suicide wish.

Two of our seven-year-old children were reported to be particularly pampered by their parents, and reacted with suicidal attempts to what appeared to be an insignificant disappointment. Subsequent studies, however, showed that the home situation was very threatening in both cases. One mother was violently epileptic, and dangerously threatened her other children while favoring this boy. Eleven-year-old Ruth obviously felt rejected by her mother, and had developed particular hate against a newborn half-brother. Her suicidal tendencies disappeared when she found a mother substitute, first in the ward nurse, and later in an aunt; she finally adjusted well, in the circus role of the woman that is cut in two. The Negro boy, with the suicidal dreams, obviously felt rejected by his father. He, himself, was inadequate and desperately needed an accepting and supporting father. Thirteen-year-old Jean lost her mother when she was three and her father when she was twelve. She felt unloved, started to give too much attention to her body, and attempted to mutilate her disfiguring breasts. A suicide attempt occurred when a boy refused to let her call him her boy friend. She subsequently accepted her unloved role in life, by becoming dull and undemanding. Fifteen-year-old Helen felt deprivation of love, because of mental disease in her mother and the indifference of her father. Helen was the only definitely schizophrenic individual in the series, although Jean had a long period of hospitalization when the diagnosis of schizophrenia was considered. Anthony seemed, to some of us, to be schizophrenic, but did not need state hospital care. Zilboorg (1936) —after referring to the medieval view that suicide was a sin and the work of the devil, and since "Many works of the Devil have come down to the present in the guise of severe neuroses and psychosis"—sought for dynamics common to the severe neuroses and psychosis, and the "pathological depression" which occurs with suicide.

In Chapter VI it was shown that deprivation of love increases the aggressiveness of children. In most of these children, disappointments provoked aggressiveness. In some cases, the increase in aggressiveness was not provoked merely by rejection, but the children came from extremely aggressive families, and an identification with aggressive parents and siblings took place. Aggressiveness, prevented from expressing itself against others, is often directed against one's self. One punishes the aggressor by acts directed toward one's self, when one identifies one's self with the aggressor. This is obvious in the case of the Negro boy, who dreamed that he was hanged instead of his father who committed a murder. The motives of spite have a close relationship to this problem. The feeling of guilt for aggressive actions is connected with the deeper motives for aggressiveness. In one seven-year-old boy, sadomasochistic fantasies and storytelling were outstanding. The strength of aggressive impulses is dependent on the family history, as well as on the drives of the individual. As noted before, we again refer to the chorea case, and also point to the fact that a tendency to run away, as an expression of restlessness, was frequently present in our suicidal cases. This factor may also explain why children of this type so often expose themselves to accidents, and are reckless, especially in relation to big cars. Analysis of adults who showed this reckless behavior in childhood very often shows that sadomasochistic attitudes against the parent combine with constitutional and organic factors.

The child reacts to deprivation concerning love by aggression which punishes the parents if they are considered responsible. It is destructive against both the parent and self. In this connection, death may mean destruction. We have mentioned that death is also an escape for the child, and a return to a more peaceful existence. This peaceful existence also means being reunited with the parents. This may be especially true in cases where the parents are dead. The object relation to the dead precedes identification with the dead person, which Zilboorg stressed as an unconscious motive for suicide. Only two of our cases showed this mechanism. We did not find any hints of this in other cases, although it may have played a part in some of the other orphans. The suicidal threat, and the death wish, unite the child with the ideal parent of his fantasy and gain for him the love and forgiveness of the surviving parent.

There was a conspicuous trend for the child to try to identify with parents who were either aggressive, psychotic, narcissistic, or rejecting. These mechanisms stood out plainly, and indicated the child's violent reaction with resentment, hopelessness, or confusion, when such attempts were unrewarding. For example, Armand (especially later when his mother was more psychotic) failed in his repeated efforts to get close to his mother, even though she favored him. Joseph apparently accepted and reflected his mother's idea that she "saved his life a hundred times" from self-destructive behavior, while actually, she may have exaggerated, as no one but herself saw much of it. His sister even more clearly expressed this mechanism, by refusing to eat as much as her mother urged, saying that she would not be a "fat slob" like her mother. Defective Peter, John, and Ed all failed, because their fathers were not satisfactory father-images for identification, and all had fearful fantasies and dreams which expressed this problem. In these boys, there was a strong compulsive tendency to repeat the aggressive, self-destructive pattern of behavior.

Death also means to be pardoned for one's aggressiveness. We find no better illustration for this than the analysis of an adult with a depression of mild degree, in which hate against the father and mother, and against the wife, was paramount. He protested against the demands they made on him, and was particularly incensed because his mother demanded of him, from earliest childhood, that he should be grateful for the life she had given to him. Between the ages of nine and eleven, he repeatedly decided that he would kill himself and give his life back to his mother. He decided that he would go into a muddy creek and suffocate. He never made a suicidal attempt, but occasionally ran away from home. In his fantasies, he was often afraid of being buried in quicksand. The suicidal fantasies were a symbolic return to the mother whom he consciously spurned.

This last observation leads us to examine the methods the children used in their suicidal wishes and attempts. Usually children threaten to jump out of the window, which is seemingly the simplest way of escape. It is a way out. Our material does not offer any conclusive proof that jumping out of the window represents rebirth fantasies. When the aggressive motives are stronger, cutting oneself, stabbing and more violent methods of suicide may play a part. Two of the children tried to choke themselves. Running in front of automobiles represented the masochistic side of the problem. Several of the older children took poison. Our material was not sufficient to explore the symbolic meaning of this type of suicidal attempt.

One cannot understand suicidal attitudes unless one keeps in mind what death means to the child and the adult. The studies of Bromberg, Wechsler and myself (Chapter IV) have tried to elucidate the various meanings of death: (1) An escape from an unbearable situation—in death, one lives a new life, without any of the difficulties of the present life; (2) a method to force others to give more love than they are willing to grant in life; (3) an equivalent for the final sexual union with the ideal mate; and (4) the final narcissistic perfection, which grants eternal and unchallenged importance to the individual, the gratification of masochistic tendencies. This is true for the adult. In the child's conception of death, the idea that death is provoked by violence has a greater importance. Furthermore, death is not considered an irreversible deprivation. The wish for perfection obviously plays a less important part in the child's conception of death. It is, furthermore, obvious that aggressive and sadistic attitudes play a more important part in suicidal attempts which involve violent actions, in children as well as in adults.

On the basis of these studies, we came to the following formulations concerning suicidal tendencies in childhood. The child reacted to an unbearable situation by attempting to escape. Mostly, these unbearable situations consisted of deprivation of love, or, at least, the child assumed that the love was insufficient to meet his needs which, in some of these cases, were especially great because of an organic inadequacy or social deprivation. The deprivation provoked aggressive tendencies, which were primarily directed against those who denied love. Under the influence of feelings of guilt, these aggressive tendencies were turned against the self. The aggressive tendencies may have been increased by constitutional factors, by identification with an aggressive parent or other aggressive member of the family, or by another of the factors which increase aggressiveness (as we have described them in Chapter VI). There was also a strong, compulsive repetitive tendency to re-enact aggressive behavior observed in the parents, or an impressive childhood incident, such as falling out of the window. The suicidal attempt also constituted a punishment against the surroundings, and served as a method for getting a greater amount of love. The suicidal death also represented a reunion with the love object, in love and peace. Suicides which follow disappointments in love, in children, are, again, attempts to regain the love object, which in the deeper sense is always one of the parents. Klein (1934) discussed suicide in similar terms, saying that the "fantasies that underlie suicide aim at preserving the internalized good object and also destroying the part of the ego that is identified with the bad object. Thus the ego becomes united with its love object."

In the subsequent careers of these children, who fantasied, threatened, and attempted suicide, it became progressively more evident that they were threatened by turmoil, both from within themselves and from their outside situations, which became increasingly difficult. In no instance, however, in the course of more than fourteen years, when all of these children had become adults, did any of them actually kill themselves. Furthermore, they tended either to direct their aggression against the environment in asocial and delinquent behavior, or to submit to the intolerable situation, suffering emotional and intellectual flattening, and, in many instances, accepting refuge in institutions.

## NEUROSIS FOLLOWING HEAD INJURY[28]

Traumatic neurosis following head injury is not necessarily based on the anatomical consequences (and their psychological reflections), but may merely be related to the psychic experience of the trauma or the psychological attitudes pertaining to injuries of the head in general. Attitudes of the personality, in connection with life problems, may transform the concussion syndrome into a unit colored by personality tendencies.

Children may present pictures of this type.

Arthur, twelve years old, was admitted to a general hospital after being struck by an automobile and landing on his head. On admission, he was conscious, and drowsy, but he answered questions clearly. He told a fantastic story in relation to the accident, complained about pain in his head, right shoulder, and right chest, and vomited shortly after admis-

[28] From Schilder (1940a). Only those parts of his paper dealing with children are quoted here. For a discussion of adult case histories see the original paper.

sion. There was a large hematoma over the left parietal and right frontal regions. There were bilateral Babinski toe signs and ankle clonus. The spinal fluid was bloody. Throughout the patient's stay in the hospital, he was difficult to control, tried to get out of bed, pleaded to go home, and stated that his father or mother would die if he did not go home. He threatened to cause the doctors and nurses to disappear by magic. Nine days later, he was transferred to Bellevue Hospital (Psychiatric Division). At that time, he was oriented and gave a rational account of his accident. However, he was dominated by anxiety and restlessness. He showed quick changes of mood, called continually for his mother and father, and did not stay in bed. He reported dreams in which he was an aviator who crashes and gets killed; also that he put a bear trap in the chimney to catch Santa Claus. The X-ray examination revealed a vertical fracture of the squamous portion of the temporal bone on the left side. There were bilateral Babinski toe signs and a dropping of the left arm. Two days later he was tense and overalert, very anxious to hold his contact with persons around him, and continually seeking assurance. He now described the accident in the following way:

He was playing in the park with other boys, and told them, "Well, I will go home," and he thought about it and hoped it wasn't late because to warm up dinner again would make trouble for his mother. He remembered that he crossed the street half-heartedly and did not look at the lights or notice that a car was coming. The next thing he remembered was that he awoke in the hospital. He said that it is very bad to be hit, and if he ever finds that he is hit by an automobile again, he hopes we will "sock" him in the eye. He certainly will be careful in the future. He had thought about other boys who were "hit by automobiles and were run over their stomachs and crushed their heads and they were dead." When telling this, he started to cry and wanted to go home to his mother (the day before he had called the nurse "mother"). "I wanted to get to my mother and had a feeling that whoever was taking care of me was my mother." The boy asked constantly to go home and to get to his mother. It seemed as if he would be sure he was not dead, and nothing could happen to him once he could get to his mother or father. In the first hospital, he had been told that his mother and father were dead. He said, "I awoke in the hospital and I saw my father and he told me what happened. My father said there was no blood. If I bled out of my nose and ears I would have had a hemorrhage and it would have been bad." His death fears and anxieties expressed themselves in restlessness, talkativeness, and a continuous wish to go home. At the same time, he reassured himself continually. At the time of discharge, a month later, the restlessness had completely subsided and there were no obvious fears and anxieties. He proved to be very dependent on his parents, especially his mother. He had an average IQ.

Immediately after the accident, Arthur showed the psychotic picture described by Blau (1936). As his illness developed, the psychotic picture retreated into the background and a neurotic picture appeared, filled with fright and anxiety. It is interesting to note that, in this fear and fright, he had a particularly strong longing for his parents and parent substitutes. Furthermore, he reassured himself continuously. There is no question that a brain injury was present, and organic factors may have played a part in the initial psychosis and in the neurosis. However, the picture is essentially a picture of fright and subsequent restlessness, and an attempt to escape the fright and fear of death.

According to Huddleson (1932), traumatic neuroses are rare in children. He quotes several observations by Oppenheim (1889), Fettermann (1928), Gabrio (1920), and others. Most of these observations were not concerned with head injuries. In a discussion of Wechsler's paper (1935), Hall even denies the existence of neuroses in children following head injuries. I think that, in children, acute fright reactions following head injuries have been overlooked. I believe they are not uncommon and have convinced myself of the long-lasting effects of injuries in children, especially head injuries, through my analyses of adults. Acute fright reactions bear a close relation to the psychotic cases described by Blau. It is an open question whether such experiences might not lead to behavior difficulties later on. It might be very difficult to differentiate such situations from the behavior difficulties found in children, following head injuries dependent on an organic basis (Kasanin, 1929).

A boy who was psychologically quite accessible, was seen on the children's ward.

Frederick, eleven years old, was of low average intelligence. His IQ was 92 on the Bellevue adult test. Educational tests showed that he was able to do fifth grade work. He was a normal boy until, at the age of nine, he fell on his head, when he was playing on a freight train. He was temporarily dazed, but got up and walked home, then he lost consciousness, regaining it before the ambulance arrived. In the hospital, he became unconscious for the third time. He was diagnosed as having a depressed fracture of the skull in the right posterior parietal region, with additional fissure fracture in the temporal bone around the mastoid, involving the base of the skull. He was operated on, on the second day, and the depressed pieces of bone were removed. The present X-ray findings show evidence of a resection of an area above the right mastoid two and one half inches in diameter. Since the accident, the boy has been emotional, unstable, and liable to outbursts of irritability, during which he attacks other children. He even choked a boy with a rope. There were also headaches, which developed in the region of the injury when there was a change in the weather. He described these headaches as maddening, at times. There were vestibular phenomena in which he felt dizzy, things whirled about him, he became nauseated and vomited, and felt hot and as if the bed were moving in wavelike motions. There were also petit mal episodes, in which he felt that his mind left him for a minute. He was extremely sensitive, and terrified by his condition; he felt that he could not fight because of the opening in his skull. He was acutely distressed by the sequelae of the accident:

"Yes, I used to say I wanted to die. I don't know why. . . . Yes, I wished it before the accident. Sometimes I would not feel it when stuck with pins. I used to feel hot and cold. Things look different before my eyes . . . . different colors, black and white. I would see black spots when I was reading, and colors also. Things would move back and forth before my eyes. The bed would move up and down. . . . Yes, I would lose my memory for hours. . . . Yes, I had my appendix out a few months ago. I was more afraid to have that scar touched afterwards than to have my head hit."

The psychotherapeutic approach revealed a deep underlying fear concerning the defect in the skull. On March 16, a plastic operation was done, with good results. He was seen on May 17, and said he felt much better. His irritability had diminished, and he adapted well to the school situation.

Although this case undoubtedly shows an organic concussion syndrome, there was deep concern of a hypochondriac type in relation to the cranial defect, and his behavior disturbances were not on a purely organic basis.

The largest group of neurotic pictures, following head injuries, is made up of hysterias. Most of the cases reported in the literature, for instance by Strauss and Savitzky (1934), are hysterias, as far as they are neurotic. It seems that hysteria, following head injuries, can occur without any organic residuals due to the head injury as such.

We may get a deeper psychological insight by studying the case of a child in which an hysterical picture followed a head injury.

Oliver was a ten-year-old Negro boy, referred to the hospital by his school, with the statement that he was subject to violent outbursts of temper, when he would "shoot spitballs." Once he attacked a child with a pocketknife. The teacher stated that "although he is considered bright in school, he constantly beats and threatens other children and he can close his mind like a door and will not learn the things he doesn't like. He even closes his eyes and stuffs his ears with his fingers. He rarely plays with other children, preferring to work on little projects of his own." The father stated that there was nothing wrong with the boy until he suffered a skull fracture two years before. "When the moon is full, Oliver always acts up," he states.

The history is as follows. The father and mother had been separated for three years. The father was fifty-seven years old. At one time, he appeared to be a fairly capable person, but he had been gradually deteriorating in his social standing and working ability. He drank to excess. The mother was much younger and worked as a domestic in a suburb. There were two children by this marriage, Oliver and his sister (who was eight years old). The mother was responsible for the girl and either kept her herself, or boarded her out in a pleasant home. Oliver lived with his father, practically since the time of his parents' separation, and, as indicated above, they lived in squalid surroundings. There seems to have been too close an attachment between Oliver and his father. Frequently, during the boy's stay in the hospital, the father visited him, usually under the influence of alcohol, at which times he would become lachrymose, assuring us that he was more than a father to Oliver; in fact, the two of them were more like brothers. He also stated that he could not live if Oliver were taken away from him. In addition to these squalid surroundings and inadequate care, Oliver also had to share the bed with his father's paramour, on occasion. His schoolteacher noted that he was always in a more dazed and irritable condition on Monday morning than on other days of the week.

His birth and early development were normal. There had been no severe illness until he was struck by a taxicab and suffered a severe cerebral concussion, serious injury to the right leg, and fracture of the right clavicle. He was then eight years old. Skull X-rays taken in the local hospital showed no fracture. Head X-rays taken in Bellevue were also normal. He seemed to have been unconscious for a few hours following the accident. When he awoke he thought he had saved a girl from fire, but

330

did not know anything about the accident. He was drowsy and semiconscious for several days. He was discharged after ten days. Both the school authorities and the father date his behavior disorders from this accident.

Our examination disclosed a mental age of eleven and a half, with an IQ of 115 on the Stanford-Binet. He had a 4A school placement, where he was doing third grade reading, arithmetic, and spelling. During the psychiatric examination, the child was friendly and talked freely, giving the following information. He had feelings of inferiority because he was colored (it should be added that the father ascribed a great many of Oliver's difficulties in school to the fact that he was colored). He described "spells" over which he had no control, and during which he felt dizzy and nauseated. He would look at an object, and it would suddenly become very large and close to him. At other times, the object would become very small and far away. He sometimes had feelings of heat in his head, or of being suffocated. Sometimes he felt his brain "separated in the middle and going back and forth"; sometimes it lifted off the skull or "went to the top." He also saw colored spots before his eyes. He wished he were a girl because he liked girls' dresses, bright colors, and partly because his sister received much better care and had more things than were given him. He spontaneously complained of not being able to defend himself against other children, and of being afraid of aggression in other boys. It has since been reported to us that, during his summer in the country, he was said to have been constantly afraid that other boys would do him bodily harm, and he ran to the director for protection. He still is entirely dependent on other people, particularly his father. He also had a masturbation complex, and feelings that he was sexually weaker than other boys his age.

He made a very good adjustment on the ward. There were a few periods of instability, but taking him away from the group and giving him assurance was sufficient to ward off one of his attacks. He had no hysterical features while there.

There is reason to believe that there were organic changes, in this case, since there had been a severe head injury with unconsciousness. We may suppose that his spells of dizziness and nausea were of organic origin. The described vasomotor phenomena may belong to Friedmann's vasomotor symptom complex or, in other words, to the organic concussion syndrome. However, whether we believe in such an organic nucleus or not, the picture gets its final meaning through an interpretation of the psychological problems related to the boy's attachment to his father, toward whom he felt completely passive. There was a hysterical symptomatology, consisting of micropsia and macropsia. Furthermore, there were behavior difficulties, the expression of the fright to which he had been exposed, which had accentuated the feelings of passivity and helplessness.

## FUNCTIONAL PSYCHOSIS ON THE BASIS OF ORGANIC INFERIORITY OF THE BRAIN[29]

It has been the general opinion that functional psychoses in children are of rare occurrence. Manic-depressive psychoses in children are very rarely observed. Schizophrenia has more often been reported as occurring in early childhood. On the other hand, it is very well known that organic brain diseases play a prominent part in childhood. Encephalitis is of very common occurrence in children; not only epidemic encephalitis, but almost every infectious disease may lead to encephalitic processes.[30] Encephalitis after measles (A. Meyer, 1927; Byers, 1928), and after smallpox inoculation, has attracted a good deal of attention. Wohlwill (1922) has described destructive processes of encephalomalacia in the newborn. Congenital encephalitis doubtless occurs. In addition, one has to consider that a birth trauma very often provokes more or less severe destruction of the brain, through hemorrhage, contusion, and anoxia.

One might expect that organic lesions of the brain would produce pictures fundamentally different from those observed in the functional psychoses, but this is not the case. Even in the adult, as Wagner-Jauregg, Stransky (1911), and Ritterhaus (1921) have shown, head injuries often lead to pictures that are very similar to manic-depressive psychoses. I have discussed the effects of head injuries on children. It is to be expected, however, that we will find irritability, hyperexcitability, and flightiness after early head injuries. We must bear in mind that even normal children show

[29] From Schilder (1935b).

[30] This statement was true in 1935 when this paper was written, but since then schizophrenia has been more readily and frequently recognized, encephalitis lethargica is rare, and the infectious diseases of children are less common and better controlled, especially by the antibiotic drugs.

trends that we would call manic in the adult. There are hyperactivity, wandering attention, and quick changes in emotions, all so characteristic of manic behavior. Hartmann and I (Hartmann and Schilder, 1924) have reported the case of a postencephalitic child who did not show the usual type of hyperkinesis observed in postencephaliuc children. The picture corresponded in all details to the picture of mania. Such cases are certainly rare. In the majority of cases, one does not find manic hyperactivity, but restlessness of a more aimless or more destructive type, or, in other words, the picture of hyperkinesis as a consequence of epidemic encephalitis, with which we are so familiar.

Hyperkinesis is one of the most common pictures in children. Kramer and Pollnow (1932) have tried to describe it as a definite disease, and report that they have found changes in the brain stem, in one of their cases, that were not of epidemic encephalitis, but another type of encephalitis. Clinical experience makes it rather doubtful that hyperkinesis is a specific entity. Not uncommonly, one sees children with endocrine disturbances who show a similar pattern in their behavior. Any kind of organic or toxic disturbance, affecting the central nervous system of the child, probably may lead to hyperkinetic pictures, if the disturbance is not too fargoing. If the hyperkinesis is not very outspoken, the picture will more and more resemble a manic one, but certainly it does not have the same significance as the manic attack of the manic-depressive psychosis. Of course, it is an open question whether this hypothetical organic or toxic disturbance must be localized in order to produce pictures of this kind, or whether a more or less diffuse disturbance will not produce the same picture which, after all, belongs to the typical reaction types of the infantile brain.

It is well known that mental defectives often show such restlessness. We know very little about the etiology and pathophysiology of feeblemindedness. We should be extremely careful, in all children in whom there is low intelligence, before we make the diagnosis of manic-depressive psychosis. Kasanin (1930) has reported a series of manic-depressive psychoses in children. In the first of his patients, the IQ was 78; in the second, the IQ dropped from 118 to 66 in the course of the disease. We might venture the hypothesis that, in both cases, an organic background was responsible for the mental picture.

333

In another case, there was a history of hereditary syphilis. With one exception, all of Kasanin's cases were about fifteen years old. In discussing case 5, the author spoke of a reactive depression in a feebleminded individual. Case 9 had a borderline defective intelligence, with signs of old poliomyelitis and a hypomanic picture. Kasanin, himself, stated that he had not observed affective psychoses under the age of ten. A case of a boy of eight with a depressive picture, continued self-accusations, and feelings of guilt was observed in Vienna. The nature of the case could not be clearly determined.

We do not doubt that affective psychoses occur close to the time of puberty, but it is extremely doubtful whether they occur much before that period. If one analyzes adult manic depressives, one never gets the impression that their childhood difficulties had a similarity to manic-depressive attacks. We therefore conclude that pictures which resemble manic-depressive psychoses in childhood generally do not belong to the group of the manic-depressive psychoses, but are, rather, connected with more or less organic disturbances in the brain, with toxic influences, and with a constitution which is not that of the adult manic depressive.

An excursion into the general psychology of the child is necessary, when we come to a discussion of the question of schizophrenia in childhood. A study of the attitudes of children toward death was made by D. Wechsler and myself (Chapter IV), and led to some conclusions concerning the way in which children think. There is a definite tendency toward realistic observation, in a matter-of-fact way. Children describe exactly what they have observed when a person dies and is buried. They even make an attempt to differentiate between what they have been told and what they have observed. Six-year-old Edward said, "How should I know that my parents are in heaven? I am not a fortuneteller. I heard somebody say the angel takes the soul, but I am not sure about it. They read it out of the Bible. I did not see it myself. But I am sure they are lying under the ground."

Children very often accept the conventional view and then become unable to solve the contradiction between this view and their own observations, but they also show no tendency to attempt to do it. Six-year-old George said, "Dead people go down in a big hole and then they put a lot of sand on. They don't feel anything. When we are good we go to heaven. We don't feel nothing up there. The hole that they put the people in is near to heaven, right next to it. If you are bad you go to hell and burn up. It hurts but you don't know if you are hurt or not."

The knowledge that the child has about many topics is dependent on what he hears by chance. It is, therefore, rather scattered and unreliable. The child generalizes his casual knowledge. There is undue generalization. For one child, all diseases are pneumonia, while according to another, all human beings die from throat disease. Children are almost unanimous in stating that they do not want to die, even when they have just declared how nice it is in heaven. At the same time, they have no clear idea of what dying means. For them, the word is seemingly a shell which contains something agreeable or disagreeable, although its exact content and meaning is not known.

These few remarks are, of course, not intended as even an attempt at a solution of the problem of children's thinking processes. They merely underline what Wildermuth (1923) has also stressed: that schizophrenic thinking and the thinking of the child have many points in common. We may assume that organic disease processes or organic deterioration will emphasize these features. In defective children, where the IQ is 60 or less, one can hardly fail to find indications of disturbed reactions, and signs of apparent dissociations which are not clearly understandable.

Bromberg (1934) studied a number of children, at Bellevue Hospital, whose personal and familial histories pointed to an organic deficiency symptomatically similar to schizophrenia. The IQ in these cases was low. In some cases, there was a definite organic hint in motility. In one group of cases, with definite mental deficiency, the clear-cut conflict led to primitive symbolizations, which corresponded very closely to schizophrenic behavior.

In order to understand cases of this kind, we must remember that when we talk about mental deficiency, we are using a very nonspecific term. The assumption that the emotions of a mentally deficient person are normal is one that is disproved by our every experience. When we study such cases carefully, we see that the emotions of the mentally deficient person are also defective. There

335

are flat inadequate emotions or sudden and violent outbursts of rage. There is apathy, indifference, lack of impulses, sudden epileptoid changes, and sudden outbursts. In other words, we have organically determined aberrations in the emotional sphere. Conflict situations in life are, therefore, conceived from the beginning in a different way, and accompanied by abnormal reactions in the emotional sphere. Since the ego system, the emotional control, is impaired, the conflicts will have a more lasting effect, as the outbursts will be uninhibited. Incomplete verbal facilities will lead to a frequent use of incompletely understood words or word shells. The vivid function of fantasy, the play instincts, will be increased, and the primitive drives, especially the sadistic ones, will come into the foreground uninhibited.

There are, therefore, four components: (1) An intellectual inferiority and the consequent frequent use of word shells, undue generalizations, and insensitivity to contradictions; (2) an unregulated emotional system, which reacts in an inadequate way to every problem; (3) the system once created will not be corrected; and (4) primitive drives will come strongly into the foreground.

One can see how great the similarity is between these pictures and schizophrenia. The minor degrees of mental deficiency will be particularly apt to provoke such pictures; but mental deficiency, stupidity, or dull mentality are not always so far apart. One should, therefore, be particularly careful in making a diagnosis of schizophrenia in children with low IQ.

There is no doubt that schizophrenia does occur in childhood. The observations of Potter (1933) are particularly persuasive in this respect. We must, however, consider the effect of mental deficiency and organic brain disorders on the emotional life of the child, before we make a diagnosis of schizophrenia. A very careful neurological examination, with special consideration given to tone and posture, will also be necessary. Neustadt (1928) has pointed out that there are psychoses in mentally defective persons which, in spite of their resemblance to schizophrenia, are not schizophrenia. These investigations also shed a new light on the problem of Propf schizophrenia, or schizophrenia superimposed on mental deficiency. Many of these cases will turn out to be schizophreniclike reactions, in the sense described above. A combination of mental deficiency and schizophrenia may occur, but, of course, is difficult to diagnose.[31]

It may therefore be concluded that pictures which resemble schizophrenia in childhood are often not schizophrenic but organic. They are schizophrenic reactions, in connection with organic processes and defects of the brain. It may also be supposed that dementia precoccissima (De Sanctis) and dementia infantilis (Heller) are not the same as schizophrenia, but are organic processes. Greene (1933) has conclusively shown how common psychotic manifestations are in mentally defective children. If we consider the discussion presented here, we come to a better understanding of these psychoses. There is also no evidence that the deteriorating processes, that are associated with organic signs and mental deficiency in children, are in any way related to schizophrenia.

A few illustrative cases, children from the wards of Bellevue Hospital, 1933-1934, are here quoted.[32]

Theodore, eleven years old, Stanford-Binet mental age 7-2, was fearful, with sudden sadistic outbursts. He said, "I will kill you. I will kill you. I want to take the poop out of his head and make it clean. I am going to fry him, he will fry all day until he gets finished." He drew a picture. "He is cooking the boy's head in the pot, the pot is turned upside down and the head is coming out." Here, again, the words were used in an emotional, rather than a logical, sense.

\*    \*    \*

Lawrence, eight years of age, Stanford-Binet IQ 81, said, in a playful way, "I am a rabbit. You are a snake. I'll throw you out of the window." Why? "Because you have big pants." He said to the examiner, "You pancake, I'll cook you in the oven." Besides this primitive identification of human beings with animals and inanimate objects, there were open outbreaks of sadistic actions against other children and the examiner. He

[31] The situation regarding the relationship between organic brain disorders, mental deficiency, and schizophrenia, in childhood, is quite different today than it was in 1935, when Schilder wrote this. Thanks to many concepts and examination methods taught by Schilder, we are able to differentiate between these conditions much more readily, and also to determine whether two, or all three, exist together. Nevertheless, the gist of the argument presented here still holds. The difference between the mentally defective and schizophrenic child is still important and cannot always be readily determined.

[32] Bromberg (1934). Unfortunately, the children from this early period could not be identified and located for follow-up.

used words as shells. The emotional content, and the direction of striving expressed in them, are more important than their logical meaning.

\* \* \*

One mentally defective boy was often found standing at a window, waving a handkerchief and saying "I surrender." He had taken this word, and the situation, from a book, but his whole attitude was a masochistic one. Indeed, he was always ready to surrender. The word "surrender" is, again, a word shell for an important instinctual drive.

\* \* \*

In the case of a thirteen-year-old boy with an IQ (Stanford-Binet) of 68, overcareful training had given him verbal facilities beyond his intelligence. This also led to the use of words in an instinctual, rather than an intellectual, way: "I think it is lack of control. You sort of can't control your emotions. You don't know how. You sort of can't control yourself and have to go to people for help." Severe self-reproaches concerning masturbation and degeneracy were behind his utterances. He wanted to be sterilized. Unable to cope with his instinctual drives, he got into a long-lasting state of restlessness and excitement.

In conclusion, the emotional patterns of children have, in themselves, a similarity to manic pictures. The incompleteness of the intellectual apparatus in connection with strong drives, in thinking as well as in action, may lead to results which are, in many respects, similar to the results of schizophrenic thinking. Inferiority of the brain, acquired or constitutional, often leads to an increase in emotional and intellectual peculiarities in children's behavior. Pictures of psychoses will occur that are similar to those of schizophrenia and manic states, although they are not identical with these disease entities. Every organic inferiority of the brain may also have an immediate influence on the repressive forces. Primitive drives and emotions, as well as primitive motor tendencies, will therefore come out in a much more open way. In addition, the reaction to conflicts will be less controlled, deeper lying, and longer lasting. Pictures resembling functional psychosis, in childhood, may be the reaction of a psychophysiological organization that is undeveloped, and that suffers from a weakness in the ego system; or, in the language of physiology, these are reaction types of an undeveloped and pathologically inferior brain organization.[33]

[33] A counterargument could now be presented that, since schizophrenia in childhood has so many features like the psychoses associated with organic brain disorders and mental deficiency in children, they have something basically in common, or at least, that the child reacts to these underlying conditions in a similar way.

## Schizophrenia[34]

One might hope that the analysis of schizophrenic children would lead to a clearer insight into the problem of schizophrenia. However, schizophrenic children are rare[35] and no complete analysis has been published so far. Klein (1930) once reported the analysis of a four-year-old schizophrenic; however she later changed this diagnosis and spoke merely of psychotic positions in childhood, in which the child feels particularly threatened by the "bad objects" inside himself.

In the material of schizophrenic children, studied on the children's ward at Bellevue Hospital by Bender, no definite psychogenic factors could be elicited; however, a dissociated cruelty appeared again and again, and, in the contents, the complaint of being rejected and attacked by the parents also appeared repeatedly. It seems at least possible to come to a consistent theory of the schizophrenic symptomatology from a psychological point of view. However, it must be conceded that the material is not sufficient, especially concerning psychogenesis.

A schematic psychology has shown, in earliest childhood (or uterine existence), a pretty uncomplicated state of satisfaction, to which the persons around the child become contributory. Generally, one may be doubtful concerning all too-simple formulations. At any rate, in schizophrenics, one sees not only the state of bliss, but also very different primitive attitudes, including the attitude of indifference. The individual shows that it is obviously not worthwhile to have any particular strivings. It is very probable that this indifference is very closely related to the feeling of self-sufficiency, which basically is the feeling that someone will take care of one's needs. Such an attitude may culminate in a stupor which may be connected with catalepsy. Closely related to the catalepsy is the so-

---

[34] From Schilder (1939b).

[35] It is difficult for me (Bender) to realize that the rather extensive work on childhood schizophrenia, done by my co-workers and myself, was accomplished after Schilder's death. This is because it is so evident that his contributions made it possible for us to reach the understanding which we have, in regard to this condition. I refer to his contributions to the problem of the development of motility and the relationship of motility to perception; body image concepts; the vestibular disorders and the relationship of clinging to equilibrium problems; and the concept that these were all of biological origin, while, at the same time, the child struggles psychologically to reorient himself in the world of reality, and reacts to his internal anxiety with a defensive neurosis (see Bender, 1947).

called autonomic obedience, the indifference toward pain, and, finally, the tendency for the schizophrenic to give in completely to postural tendencies. Two symptoms, I have observed with Hoff (Hoff and Schilder, 1927), belong here: The schizophrenic gives in to his postural tendency toward divergence of the outstretched arms, and also to the postural tendencies which occur after turning the head. One can easily turn the schizophrenic around his longitudinal axis, by putting a hand on the top of his head and twisting it slightly, but persistently, toward one side, which causes the schizophrenic to start whirling around his longitudinal axis.

A further type of schizophrenic reaction is a leveled and diffuse defense, by the patient, against everything which is done to him. This defense may be purely muscular (negativistic tension); but it may also be connected with an extreme degree of fear and anxiety. It is characteristic of such reactions that almost everybody who approaches the patient is reacted to in the same way.

Although we do not know any organic data pertaining to catalepsy, we do know that the automatic compliance, changes in postural reflexes, and, finally, the negativistic reactions, have clear-cut relations to mechanisms in the central nervous system, which, according to our knowledge, are accessible only to so-called organic agents. This does not change our opinion that we deal with primitive reactions from a psychological point of view; however, these are primitive reactions based on organic changes within the central nervous system.

Gestalt drawings by schizophrenic children are particularly instructive in this area. Bender (1938) has collected such drawings. One by Francine (see Figure 5), age eight, shows that she is capable of copying the gestalt figures, but immediately reverts from this developed perceptive world and adds loops and extensions, until the primary pattern is completely destroyed. In every one of her gestalt test drawings, one can see how she shrinks back from the world of clear-cut forms. It is also interesting that she often attempted to tear up her drawings. The reversal to primitive forms comes out particularly clearly, in one of her abstract drawings, into which the primitive formal principles come into clear expression. In describing parts of one of her pictures, she said "This is a roni, but not a macaroni."

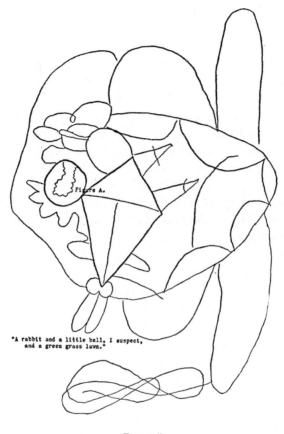

"A rabbit and a little ball, I suspect, and a green grass lawn."

FIGURE 5

It is not surprising to find the same primitive tendencies in the emotional sphere, as we have found in the perceptive, motor, and conceptual spheres. A varying process of going back to primitive experiences, with continuous impairment of the fundamental motor, sensory, and conceptual functions, is characteristic for all these varying functions. The various processes of projections, identification, the various defense mechanisms, and the libidinous trends, have been described by Freud, Jung (1911-1912), Bleuler (1911), Ferenczi (1913), myself, and others. Sinking down to the deepest level of libidinous development, the schizophrenic clings to those stages of his development where he has strong infantile experiences and retains some of his object relations of higher level in the hetero-

341

sexual, homosexual, anal, urethral, and oral spheres. He uses the same object relations as steps in the ladder to come back to his previous heights of adaptation, to reality.

It goes without saying (Schilder, 1928a) that the actual cause of every psychosis is the product of the external event plus the inner constellation.

Much more difficult, however, is the determination of the fixation point in schizophrenia. We have already indicated that we must look for this fixation point in the sphere of magical experiencing, in the realm of narcissism, at a level where the self and the environment are not very sharply differentiated. But when we speak analytically of points of fixation, we must demand that the events which caused the fixation, or the experiences in connection with which the state of fixation has occurred, should be demonstrated. We know nothing of the specific experiences of the schizophrenic, at this level of development. Shall we search for them in peculiarities of the foetal life, birth, or the suckling period? At any rate, it is hardly probable that, from the observation of these phases of an individual's life, any very definite and conclusive psychic experiences can be demonstrated. (In this connection, see White, 1917.)

Thus, we get nowhere with the assumption of a narcissistic, magical point of fixation in schizophrenia. Altogether apart from those rare cases in which one can demonstrate a fixed pupil (thus an increase in the brain volume, an undoubtedly gross organic disturbance), the psychology of so-called catatonic manifestations furnishes us with much matter for thought. Among these manifestations, one finds marked muscular tensions of various kinds, and an exaggerated motility, which reminds one of chorea minor (Saint Vitus's dance), and of the hyperkinesis of certain encephalitics. But we find a number of cases in whom these manifestations are the direct expression of certain psychic constellations, and can be understood only as the effect of these on certain brain mechanisms. In other cases, there can be found nothing indicative of such psychogenesis, and we must assume the existence of a disorder of those cerebral mechanisms which regulate muscular posture and tension. In the center of these brain structures stands the strio-pallidal system, gross organic disorders of which actually give rise to manifestations which, if not entirely identical with those of catatonia, at least resemble them very closely. We have in mind, for instance, the manifestations of catalepsy, which we meet with in catatonics, as well as in certain encephalitics.

The point might be stressed that one is here dealing with disturbances of a more primitive motility, since the central nuclei are undoubtedly, phylogenetically, the older portions of the brain. One might be justified, therefore, in associating these disturbances with a regression to the embryonal stage. Tausk has actually maintained this point of view. Nevertheless, it must be stated at once that the embryonal postures in no way resemble those of catatonia; and the embryonic movements, which Minkowski (1928) studied more carefully, differ materially from those of the catatonic.[36] The movements of the embryo are slow, difficult, and uncoordinated. In the motility type of catatonic, stiffness and explosiveness of movement predominate. It is only from the point of view of phylogeny, and not ontogeny, that one is able to bring the postural disorders of the schizophrenic into relation with the concept of regression. But even if one were to ignore these differences between the catatonic and embryonal motor phenomena, perhaps on the assumption that the stiffness of catatonic postures and movement is a reflection of the impediments of embryonal movements, the question of the psychological nature of a developmental period in which such movements predominate, would still remain unsolved. It is a question which can presently only be approached through speculation.

The schizophrenic, threatened in early childhood, withdraws into a more secure position. He tries to heighten the importance of the strength of his own personality. Furthermore, he uses primitive methods of defense, either by giving in to immobility or catalepsy, or by negativism. He may also use the method of violent attack. He does not dare retain higher forms of object relations. Primitive types of libidinous development occur. In addition, we find primitive stages of ego ideal development. The primitive attitude also appears in the formation of language and thought processes. Symbolism, projection, and renewed identifications belong to this sphere. The primitive threat is revived by the dangerous situ-

---

[36] The later work of Gesell and Amatruda (1945) shows a close parallel between the behavior of the fetal infant and the schizophrenic child. See Bender and Freedman (1952).

343

ations of everyday life. The threat of being destroyed leads to outbursts of aggressiveness, which appear particularly clearly in the schizophrenia of children. Many of these manifestations of primitive motor defenses and obedience have close relation to organic brain mechanisms. However, the perceptive faculties and the motor faculties are disturbed in a sphere which is not the same as in gross lesions of the brain.

### CONGENITAL ALEXIA AND ITS RELATION TO OPTIC PERCEPTION[87]

The practical importance of congenital alexia, or congenital word blindness, has been notably appreciated by Hinshelwood (1917), in England, Warburg, in Germany, and Orton (1928, 1930), in this country. Monroe (1932) has made an extensive study of cases of reading difficulties in children, and has compared normal and retarded children in this respect. Orton has developed an interesting theory concerning the genesis of congenital word blindness, especially emphasizing the interference of left and right cortical impulses.

But the theoretical importance of so-called congenital word blindness, in its relation to the present aphasia discussion, has not yet been fully considered. Investigation of seven cases has been made on the nature of congenital word blindness, from the point of view of its position in the system of aphasias and agnosias. The examination consisted of presentation of letters in correct and reversed position, numbers, and short and long words and sentences. The letters and words were both printed and written. The examination also included letters, numbers, words, and short sentences, written spontaneously and from dictation, and the copying of printed and handwritten words and sentences. Pictures were presented to the subject and a description was elicited. Letters, words, numbers, and figures, used by Orton in his test, were presented to every subject. Pictures, drawings, words, numbers, figures, and all the other material used by Orton, were also presented tachistoscopically. The subjects were not only asked to report what they saw, but also, in many instances, to reproduce the material by drawing or writing. The pictures varied from relatively simple outline figures of houses,

[87] From Schilder (1944).

trees, and heads, to somewhat complicated landscapes, one of them having a cluster of trees, a church spire, and a road. The numbers and letters were the three-quarter-inch gummed letters used in making posters. Some written words were also included. Subjects were also examined on their perception of movements which were exposed to them for a very short time. The tachistoscope was a shutter model, making an exposure of about 1/35 of a second, or longer, when so desired. Several examinations were given to each subject, as the children tended to get tired after thirty or forty minutes of work.

In the following seven cases, specific reading disability was brought to light in connection with the routine psychological examination of the psychiatric service at Bellevue Hospital. They were either ward patients in the hospital, or mental hygiene clinic patients admitted to one of the wards for a brief period of observation. Six were boys and one was a girl. The youngest was eight years and two months old, the oldest was fourteen. Two of the boys were Negro, one born in the United States, the other in Puerto Rico.

J.S., a twelve-year-old boy, was sent in by the children's society, because of a poor school record. His mental age, on the Stanford-Binet scale, was 10-5; on the Army Performance scale, 11-9; and, on the Healy P.C. I, 9-5. He showed no difficulty in the recognition of letters and in copying, with special reading material. There was considerable difficulty in recognition of longer words, but he had learned to read simple words and sentences fairly well. He had no difficulty with numbers, and his copying was invariably correct.Tachistoscopic exposures were readily recognized, unless the stimulus was a rather long or unfamiliar word. No trouble was encountered with simple and familiar words. He tried to read longer words by sounding the letters. Often, he would sound one letter and then make errors in the adjoining letters. There were almost no reversed letters. Words printed mirrorwise were recognized as "turned around," and were read with great difficulty. It was easier for him to assemble words than letters. There were occasional optic mistakes (Table 1).

When "1" is read instead of "I," the difficulty is apparently in optic perceptions; also, when "doy" is read instead of "dog," the trouble lies in the perception of a single letter. It is the same type of difficulty in mistaking "M" for "N." Otherwise, it was remarkable that this boy succeed-

| TABLE 1 | | |
| --- | --- | --- |
| Test Material | | |

| Presented in Print | Read | |
| --- | --- | --- |
| At | Correct | |
| You | Correct | |
| Long | Correct | |
| In Brooklyn | Correct | |
| News of | News of - - News of | |
| Local interest | Inter - - | |
| Territory | Teri - - Tart - - | |

| Dictated | Written | |
| --- | --- | --- |
| Sixty-nine, one, two, three | Correct | |
| (Own name) | Correct | |
| I have a little dog | I have a litter dog | |
| I like to go to school | I like to go to sch - - so - - st - - school | |
| We are going to have some candy | We are going to have some car - cac - kn - can | |

| Dictated | Spelled verbally | |
| --- | --- | --- |
| Dog | D - O - - I had it a minute ago. I had it on my mind. I can't say it. It isn't W, it isn't C | |
| Little | L - I - T - R - E . . . I left out the E | |
| Dog | I got it now: D - O - G | |

| Tachistoscopic Exposure (Print) | Read | Written |
| --- | --- | --- |
| q | "P backwards" | Correct |
| D | Correct | Correct |
| Walter | "W - E -, That was some word. I couldn't get it. A - L - K - E, a couple of E's" | |
| (Second exposure) | "W - A - E - R" | |
| (Without tachistoscope) | Correct. "That wasn't the same word." | |
| Beat | "B - E - E - T, B - E - T - T B - E - T" | Bett, Bat |

ed in the synthesis of only the first part of long words and his separation of the word "Beat" into two halves.

*  *  *

P.F. was a thirteen-year-old boy, with a mild Froelich syndrome (pituitary infantilism), pudgy hands and features, soft skin, undescended testicles, and a BMR of plus 6. He scored a mental age of 9-6 and an IQ of 70 on the Stanford-Binet scale, and a mental age of 10-2 (IQ 75) on the Army Performance Scale. His problem was inability to learn, throughout childhood, with poor concentration, poor memory, and difficulties in reading and writing.

With the special reading material, he showed marked difficulty in the reading of simple words. He read reversed letters as readily as those correctly printed, and recognized mirror words at least as quickly or possibly faster than ordinary words. There was, however, hesitation and slowness in the identification of mirror-written words, as such. He had no difficulty in spelling words, but there was a marked hesitation, and inability, in putting letters together into words. The patient was unable to read words that he did not know. He wrote from left to right, and, in work with anagrams, used the correct order of placing letters. There was marked difficulty in writing words from dictation, but copying was consistently correct.

This patient made many more optic mistakes, in single letters, than did others of the group studied; however, he made similar mistakes in the reading of words. Errors with the tachistoscope were just as frequent as when words were directly presented.

Unlike the other patients studied, this boy had considerable difficulty with numbers, which he frequently misread, when they were shown to him tachistoscopically. The errors often seemed quite unrelated; for example, 181 was read as 840, and 373 as 180. He had, however, no trouble in writing numbers from dictation (Table 2).

TABLE 2

### Test Material

| Presented in Print | Read | Spelled |
|---|---|---|
| SEE | "ESS-SEE" | |
| ASS | Correct | |
| NO | "ONE" | N-O |
| ON | Correct | |
| SAW | "I don't know - -ASS" | S-A-W |
| WAS | "HIS" | W-A-S |
| DO | Correct | |
| BOY | "DOG" | D-O-G |
| UP | "Don't know what the letter is" | U-P |
| 800 | Correct | |
| BAT | "Don't know - -BUT" | B-A-T |
| (Second test period) | | |
| DOG | Correct | |
| YOU | "Can't read it" | Y-O-Q-U |
| AT | Correct | |
| SEE | Correct | |
| ME | "Can't say it" | M-E |
| ON | Correct | |

TABLE 2 *(cont'd)*

| | | |
|---|---|---|
| BEAT | "Can't say it - -DEAT" | D-E-A-T |
| HEM | "DEM" | Correct |
| MAMA | "MAN" | M-A-N-A |
| ASS | "SEE" | M-S-S |
| 404 | "400" | 404 |
| 373 | "373" | |
| 1551 | "155-1" | |
| 649 | "6-40-6" | |
| 800 | "80" | |

| *Dictated* | *Written* |
|---|---|
| CAT | Correct |
| DOG | Correct |
| LITTLE | elttli |
| BIRD | Bef |
| ON | No |
| AT | Atn |
| SEE | Correct |
| ASS | af |
| GOOD | go |
| DOG | Correct |
| ON | am |
| WEATHER | of |
| MAN | anam |

MAMA, BEAT, ON, and COST were presented in print and copied correctly.

| *Tachistoscopic exposure (Print)* | *Read* |
|---|---|
| ON | "ON-I am not quite sure" |
| Cost | "C-COE" |
| 181 | "181" |
| DOG | "DOY, BOY" |
| ME | "Me; Spells M-E" |
| SEE | Correct |
| AT | "E, A-T, at" |
| You | Correct |
| Walter | "W-EA" |

This patient, too, made mistakes between B and D, N, A, M, H, and D. He also copied A instead of S. It may be supposed that these are optic difficulties, especially as there are also mistakes in copying. During other test periods, he made mistakes between B and D, Q and G, and P and D, and showed several instances of mirror-reading. It is remarkable how he was able to substitute a word that he knew for an unknown one, even when there was not more than one letter in common with the word offered.

\* \* \*

W.B., an eight-year-old Negro boy, was referred to the clinic for admission to the hospital as a behavior problem. He had a congenital infantile paralysis of the right arm and leg. His mental age, as measured by the Stanford-Binet scale, was 6-6. His vision was 16/25 in each eye.

When presented with the special reading material (Table 3), he displayed no difficulty in the recognition of letters, spontaneous writing, copying, tachistoscopic reading of letters, numbers, or short words. However, he was unable to read long words or to write them from dictation.

TABLE 3

Test Material

| Presented in Print | Read | Written* | |
|---|---|---|---|
| I GO | "L-G-O, that's No" | | |
| OG | "D-O, that's No" | | |
| WALTER | "W-A-L-T-E-R [after some hesitation] - - Ah ha! That's my name. I knew you were going to fool me. It's Walter." | | |
| NO | | NO ← | (R) |
| | | WO ← | (L) |
| SEE | "Eyes," (Spelled: | SEE ← | (L) |
| | "S-E-E-E") | ƎƎS → | (R) |
| DOG | "D-O-G, Is that dog? | DOG ← | (L) |
| | Yes sir, it is" | ƆOᗡ → | (R) |
| OG | "Oh, it's dog again, only this time it's this way." | GOᗡ ← | (L) |
| | | ᗡOƆ → | (R) |
| GO | "That's OG" | OƆ ← | (L) |
| | | OƆ → | (R) |
| WALTER | "That's my name [Starts printing from right to left, then writes from left to right]" | W-A-L-T-E-R (L) ← | |
| GO | "GO- - now it's O-G" | GO     OG | |
| OD | "D-O" | D-O → | |
| 3 | "3" | 3 | |
| 61 | "Nineteen" | 19 | |
| 41 | "Fourteen" | 18 ← | |
| 12 | "Twelve" | 12 ← → | |

* R = right hand; L = left hand; arrows indicate direction of writing.

TABLE 3 *(cont'd)*

*Tachistoscopic exposure (Print)*

| | | |
|---|---|---|
| YOU | "You, I only seen U, I didn't see the rest" | U<br>U O<br>→<br>U O |
| BOY | "V-O-Y--B-U-O-Y" cannot read it | ← B O Y → |
| ME | "E"--cannot read it | M E → |
| MAMA | Does not know | M |
| DOG | "DOG, D-O-G" | DOG → |
| ASS | "S-E-E-E, Eyes" (when repeated, he says: "Again S-E-E-E, of course.") | |
| 373 | | E--, then 37--, "I wonder what's the other one? --373." |
| 88 | "Thirty-eight" | 38 ← |
| 81 | Does not know | 8 1 1 → |
| 181 | Does not know | 1 8 1 ← |
| 181 | "One-eight-one" | 181 → |
| 699 | "Six-nine-nine" | 996 |

* R = right hand; L = left hand; arrows indicate direction of writing.

He recognized reversed letters. He made frequent mirror mistakes when writing spontaneously, and showed a marked tendency to write from right to left. This tendency was as marked in the writing of numbers, and work with anagrams, as it was in his writing of letters and words. These mirror mistakes only appeared in spontaneous work or during dictation, but were not present during the copying of words or letters.

Single words were almost always spelled correctly, but could not be read by him. The tachistoscopic performance was somewhat worse than his performance with the usual time span. The recognition of objects, pictures, and movement was uniformly good, whether the stimuli were presented tachistoscopically or not. Right and left confusion was confined to reading and writing. Practically all writing was done with the left hand, due to right-handed hemiplegia. Right-hand writing was helped by, and determined by, the left hand. Left-hand writing was done with the arm encircling the paper above the writing.

In anagram dictation, he was given cut-out letters, and asked to pick out the correct letters to form the word DOG. While he spelled vocally, "D-O-G," he joined the letters G and O, and then reversed the entire word. For CAT, he selected C and T, spelled out "C-A-T" vocally, found A, and placed it correctly. For RAT, he placed R-T, spelled out "R-A-T" vocally, and was satisfied with an incomplete anagram. UP, BOY, and NO were joined correctly. He seemed to have little difficulties in the orientation of letters after the first word. He always began with the first letter, spelled the word orally, and worked out the problem by finding the letters consecutively. But when told to place the letters B-A-T or H-A-T, he could not read the found word.

* * *

A.S., an eleven-year-old boy, was referred to the clinic by an orphan home where he had been for eight years, with the report that he was annoying and quarrelsome in school, and unable to keep up with his grade work. His mental age was 8-10 on the Stanford-Binet scale, 8 on the Pintner-Paterson Performance Test, 10-9 on the Healy P.C. II, and 12 on the Porteus Maze. His eyesight was normal.

In his work with the special reading material (Table 4), he had difficulties with combinations of letters. He recognized individual letters, could pick them out, copy them correctly, and spell short and long words, without hesitation. There was slight difficulty with two and three letter words, but with words of more than three letters the patient was completely lost, unless the word happened to be the one he had especially learned. He knew his name, both first and last, could write them from dictation, and recognized them immediately in either print or written form. Most words of four or five letters, however, were impossible for him, and he would respond by saying "I don't know" or "I can't." When urged, he would attempt to sound out the word, usually getting the first letter correctly, without being able to synthesize the entire word. For example, "mama," after eight seconds of effort, was called "man." After being spelled out, and after he was told that this is a boy's name, "Walter" was read as "Wallace." This boy had no difficulties with numbers.

When shown drawings, words, numbers, and designs, tachistoscopically, there was no difficulty in perception of anything but words, and even the recognition of simple words seemed to be somewhat facilitated by a brief exposure. It seemed as though tachistoscopic presentation tended to assist the putting together of the letters into a single word, if the word presented was not a long one and was familiar.

Copying, either with anagrams or with pencil, was done without error, though often the patient could not read what he had just written.

TABLE 4

Test Material

| Presented in Print | Read |
|---|---|
| Once | "O-N-C-E" (cannot read) |
| there | "T-H-E-R-E" (cannot read) |
| was | "W-A-S--Where" |
| little | "L-I-T-T-L-E" (cannot read) |
| so | "so" |
| CANDY | "C-A-N-D-Y" (cannot read) |
|  | Do you want to have it? "Yes, sir." |
|  | Is it a dog, cat, elephant? "No." |
|  | Is it candy? "Yes." |
| THIEF | (cannot read) Is it thirst, thunder, Thursday, murderer, house, or thief? "It is thief." |
| As | "As" |
| Cat | "Cat" |
| Candy | (now reads correctly) |
| TABLE | (cannot read) Is it clothes, shoe, ear, eye, threatening? "No." Is it a chair? "Yes." Are you sure? "Yes." |
| 1284 | "Twelve-hundred-and-eighty-four" |

| Tachistoscopic exposure (Print) | Read | Written |
|---|---|---|
| CANDY | Correct |  |
| CAT | Correct |  |
| Monkey | "I don't know how to spell it. I don't know what it is." |  |
| Third exposure | "Monkey" | M-O-N-K |
| Ass | Correct |  |
| THIEF | "Thie" |  |
| Shoes | "Stockings" | S-E-T |
| LION | Correct | L-O |
|  | What is the last letter? "N" |  |
| Stick | "Stockings" |  |
| Frog | "Don't know what it is or how to write it." |  |

| Anagram Dictation | Put together | Spelled verbally |
|---|---|---|
| ALBERT | Correct |  |
| ON | O-N-G |  |
| DOG | GOD | "D-O-G" |
| HOUSE | HAST | "H-A-S-T," reads "House" |
| ME | Correct |  |
| Cow | KIAT | "K-I-A-T," reads "Cow" |
| CAT | Correct |  |
| DOG | "GOOD," reads "Dog." What is the first letter? "G." Read it. DOG |  |

TABLE 4 *(cont'd)*

| | |
|---|---|
| Up | Correct |
| BOY | "BOUT," reads "BOY" |
| GOD | Correct |

There were a few mirror mistakes, in the writing of single letters shown tachistoscopically, and occasional mirror reversals in the use of anagrams. These, however, were not frequent and formed but a small part of the reading errors. There was no tendency to mirror-writing or left-handedness.

It is remarkable that the patient occasionally had a vague general idea concerning the contents of words he couldn't read. This is especially outstanding concerning the word "Candy." It is also remarkable that he chooses the word "Stockings" for "Shoes." One could believe that it is only the similarity in the first letters, but then he selects the word "Chair" for "Table." When he chooses the word "Lung" for "Lion," there is only the similarity in first letters to warrant the choice.

When he has incorrectly put together a long word, in anagram dictation, he spells correctly what he has put together, but reads it as the word asked from him.

\* \* \*

C.A., a boy aged eight years, two months, was referred by the children's court, with the complaint that he acted like a mental defective. He was restless and disobedient on the ward. His mental age was 8-8, on the Stanford-Binet scale, 10 on the Pintner-Paterson Performance Scale, and 7-4 on the Healey P.C. II. His eyesight was normal.

In the work with the special reading material (Table 5), he was found to have considerable difficulty in the recognition and writing of letters. He knew the names of many letters, but seemed to encounter trouble in associating them with the appropriate letter forms. For example, when working with anagrams and trying to write his name, he would say "P, P, where is P?" fingering over many of the letters in front of him, passing again and again over the letter for which he was looking. Though this occurred especially frequently with such letters as D, B, and P, it also took place with W, S, V, and other letters.

There was much less difficulty with numbers; in fact, he made few errors with them, except in the reading of longer numbers presented tachistoscopically. Though there were mirror mistakes in recognition, in reading letters, and a few mirror mistakes in such words as "on" and

TABLE 5

Test Material

| Presented in Print | Read | Written |
|---|---|---|
| DOG | No response | Doc, D-O-C |
| ASS | No response | Ace, A-C-C. "It is an S, it is the first letter of my name." |
| M, R, S, and E were read correctly | | |
| G | "C" | |
| P | "B, P" | |
| D | "D" | |
| ON | "DO" | ON, O-N |
| ME | "I don't know the whole word" | N-E |
| DOG | "It is the same word, I don't understand it good" | D-O-C |
| 37, 811, and 181 were read correctly | | |
| 1551 | One-hundred-five-hundred-fifty-one | |
| 18,152 | One-eight-one-five-two | |

| Tachistoscopic exposure (Print) | Read | Written |
|---|---|---|
| ME | "I don't know what it is" | N |
| 2nd exposure | | M-T, N-T |
| 3rd exposure | "Same word. I saw it twice." | F |
| ASS | "It's A." | a-s-s (uses written letters) |
| NO | | To-N-O, To |
| UP | "Up" | P-U |
| BOY | "There is an 'R' at the beginning" | |
| 2nd exposure | "I only saw the last letter" | Y |
| 337 | 7-3-7 | 7-3-7 |
| 2nd exposure | 3-3-3 | 3-3-3 |
| 3rd exposure | 7-3-3 | 7-3-3 |
| 4th exposure | 3-7-3 | 3-7-3 |
| 83 | 83 | |

| Anagrams | Put together | Read |
|---|---|---|
| BOY | Y-O- | |
| Girl | "L, where is L, where is G?" Puts together F-C, and does not find the rest | |
| DOG | C-O-R | "D-O-G, Dog" |

| | Anagram Copying | |
|---|---|---|
| HEN | T-H-E-N, T-H-E-H-E-N | |
| THE | T-H- | |
| BAG | Correct | |

"saw," this formed a relatively small percentage of his total errors. Tachistoscopically, he had no difficulty with perception of objects, faces, and directions. Even the most complex of the presented pictures were accurately reported. He was also able to describe, correctly and in detail, pictures that were presented nontachistoscopically. He seemed to have no difficulty in the recognition of directions.

Copying, either with anagrams or pencil, of short or long words, was done without error, but spontaneous writing of words, and the reading of either long or short words presented on a card or presented tachistoscopically, was impossible for him. Numbers were hardly any problem for him. In reading numbers, writing them spontaneously, or copying them, he showed no errors, and only a few mistakes were noted for numbers read tachistoscopically.

Of the entire group studied, this boy was the most difficult one to work with. He easily became irritable and often refused to continue. He used his right hand exclusively. No tendency toward mirror-writing was noticed. He often read S as C, G as C, and P as B, mistakes which point to difficulties in optic perception.

*  *  *

R.T., a Negro boy of nine years, eleven months, was referred to the clinic because he was disobedient, restless, and beyond control. He had started school at the age of six, but could not make progress, and had been placed in an ungraded class. His mental age was 7-6 on the Stanford-Binet scale, 10 on the Pintner-Paterson Performance Test, and 8-10 on the Healey P.C. II.

During the examination (Table 6), he was alert and responsive when presented with nonverbal material; but he became restless and distractable when confronted with verbal material for any length of time. In work with the performance material, there was a tendency to use the left hand.

During the experiment with the special working material, he had no difficulty with spontaneous writing of letters, copying with pencil or anagram, letters or short words. There was an occasional difficulty with the recognition of letters, considerable difficulty with short words, and complete inability to handle long words. The difficulty with letters was not noted when letters were presented tachistoscopically. The difficulty with short words was present, but seemed slightly less marked. His trouble with long words was unaffected by tachistoscopic presentation. This boy had greater difficulty with numbers, both in copying and writing from dictation, than most of the cases studied.

He wrote mirrorwise with his left hand, and normally with his right hand, with nearly equal facility. His errors were of the same sort and as frequent in his left handwriting as they were in his right handwriting.

TABLE 6

Test Material

| Presented in Print | Read | Spelled | Copied |
|---|---|---|---|
| as | "at" | correct | correct |
| it | "it" | correct | correct |
| left | "little" | correct | correct |
| ball | "black" | D-A-L-L | dall |
| pod | "dog" | P-O-D | God |
| balk | "black" | B-A-L-K | dalk |
| pig | "pirl" | P-I-G | dig |
| plea | refused to read | | glea |
| Bed | refused to read | | ded |
| Plea | refused to read | | clea |
| Boy, Cat, Man, were read correctly | | | |
| The boy has | "The boy has" | | |
| a dog | "a ball" | | |
| HAS | "his" | has | |
| HORSE | "Hees" | | |
| THE | "There, the" | | |
| WAGON | "woke" | | |

| Tachistoscopic exposure (Print) | Read |
|---|---|
| YOU | "Y-O-T" |
| GO | correct |
| BAT | "B-O-L" |
| HEM | "H- I did not see it so good" |
| ASS | "A- What's the other?" |
| 2nd exposure | "A-B-S, bass" |
| 69 | correct |
| 800 | correct |
| 482 | 23 |

| Anagram dictation | Put together as | Spelled |
|---|---|---|
| GO | og | |
| BOY | bog | |
| G | correct | |
| Y | correct | |
| 19 | 92 | |
| BOY | dog | |
| 354 | 3054 | |
| TODAY | todog | "D-O-G" reads "today" |
| weather | water | "I can't spell it" |
| 24 | | |
| 61 | | |
| 192 | 0042 | |
| 354 | 3054 | |
| Has | us | |
| on | mot | |

In spontaneous dictation, and in copying of print, he changed b to d, p to d, and p into g. There was trouble with his spelling, but he was more easily able to overcome this. In reading, he correctly read only words that he knew, and changed unknown words into known words. He was unable to put single words together. The letters were spelled correctly, but he could not put them together unless he knew the word. The difficulty with right and left appeared only with single letters. There was no tendency to mix the order of the letters.

\* \* \*

C.M., a fourteen-year-old-girl, was referred to the clinic because she was unable to concentrate on or remember anything pertaining to schoolwork; but she was handy in manual activities. She had a mental age of 9-4 on the Stanford-Binet scale, 15 on the Pintner-Paterson Performance Test, and 10-10 on the Healy P.C. II.

In her work with the special reading material, she was able to read single letters and numbers without difficulty. Simple words were read slowly, in spelling fashion. There were many errors in writing. For example, Brooklyn was written Brooklny; Little was written Litter. In writing from dictation, words were omitted or written with great difficulty, and with frequent mistakes. When letters and numbers were shown tachistoscopically, she seemed to have no difficulty in recognition, on the whole, though there were occasional mirror mistakes, such as reading a capital E as 3, or reading the word "no" as "on." Longer words were not read at all, though they were recognized as words. Relatively long numbers were read correctly. Recognition of pictures was excellent. This patient showed the same general tendencies that the others did, as far as the examination went. Examination was not completed because she was taken to Chicago by her mother.

In general, all of the cases studied showed the characteristics reported by Orton, in his case studies of word blindness. Letters of the alphabet, either printed or written, were generally well recognized. There were numerous mistakes between B and D; b and d; g and p; Y and G; p and d; M and N; m and n; b and g; A and S; d and t; C and S; A and M; I and L; T and L; and H and D. It is true that these mistakes were much more outspoken when the word was presented as a whole, and rarely occurred when the single letter was presented. The same mistakes were made in spontaneous writing and in writing from dictation. There were fewer mistakes concerning Arabic numerals. Spelling of presented words was generally good, and only those mistakes were made which also appeared in reading of single letters. The difficulties varied in the different cases. There was also a variation of mirror mistakes, conspicuous only in two cases. The tendency to sound one or two of the initial letters of a word, and then jump at the rest, was most marked in two cases, where there had been the greatest amount of school training. The following tendencies were noted:

1.  In practically every case, the difficulty was confined to letters and words. Four-digit numbers were recognized and reported correctly, where four-letter words were not recognized at all. The four digits could even be read as a continuous number, as for instance, "twelve-hundred-and-eighty-four." Of the seven cases studied, only one showed difficulties in the recognition of numbers, but, even there, there was less hesitation than in the recognition of words.

2.  Mistakes concerning the Orton pictures were rare, and only outspoken in Case 3, which showed the greatest amount of mirror mistakes. Otherwise, the recognition of pictures was very good, even when the details of the pictures were rather complicated. Tachistoscopic presentation of pictures revealed prompt recognition of the parts of the pictures. Within the limits of the tachistoscopic perception of normals, the pictures were perceived as a whole, in practically every case. We never observed mirror mistakes in the permanent or tachistoscopic presentation of pictures. The accuracy of picture recognition was in marked contrast with the difficulty in word recognition.

3.  On the whole, tachistoscopically presented words were as readily recognized as permanent exposures. Familiar words seemed to be, at times, more readily recognized tachistoscopically. One can say that the tachistoscopic presentation did not increase the difficulty.

4.  Difficulties with reading, spelling, or writing words were present in all the cases studied, even when the single letters and sounds did not offer any trouble. Noted tendencies toward mirror writing and reading were found in two cases. In the others, mirror writing was entirely absent. Mirror mistakes in reading were either absent or played a very unimportant part, quantitatively.

5.  The optic perception of movements and their directions was

excellent even when the movements were exposed only in the tachistoscope.

6. All of our patients could differentiate well between their left and right side, perform movements with either hand if asked, and were also able to touch the right part of their bodies with the left hand and vice versa, according to given orders.

Orton (1928, 1930) emphasizes the importance of mirror mistakes for the genesis of reading and spelling disabilities. He supposes that the process of learning to read entails the elision, from the focus of attention, of the confusing memory images of the non-dominant hemisphere, which are in reversed form and order, and the selection of those which are correctly oriented and in correct sequence. According to this theory, in reading disability there has been an incomplete elision of the memory patterns in the non-dominant hemisphere, and, therefore, left or right sequence may be followed in attempting to compare presented stimuli with memory images. This leads to confusion or delay in selection. "Our analysis points to confusion because of reversals in the memory images of symbols, resulting in a failure of association between the visual presented stimulus and its concept." He points out that children with these confusions see as others do, but fail to learn to elide completely one of the two antitropic anagrams registered as a pattern for a later comparison, which forms the basis of recognition. Orton distinguishes between static reversals, which occur in the single letter (for instance, in the mistake between b and d, and p and q), and kinetic reversals, where there is a tendency to assemble the letters in sinistral, alternating sinistral, or dextral order. In reading disability, this tendency may exhibit itself in only a few letters of a word, in a syllable, or in a whole word. In this way, Orton is inclined to explain all changes in the order of letters. In the in-and-out reversals, the child may spell in both directions; "how" becomes "wow," and "rag" is spelled as "raggag." A good instance of this occurred in Case 2, where "little" was written as "elttli."

Cases 3 and 6 of our study showed a marked left and right disorientation, but in the majority of our cases, the left and right mistakes did not play an important part, and may be completely absent, as in Case 1. This makes it, at the very least, improbable that Orton's theory covers the whole field. It is worthwhile to discuss whether even extreme difficulties in the left and right orientation of letters and words can produce the enormous difficulties children have in coordinating the reading of the sounds of two letters, which are, as such, very well known to them. One would at least expect that, when a child can read u and p, he should be able to make one word out of these sounds. In our Case 3, the boy correctly copies "m-e," but still is not able to make a word out of it. It is hard to believe that difficulties of this kind should be merely secondary to the difficulties in right and left orientation of the letters. However, Orton is certainly right when he supposes that the difficulty in visualization of words by mirror mistakes may drive the child to phonetic spelling, and phonetic mistakes in spelling and writing.

We find, in addition, in cases which do not show mirror mistakes, difficulties in reading single letters, which can hardly be explained in any way other than as a primary difficulty in the optic perception or imagination of letters. Here belong the mistakes between L and I, T and L, and g and y; or, in another case, between C and S. I believe, therefore, that primary optic difficulty in the perception and use of letters exists in at least some cases. The mistake between M and N, and m and n, probably belongs in this category, although definite proof was not possible. But there is no question that even the optic mistakes, in these cases, are very different from those one finds in the cases of so-called pure alexia in adult persons, in which (at least in one group of cases) not only the wrong letter is perceived, but also the form of the letter is distorted. The condition of the eyes is not responsible for such mistakes. We observed trouble in refraction only in Case 3. In Case 2, there was some impairment of the eyesight, in connection with a hypophyseal condition. But, even in those cases, the impairment of the eyesight was certainly not responsible for the difficulty in the perception of letters. Case 2, by the way, is the only case in which there was some difficulty in the perception of numbers, more than simple reversals.

Certainly, the optic mistakes, concerning the letters, cannot be taken as the cause of the reading disability. They are merely an indication that we deal with primary disturbances in the perceptual optic sphere, which are not merely due to a difficulty in the dominance between left and right.

But in all these cases one difficulty was outstanding, and that was the difficulty of coordinating the sounds which are more or less correctly connected with the single letter, with the sequence of letters in the rewritten word. This inability was especially evident in short words, such as me, up, was, bat, and hem. It is hard to see how this inability, which occurred in reading as well as writing, could be secondary to any other disturbance, either in the optic sphere alone, or in the left and right correlation. When severe cases of that kind are able to read the whole word, it is because they have learned the word as a whole, but they are absolutely unable to analyze the word. Even the attempt at analysis causes great disturbance. This seems to be the reason why these words are sometimes pretty well perceived in tachistoscopic exposure. It also explains why, sometimes, only an identity of one more-or-less important letter causes misreading of one word for another. One child read "stockings," instead of "shoes." Sometimes, as in Case 4, one gets the impression that there is vague knowledge of the concept of the words which cannot be read. All this leads to the conclusion that we deal with a primary disturbance concerning the sound structure in the written words. This disturbance can be compared with the difficulty with the spoken word, as observed in some aphasias. In some aphasias, we find that sounds are not put in the right place, that they change their positions in the whole of the word. Reduplication takes place. We are not justified in believing that all these mistakes of sequences in sounds are due to interferences between the right and left hemispheres, although interferences of that kind may also be of importance in aphasia. The lesion of a center of the left hemisphere certainly pushes the function back to a level of lower integration. The disintegration between left and right impulses may be one part in this disturbance.

We know that the destruction of the left practic region may liberate mirror tendencies in the left hand, and even improve the left-hand mirror writing. But the destruction of the left region, which alters the dominance, at the same time changes the inner development of action, generally, and writing in particular. The change in the dominance of the hemisphere, although important in itself, is not sufficient to explain all the other disturbances. The German literature on aphasia has repeatedly tried to explain the paraphasias of the so-called sensory aphasia as the expression of the activity of the right brain. In the so-called sympathic apraxia, which occurs on the left side, when either the left practic region or the connection between the left and right practic region (*corpus callosum*) is impaired, we find the motor activities of a more primitive type. But, even in this instance, the removal of the dominance of the left hemisphere provokes a type of reaction which is identical with the lower type of integration which results from every lesion of a cortical center of high order, and is not merely due to the tendency of mirror reversal.

In congenital reading disability, there are sufficient hints—in the so-called optic mistakes, inability to coordinate the single sounds with the whole word and differentiate the whole word into the single sounds, and in their written expression—that we deal with a primary inability and insufficiency of centers. This primary inability may release the mirror tendencies. This mirror tendency certainly can have a disturbing effect on the process of reading, writing, and spelling, but the mirror tendency, in itself, is insufficient to explain the whole picture. We come, therefore, to the formulation that the congenital reading disability is due to an incomplete function of centers. It is the inability of the patient to differentiate the spoken word into its sounds and to put sounds together into a word. It makes the word have meaning only as a whole. The sound has a meaning of its own. Single sounds are connected with a written letter, but the written letter cannot be put together into a whole. The written word, even when connected with the object named, cannot be separated into its single sounds and letters. The letters correlate with the sound within the word.

This formulation agrees pretty closely with those of Monroe (1932), Illing (1929), and Bachmann (1927). It differs from the formulation of Orton only insofar as Orton thinks that this disturbance, which he too emphasizes, is secondary to the disturbances in the dominance of the hemispheres, which increase the mirror tendencies; whereas, according to our opinion, the disturbance is primary and the release of the mirror tendencies is secondary. The released mirror tendencies (insofar as we agree with Orton) may increase the difficulty. It is worthwhile to give some consideration to Case 3, from this point of view. According to the history, this child had not only a birth paralysis of the right arm, but also a subsequent encephalitis, with right side hemiplegia. One is astonished to see that, in this case, the mirror tendencies have remained outstanding, and that static and kinetic reversals are in the foreground. But, even in this case, the difficulties in putting together the sounds into a word are so great that the mirror tendencies do not explain the whole difficulty. We do not deny that mirror tendencies are a factor of enormous importance. One could be tempted to range this case with the rare cases in which congenital reading difficulties are connected with organic lesions (Guenther, 1928; Currier and Dewar, 1927). In our case, as well as in the cases of the literature, it is doubtful whether the focal lesion provokes the reading difficulty; it is probably a factor which adds to reading disabilities which are based on the insufficient development of those centers which guarantee the development of the faculty of reading. Orton has rightly emphasized the familial character of reading disabilities. Poetzl (1928), in this connection, has pointed to the investigation of Karplus, who found that the configuration of the gyri in the brain may show hereditary and familial characteristics. We do not doubt that congenital reading disability can and must be interpreted from a neurological point of view. Therefore, we consider the opinion of Gates (1929), that reading disability is due to faulty habits in learning, as contradictory to the facts.

We deal with a trouble of the agnostic type, and Bachmann's attempt to separate it from agnosia and aphasia is not justified. We agree with Orton and Monroe, who point out that the intelligence of these cases of congenital reading difficulties is good, or at least sufficient for the acquisition of reading and writing. We certainly do not deal with a general lack of intelligence. All of our cases, with the exception of Case 2, were sent to us as behavior problems, resulting, to a large degree, from their inefficiency in reading. We again emphasize that we deal with a rather isolated gnostic disturbance.

It is worthwhile to remember how different congenital reading disability is from pure word blindness which results, in adults, from a lesion of the gyrus-angularis (according to Poetzl: gyrus-lingualis). Cases of that type are very often unable to recognize letters. In the less serious cases, the difficulty is restricted to the recognition of

363

words. But they are unable to copy letters and words, whereas their spontaneous writing is good. They are unable to read what they, themselves, have written. Pure word blindness is a mere optic product. In congenital reading disability, the difficulty concerns the inner structure of the word and its sounds. It is an agnostic trouble, not so much concerning the merely optic sphere, but a sphere which is nearer to the intellectual life than optic perception. It is true that every gnostic function is also an intellectual one, but the intellectual function which is disturbed, in congenital reading disability cases, is of a higher level than the function which is disturbed in cases of pure word blindness. We deal here with an isolated trouble in gnostic intellectual function.

This formulation strictly contradicts tendencies which are almost predominant in modern neurology. Head (1926) and Goldstein (1923), do not believe that isolated disturbances of gnostic and speech function can occur by cortical lesion a disturbance which impairs one gnostic function damages every gnostic function. Lashley (1929) has come to very similar formulations in his experiments on rats. Orton's and our patients did not show any aphasic trouble. There was no general intellectual impairment. Our study placed special emphasis on the careful examination of optic perception, which disclosed no pathology or functional inability. Deviations from the norm were not observed during tachistoscopic expositions of objects. We say that careful investigation did not reveal any difficulties in the optic perception; if optic perception, as such, would be disturbed, one could expect that the tachistoscopic exposure of letters and words would impair the perception enormously. As Bachmann (1927) has already shown, this is not the case. The increase in difficulties was in no case greater than the difficulties a normal child would experience under similar conditions. In Case 5, the tachistoscopic perception of words seemed to be even better than perception under ordinary conditions, but this was only true of words familiar to the subject. The tachistoscopic exposures made it easier to take the word as a whole.

Our final interpretation would be that final mastery of the written and spoken word, concerning differentiation and integration of sounds, is a very complicated function. These difficulties vary in different languages, and increase in English, where the sound of a single letter is not identical with its sound in the word. The faculty varies in different children (Monroe). These variations are probably due to a different development of those parts of the brain which are indispensable for the process of reading. In the serious cases, we probably deal with a dysfunction of a cortical apparatus. This dysfunction expresses itself in the integrating and differentiating difficulty in optic mistakes concerning letters, and in increased mirror tendencies. The inherent mirror tendencies, as well as mirror tendencies originating from other sources, and intellectual difficulties may alter and increase the primary trouble, which is an isolated trouble of gnostic intellectual function.

## Conclusions

The basic difficulty in congenital reading disability is the difficulty to differentiate the spoken word into its sounds and to put together the sounds of a word. Words and single sounds are brought into connection with a written word and written letter, but the written word and written letter cannot be integrated and differentiated. Two other independent difficulties may be present— mirror mistakes and trouble in the optic perception of letters. There are no troubles in other optic perceptions. We deal with an isolated trouble in a gnostic-intellectual function.

### CULTURAL PATTERNS AND THE FAMILY[38]

Every family is a unit of culture in a bad or good sense. Ideologies are the result of a psychological interaction of various generations of one family. They are either symbolic expressions of the unconscious libidinous situation of the family, or they are secondary elaborations and rationalizations. The real basis of ideologies belongs, in psychoanalytic terminology, to the system of the unconscious. In other words, they are continuous condensations, symbolizations, and transformations. Of course, the family structure is different in different cultures. An Australian or Melanesian family is rather different from a North American family. The family structure of the so-called "smart set," and of a workman's family, is fundamentally different. One generally has the impression that the

[38] From Schilder (1940c).

family structure, in a given primitive tribe, is identical in different families, and there is more homogeneity in family structures and in ideologies than in more developed cultures. However, this conclusion is unproved, since it overlooks the fact that a whole tribe in Australia may not have many more families than a small community in our culture. The family structure of adjacent tribes varies perhaps more than the family structures in communities of a similar size, or social sets in larger cities, which form units comparable to tribes, although they are mixed, in space, with other sets.

Let us study the ideologies and behavior of a family of which three members, a mother and two daughters (twelve and thirteen), were admitted to the Psychiatric Division of Bellevue Hospital at the same time. The mother, a woman about forty, reported that she had always been badly treated by her in-laws. Many years ago, she lived in crowded quarters with many of her relatives. At that time, she had a baby which, according to her report, was badly treated by the in-laws, pushed around, and thrown on the sidewalk, until it finally died at the age of six months. The older daughter of the patient, Vida, thirteen years old, believed this story, and added, "My mother was paralyzed every time my aunt looked at her and my sister died because my mother couldn't feed her with my aunt around." However, this woman also did not get along with her husband, whom she blamed for taking care of other people, without taking care of his own health. Her husband had died a few months previously, of a heart disease which had lasted for about ten years. At the time of the first signs of the father's heart disease, the two children were put into a children's home, where both contracted a specific vaginitis. This was adequately treated and cured, but the mother continued to give the girls irrigations. Soon, she also complained about vaginitis and, partially because of this and partially because of the husband's heart disease, their sex relations became rare; and there were no sex relations in the last seven or eight years before the husband's death.

Seemingly, the patient had little inclination for sex relations, and was preoccupied with her hostilities against her relatives, and with her vaginitis. She was a rather belligerent and active individual, who felt that people, especially her relatives, were not friendly toward her and persecuted her. The illness of the husband had become exacerbated about eighteen months before his death. Shortly after he became ill, the patient was visited by her brother, whom she had not seen for thirty years. She felt that he had an extraordinary power over her and could make her do whatever he wanted. This particular power emanated from his eyes, and she felt paralyzed when he looked at her. The patient felt that her brother forced her to neglect her husband, and that this neglect resulted in the death of her husband. The brother was described as an attractive, unmarried man, who charmed women and always tried to get something for nothing. The patient was convinced that this was true. However, this was not a true delusional system. The patient was a badly adjusted person, who was confronted with a difficult situation when her husband got sick. It is probable that the deep sexual interest in her brother was merely a revival of earlier attitudes. We have to assume that there were many problems like this in her childhood, and that she might have been less averse to sex if they had not existed. Since she did not have sex relations with her husband, the attachment to her brother took on sexual coloring. We must, however, also ask what was the husband's psychology. Husbands are generally not deterred by a vaginitis of their wives, nor by a minor ailment of their own, from having sex relations.

The patient developed her belief that people were against her. It is true that there are always people who are against you, but there are also always people who are for you. It may be the same person who is sometimes against you and sometimes for you. The attitude of others depends not only on the individual circumstances, and their own experiences, but also on the attitude which you take toward them. Perhaps the sorcerers of Dobu had a difficult struggle for food supplies. Perhaps there had once been an extended period of scarcity, and these conditions brought hatred and distrust to the foreground. Such patterns, once developed, are not so easily relinquished. They become habits which one cannot give up, even if it would be advantageous and agreeable to do so. The Dobuans had the bad habit of distrusting each other; they could not help it. The pattern perpetuates itself, since the children are brought up in the same environment. A good part of what we call culture has been acquired under specific circumstances, and persists after the circumstances have changed. Many of our institutions were alive in the past, but do not have meaning for the present. However, they persist. Consequently, our culture is filled with relics of the past, which may have become completely nonunderstandable. They are residuals from very different strata, and we may try in vain to make a unit out of different disconnected structures, of varying historical age. The relics are relics of material culture, which guarantee a set of attitudes that fit the material culture.

Let us return to the discussion of our particular family. The two girls, thirteen and twelve, were born at a time when the mother's belief that everybody persecuted her was already fully developed. The relation between the parents was already strained, and intercourse was infrequent. The girls were put into the home where they contracted the specific vaginitis, which was cured. However, as mentioned, the mother stuck to the douche pattern. The relations between the three vaginitis cases is a psychological problem in itself. The older of the two girls had an IQ of 115, and the younger had an IQ of 125. It seems that the younger child was always the livelier. She was the more outgoing and attractive personality, and received more love from the parents. It is always difficult to say why one child is more loved than another. Sometimes, this may be due to the characteristics of the child or the erotic relations between the parents. Sometimes, the firstborn does not get so much attention, because the parents are enwrapped in each other, while sometimes, the firstborn profits by the love the parents still have for each other. When the parents start to hate each other, they may take refuge in love of the child. Sometimes, when the mother is frigid, the unused sexual energy may flow to the child. Children react very promptly to every shade of libidinous reaction in the attitudes of their parents. The variability of family patterns is almost inexhaustible. At any rate, in this case, the older girl (Vida) was less loved, by both parents, than the younger one. She was always shy, reticent, and very sensitive. She was deeply in love with her father, whom she admired greatly. She felt she could not obtain the love of her father, so she consoled herself with the idea that she would become like her father, and would become a machinist, her father's trade. She always wished to be a boy.

I really do not know what a man is. It would be comparatively simple if we were satisfied to define a man as an individual with a male sex organ. That is, indeed, the only correct definition. It is probably not true that the man is more aggressive than the woman, although we have been encouraged to believe so. It is true that men are generally stronger than women, although there are some Siberian tribes where women are reported to be stronger than men (Briffault, 1927). Strength is no longer of value in our civilization. One needs great strength only in a few callings, for instance as a longshoreman. Even during the war, possession of mere strength did not prove to be of great value. When cannon are a few miles away, one cannot defend oneself against them by being strong. The concept that strength is a value, in itself, is a remainder from a long past social situation. Children generally think that strength and health are identical. However, it seems that strength and health have no correlation to each other. Strength is obviously not needed for men to protect women. Women are just as capable of protecting themselves. So, when a girl says she wants to be a man, it is very difficult to understand what she means. Perhaps she merely wants to be a machinist. However, behind that wish lies the desire to have compensation for the unfulfilled love for her father. She identifies herself with the father. Sometimes, one wants to be a man in order to have the male sex organ. Perhaps many men want to be women because they want to have female sex organs.

The psychology of masculinity or femininity, in a given culture, is the result of cultural, rather than biological, factors. In some animal groups, the males are stronger; in others the females are stronger. However, why should one go to lions, tigers, and monkeys in order to find out something about human ideologies? The sex organs and their products (spermatozoa and ova) give a clear enough indication who is a man and who is a woman. From the point of view of cultural psychology, we know what the girl meant when she said that she wanted to be like her father and did not want to marry. However, she still clung to the father, whom she endowed with magic qualities, and was therefore ready to accept the magic relation between her mother and her mother's brother (the child's uncle). She, too, believed that the uncle had hypnotized

369

her and was responsible for the death of her father. In this respect, she took a clue from her mother.

She reported "My uncle came to stay with us. He can put an enchantment over you and keep you there. He looks at you, you can't move, you turn to stone. He made believe he was working and went out." She always blocked when asked whether she was jealous of his women or curious as to his activities. "When he was there, it seemed as if a big fog was in the air. When he left it lifted, but we were all tired. When I got up in the morning and went to the door, I felt so tired my feet could hardly move. I would lie on the bed and sleep until four, then eat and go back to bed. The worker thought it was my mother keeping me home but she wasn't. I couldn't go. It seemed like everybody was watching me. It seemed like eyes were staring at me from all around, like an animal. When he left then I didn't feel so tense. My mother felt like something was driving her when he was there. Made her sick for a day and the house was dirty. Uncle thought father had some money." She stated that this tenseness and worry began before her father's death in October. Sometimes, when alone, she felt that something was boring into her skin. "I always felt he was staring at me. It felt like the eyes of an animal, tiger's eyes ready to pounce on me. He treated me nice, but I hate him. I told mother that he was the cause of father's death. I knew I hated him. I talked back to him. Hit him. [He denied that he ever made advances to any of the family.] He went away and stayed all night and never took us. I don't want to touch anything he touched."

There was no manifest sex interest between uncle and niece. However, this relation replaced, for the child, the love she could not obtain from her father. In turn, therefore, she identified herself with the father, and, unloved as a woman, desired to become a man; but she also identified with the mother, whose ideas and symptoms she took over. If similar experiences had occurred in a primitive and rather limited society, we might have found variations in the masculinity concept (compare, for instance, the study of Mead, 1935), and a belief in sorcery with rituals of protection against sorceries. It is interesting that the younger sister had accepted the mother's and older sister's belief without being emotionally preoccupied with it. Loved by her parents, she felt secure in her heterosexual attitude.

This was a family with a strong belief in psychological sorcery and witchcraft. There were no flaws in the family ideology, which was accepted by all members of the family, with more or less fervor. However, this family ideology was contradictory to the prevalent ideologies in the larger society, and the family thus came into difficulties. It may be added that the family ideology was due to the particular insufficiencies of the mother, and had only a limited subjective value for the mother herself. It was obvious that it was not of value for the community at any time. We do not wonder that such an ideology originated from a person who was otherwise rather insufficient in the ordinary tasks of life.

We may conclude that ideologies, of cultural value, must have at least once given something to the community, and transgressed the borderlines of a single family. Such ideologies, incorporated into the beliefs and actions of the whole community, would not remain merely in the psychological field, but would express themselves in the material culture, which gave them a better chance to perpetuate themselves. The ideology of a small group or of a single family, as in our case, has no possibility for the creation of a specific material culture, and merely manifests itself psychologically. Family interactions have to be considered as the origin of ideologies, and the family is the ideological unit. Some families have specific ideas about cleanliness, others about sex, and others about religion. In Clarence Day's book, *God and Father*, the father was a man who believed in God, and considered Him as good when He did what was asked of Him, but thought He was deserving of punishment and contempt when He failed to do what was expected of Him. Concepts of this type are not fully conscious, and are handed down from father to son as unconscious tradition. This represents culture in the growing. A family ideology can become the ideology of a group, if it helps to handle specific situations and fits the physical situation or economic trend of the outer world.

Culture, as it appears as a more or less complete gestalt, is more than it is conscious of, itself. It has to be deciphered, like a neurotic symptom or a dream. It has to be seen in its historical aspects, and in its relation to nature and material culture. Cultural patterns have been erected slowly, by a system of trial and error. At the time of their creation, they expressed an approximate equilibrium between the various libidinous and realistic tendencies. Once created, they have the tendency to persist, even if they have outlived their usefulness. A given culture always contains a considerable set of more-or-less antiquated and superannuated cultural configurations, which, for emotional reasons, are no longer exposed to the trial-and-error method, by which they could prove their usefulness. Reality is continually changing. Fortunately, it puts new tasks before us, again and again. A static cultural pattern and a static culture in general, lose their value. Cultural configurations are not made for eternity. We should not try to find a lasting security in cultural gestalten, which, when superannuated, are dangerous obstacles against the vital experiences which constitute the true culture.

# Bibliography

Abraham, K. (1927), The First Pregenital Stage of the Libido. *Selected Papers of Karl Abraham*. London: Hogarth Press, pp. 248-279.

Adler, A. (1917), *The Neurotic Constitution: Outline of a Comparative Individualistic Psychology and Psychotherapy*. New York: Moffat, Yard.

Allport, F. H. (1924), *Social Psychology*. Boston: Houghton Mifflin.

Bachmann, F. (1927), Ueber Kongenitale Wortblindkeit. *Abhandl. Neurol., Psychiat. & Psychol.*, 40:1-72.

Baldwin, J. (1903), *Mental Development*. New York: Macmillan.

Balint, M. (1935), Zur Kritik der Lehre von der praegenitalen Libido Organization. *Int. Ztschr. Psychoanal.*, 21:525-544.

Baudouin, C. (1933), *Mind of the Child*. London: Allen & Unwin.

Bauer, J. (1925), *Allgemeine Konstitutions—und Vererbungslehre*. Berlin: Springer.

Bechtereff, V. (1926), *Allgemeine Grundlagen der Reflexologie des Menschen*. Leipzig & Vienna: Reuticke.

Bender, L. (1932), Gestalt Principles in Sidewalk Drawings and Games of Children. *J. Genet. Psychol.*, 41:192-210.

———— (1937), Group Activities on a Children's Ward as a Method of Psychotherapy. *Am. J. Psychiat.*, 43:1151-1173.

———— (1938), *Visual Motor Gestalt Test and Its Clinical Use*. New York: American Orthopsychiatric Association.

———— (1939), Behavior Problems in Negro Children. *Psychiatry*, 5: 213-239.

———— (1940), The Psychology of Children Suffering from Organic Disturbances of the Cerebellum. *Am. J. Orthopsychiat.*, 10: 287-292.

———— (1947), Childhood Schizophrenia. *Am. J. Orthopsychiat.*, 17: 40-56.

373

———— (1952), *Child Psychiatric Techniques*. Springfield, Ill.: Charles C Thomas.

———— (1953), *Aggression, Hostility and Anxiety in Children*. Springfield, Ill.: Charles C Thomas.

———— (1954), *A Dynamic Psychopathology of Childhood*. Springfield, Ill.: Charles C Thomas.

———— (1955), *The Psychopathology of Children with Organic Brain Disorders*. Springfield, Ill.: Charles C Thomas.

———— & Schilder, P. (1933), Encephalopathica Alcoholica. *Arch. Neurol. & Psychiat.*, 29:990-1053.

———— & ———— (1936), Form as a Principle in the Play of Children. *J. Genet. Psychol.*, 49:254-261.

———— & ———— (1936a), Studies in Aggressiveness in Children. *Genet. Psycholog. Monogr.*, 18:410-425.

———— & ———— (1937), Suicidal Preoccupations and Attempts in Children. *Am. J. Orthopsychiat.*, 7:225-234.

———— & ———— (1940), Impulsions, A Specific Disorder in Behavior of Children. *Arch. Neurol. & Psychiat.*, 44:990-1008.

———— & ———— (1941), Mannerisms as Organic Motility Syndrome. *Confinia Neurologia*, 3:321-330.

———— & Woltmann, A. G. (1936), Use of Puppet Shows as a Psychotherapeutic Method for Behavior Problems in Children. *Am. J. Orthopsychiat.*, 6:341-354.

Bernfeld, S. (1925), *The Psychology of the Infant*. New York: Brentano, 1929.

Bettelheim, B. (1924), Ueber Nachgreifen bei Hirnlaesionen. *Monatschr. Neurol. & Psychiat.*, 54.

Bieber, I. (1937), Grasping and Sucking. *J. Nerv. & Ment. Dis.*, 85:196-201.

Blau, A. (1936), Mental Changes Following Head Trauma in Children. *Arch. Neurol. & Psychiat.*, 35:723-769.

Bleuler, E. (1911), *The Theory of Schizophrenic Negativism*. New York: Nervous and Mental Disease, Monograph Series No. 11.

———— (1950), *Dementia Praecox or the Group of Schizophrenias*. New York: International Universities Press.

Bond, E. D. & Appel, K. E. (1931), *The Treatment of Behavior Disorders Following Encephalitis*. New York: Commonwealth Fund.

Boring, E. G. (1933), *The Physical Dimension of Consciousness*. New York & London: Appleton-Century.

Breed, F. S. & Shepard, J. R. (1913), The Maturation and Use in the Development of an Instinct. *J. Animal Behav.*, 3:274.

Bridges, K. M. (1931), *The Social and Emotional Development of the Pre-School Child.* London: Kegan Paul.

Briffault, R. (1927), *The Mothers, The Matriarchal Theory of Social Origins.* New York: Macmillan.

Bromberg, W. (1934), Schizophrenia-Like Psychosis in Defective Children. *Am. J. Psychiat.*, 90:226-257.

———— & Schilder, P. (1932), On Tactile Imagination and Tactile After-Effects. *J. Nerv. & Ment. Dis.*, 76:37-51.

———— & ———— (1933), Death and Dying. *Psychoanal. Rev.* 20: 133-185.

———— & ———— (1933a), Psychologic Considerations in Alcoholic Hallucinosis: Castration and Dismembering Motives. *Int. J. Psycho-Anal.*, 14:206-224.

———— & ———— (1936), Attitude of Psychoneurotics Toward Death. *Psychoanal. Rev.*, 23:1-25.

Brown, T. G. (1911), The Intrinsic Factors in the Act of Progression in Mammals. *Proceed. Royal Soc. London*, 84.

Buehler, K. (1929), *Die Geistige Entwicklung des Kindes.* Jena: Fischer. *The Mental Development of the Child.* New York: Harcourt, Brace, 1930.

Byers, R. K. (1928), Tonic Neck Reflexes in Children. *Am. J. Dis. Childhood*, 55:696-742.

Canestrini, N. (1913), Das Sinnesleben der Neugeborenen. *Monogr. ges. Neurol. & Psychiat.*, 5.

Cavan, R. S. (1928), *Suicide.* Chicago: University of Chicago Press.

Clark, L. P. (1933), *The Nature and Treatment of Amentia.* London: Baillière, Tindall & Cox.

Coghill, G. E. (1929), *Anatomy and the Problem of Behavior.* Cambridge, Mass.: Harvard University Press.

———— (1933), The Biologic Basis of Conflict in Behavior. *Psychoanal. Rev.*, 20:4.

Cohen-Booth, G. (1935), Paralysis Agitans. *Nervenarzt*, 8:2.

Collingswood, S. D. (1929), *The Life and Letters of Lewis Carroll.* London: Benn.

Corré, A. (1891), *Crime et Suicide.* Paris.

Cottington, F. (1941-1942), The Treatment of Schizophrenia of Childhood. *Nerv. Child*, 1:172-187.

———— (1941), The Treatment of Childhood Schizophrenia by Metrazol Shock Modified by B-erythroidin. *Am. J. Psychiat.*, 98: 397-400.

Curran, F. J. & Schilder, P. (1940-1941), A Constructive Approach to the Problems of Childhood and Adolescence. *J. Crim. Psychopath.,* 2:125-142; 3:305-321.

Currier, F. P., Jr., & Dewar, M. (1927), Difficulties in Reading in School Children. *J. Michigan State Med. Soc.,* 26:300-304.

de la Mare, W. (1932), *Lewis Carroll.* London: Faber & Faber.

Delboeuf, A. (1901), *Grundfragen der Sprach der Sprachforschung.* Strasbourg.

Deutsch, H. (1932), *Psychoanalysis of the Neuroses.* London: Hogarth Press.

Dewey, E. (1935), *Behavior Development in Infants.* New York: Columbia University Press.

Dewey, J. (1934), *Art as Experience.* New York: Minton, Balch.

Dix, W. K. (1911-1923), *Koerperliche und geistige Entwicklung eines Kindes.* Leipzig: Barth.

Dorff, G. B. (1935), Masked Thyroidism in Children. *J. Pediat.,* 6:788-798.

————— & Stoloff, B. (1939), Abdominal Distention—A Manifestation of Possible Thyroid Insufficiency in Children. *Arch. Pediat.,* 56:291-303.

Dublin, L. I. & Bunzel, B. (1933), *To Be Or Not To Be—A Study of Suicide.* New York: Smith & Haas.

Economo, C. von (1931), Encephalitis Lethargica. *Jb. Psychiat.,* 38:19.

Engerth, G. & Hoff, H. (1929), Ueber das Schicksal der Patienten mit Schwerer Characterveraendering nach Encephalitis Epidemica. *Dtsch. med. Wochenschr.,* 55:181-183.

Erickson, M. (1937), Hypnotic Reliving of a Traumatic Experience. *Arch. Neurol. & Psychiat.,* 38:1222-1228.

Esper, E. A. (1933), Language. In: *Handbook for Social Psychology,* ed., C. Murchison. Worcester, Mass.: Clark University Press.

Fenichel, O. (1934), *Outline of Clinical Psychoanalysis.* New York: Norton.

Ferenczi, S. (1913), Stages in the Development of a Sense of Reality. In: *Sex in Psychoanalysis.* New York: Brunner, 1950.

————— (1919), *Hysterie und Pathoneurosen.* Leipzig: Barth.

Fettermann, J. (1928), Traumatic Neuroses. *J. Am. Med. Assoc.,* 91:315.

Feuchtwanger, E. (1933), Koerpertonus und Aussenraum. *Arch. Psychiat.,* 100:439-490.

Field, R. (1934), *Susanna B. and William C.* New York: Morrow.

Fischer, M. H. & Wodak, E. (1924), Beitraege zur Physiologie des menschlichen Vestibular Apparatus. *Arch. ges. Physiol.,* 202:253.

Freud, S. (1894), The Defense Neuro-Psychoses. *Collected Papers,* 1:59-75. London: Hogarth Press, 1948.

———— (1900), The Interpretation of Dreams. In: *The Basic Writings of Sigmund Freud.* New York: Modern Library, 1938.

———— (1905), *Three Essays on the Theory of Sexuality.* London: Imago, 1949.

———— (1918), From the History of an Infantile Neurosis. *Collected Works,* 3:473-605. London: Hogarth Press, 1950.

———— (1919), A Child is Being Beaten. *Collected Works,* 2:172-201. London: Hogarth Press, 1949.

———— (1920), *Beyond the Pleasure Principle.* London: Hogarth Press, 1948.

———— (1924), The Passing of the Oedipus Complex. *Collected Works,* 2:269-282. London: Hogarth Press, 1949.

———— (1926), *Inhibitions, Symptoms, and Anxiety.* London: Hogarth Press, 1936.

———— (1931), Female Sexuality. *Collected Works,* 5:252-272. London: Hogarth Press, 1950.

Freudenberg, E. (1921), Der Morosche Umklammerungs Reflex. *Muenschen med. Wochenschr.,* 68:146-7.

Friedjung, J. K. (1925), Akute Psychoneurosen in Kindheit. *Ztschr. Neurol. & Psychiat.,* 136:126-132.

Frisch, K. von (1915), Der Farbensinn und Formensinn der Biene. *Zool. Jb.,* 25:1-182.

Gabrio, M. R. (1920), A Case of Traumatic Hysteria. *Arch. Neurol. & Psychiat.,* 3:569.

Gamper, E. (1926), Bau und Leistungen eines menschlichen Mittelhirnwesens. *Ztschr. Neurol.,* 102:154; 104:49.

Gates, A. I. (1929), *Improvement of Reading.* New York: Macmillan.

Gelb, A. & Goldstein, K. (1918), Zur Psychologie des Optischen Wahrnehmunges und Erkennung Vorganges. *Ztschr. ges. Neurol. & Psychiat.,* 41:1.

———— & ———— (1919), Ueber den Einfluss des Vollstandigen Verhestes des Optischen Vorstellung Vermoegens auf das Taktile Erkennen. *Ztschr. Psychol. & Physiol. Sinnesorgane,* 83:1.

———— & ———— (1920), *Psychologische Analysen Hirnpathologischer Faelle.* Leipzig: Barth.

Gesell, A. L. (1929), Maturation and Infant Behavior Pattern. *Psycholog. Rev.,* 36:307.

———— (1939), *Biographies of Child Development.* New York: Hoeber.

———— (1940), *The First Five Years of Life.* New York & London: Harper.

———— & Amatruda, C. S. (1945), *The Embryology of Behavior.* New York: Harper.

———— & Thompson, H. (1934), *Infant Behavior, Its Genesis and Growth.* New York: McGraw-Hill.

Goldstein, K. (1923), Die Lokalization in des Grosshirn. *Dtsch. Ztschr. Nervenheilkunde,* 77:891.

———— (1934), *The Organism.* New York: American Book, 1939.

———— (1938), Moro Reflex and Startle Pattern. *Arch. Neurol. & Psychiat.,* 40:322-327.

Goodenough, F. (1926), *Measurement of Intelligence by Drawing.* New York: World Book.

Greene, R. A. (1933), Conflict in Diagnosis Between Mental Deficiency and Certain Psychoses. *Proceed. Am. Assoc. Ment. Deficiency,* 57:127-148.

Griffith, R. (1935), *A Study in Imagination in Early Childhood.* London: Kegan Paul, Trench, Trubner.

Gross, A. (1933), Zeitsinn und Traum. *Int. Ztschr. Psychoanal.,* 19:613.

Guenther, F. (1928), Beitraege fur Psychiatrie, Pathologie und Klinik der sogenannten Leseschwaeche. *Ztschr. Kinderforgang,* 34.

Hall, G. S. (1905), *Adolescence.* New York: Appleton, 1917.

Harms, E. (1936), Struktur-psychologische Korrektur am Begriffe der infantilen Sexualität. *Ztschr. Kinderpsychiat.,* 3:50-60, 88-90.

Hartmann, H. & Schilder, P. (1924), Zur Klinik und Psychologie der Amentia. *Ztschr. Neurol. & Psychiat.,* 92:531-596.

———— & ———— (1927), Koerperinneres und Bewegungen. *Monatschr. Neurol. & Psychiat.* 109:666-675.

Head, H. (1926), *Aphasia and Kindred Disorders of Speech.* Cambridge, England: Oxford University Press.

Heidegger, M. (1929), *Sein und Zeit.* Halle: Niemeyer.

Heller, I. (1908), Ueber Dementia Infantilis. *Ztschr. Erforschung & Behandl. des jugendlichen Schwachsinns,* 2:378.

Hempelmann, F. (1926), *Tierpsychologie.* Leipzig: Barth.

Hermann, I. (1936), Sich Anklammern und auf die Suchegehen. *Int. Ztschr. Psychoanal.,* 22:349.

———— (1940) Studien zur Denkpsychologie. *Acta Psychol.,* 5:22-102.

Herrick, R. (1932), *The Lewis Carroll Book.* New York: Dial Press.

Hinshelwood, J. (1917), *Congenital Word Blindness.* London: Lewis.

Hoff, H. & Schilder, P. (1927), *Die Lagereflexe des Menschen.* Berlin: Springer.

Holzer, J. (1926), Die Glienarbe im Mach-und Zwischenhirn Nach Encephalitis Epidemische. *Ztschr. Neurol.,* 104.

Homburger, A. (1922), Ueber die Entwicklung der Menschlichen Motorik und ihre Bezeihung in den Bewegungstoerungen der Schizophrenen. *Ztschr. Neurol. & Psychiat.*, 78:562.

Horney, K. (1924), The Genesis of the Castration Complex in Women. *Int. J. Psycho-Anal.*, 5:117-131.

Huddleson, J. H. (1932), *Accidents, Neuroses and Compensation.* Baltimore: William & Wilkins.

Husserl, E. (1913), *Logische Untersuchungen.* Halle: Niemeyer.

Illing, E. (1929), Ueber Kongenital Wortblindheit. *Monatschr. Psychiat. & Neurol.*, 71:297-355.

Isaacs, S. (1933), *Social Development of the Young Child.* New York: Harcourt.

Jacobson, E. (1932), Electrophysiology of Mental Activity. *Am. J. Physiol.*, 154:677-699.

Jaensch, E. R. (1930), *Ueber den Aufbau des Bewussteins.* Leipzig: Barth.

James, W. (1902), *The Principles of Psychology.* New York: Holt.

Jung, C. G. (1911-12), Criticism of Bleuler's "Theory of Schizophrenic Negativism." In: *Collected Papers on Analytic Psychiatry.* London: Baillière, Tindall & Cox, 1922.

Kahlbaum, M. (1902), Zur Kasuistik der Katatonie. *Monatschr. Neurol. & Psychiat.*, 12:22-56.

Kanner, L. & Schilder, P. (1930), Movements in Optic Imagination. *J. Nerv. & Ment. Dis.*, 72:489-517.

Kasanin, J. (1929), Personality Changes in Children Following Cerebral Trauma. *J. Nerv. & Ment. Dis.*, 69:385.

——— (1930), The Affective Psychoses in Children. *Trans. Am. Assoc. Nerv. & Ment. Dis.*, 11:88-117.

Keiser, S. & Schilder, P. (1936), Studies in Aggressiveness. *Genet. Psychol. Monogr.*, 18:361-401, 526-545.

Klein, M. (1930), Symbol-bildung und Ichentwicklung. *Int. Ztschr. Psychiat.*, 16:57-72.

——— (1932), *The Psychoanalysis of Children.* London: International Psycho-Analytic Press.

——— (1934), The Psychogenesis of Manic Depressive States. *Contributions to Psychoanalysis: 1921-1945.* London: Hogarth Press, 1948.

Kleist, K. (1923), Die psychomotorischen Stoerungen Geisteskranker. *Monatschr. Psychiat. & Neurol.*, 52.

Klüver, H. (1933), *Behavior Mechanisms in Monkeys.* Chicago: University of Chicago Press.

————— (1934), The Eidetic Child. In: *Handbook of Child Psychology*, ed., C. Murchison. Worcester, Mass.: Clark University Press.

Koffka, K. (1928), *The Growth of the Mind*. London: Kegan Paul.

————— (1935), *Principles of Gestalt Psychology*. New York: Harcourt, Brace.

Köhler, W. (1929), *Gestalt Psychology*. New York: Liveright.

————— (1931), *The Mentality of Apes*. New York: Liveright.

Korzybski, C. A. (1933), *Sanity and Science*. Lancaster, Pa.: International Non-Aristotelian Publishing Company.

Kramer, F. & Pollnow, H. (1932), Ueber eine Hyperkinetische Krankung um Kindersalter. *Monatschr. Neurol. & Psychiat.*, 82:1-10.

Lashley, K. S. (1929), *Brain Mechanisms and Intelligence*. Chicago: University of Chicago Press.

Le Maitre, A. (1910), *La Vie Mentale de L'adolescent et ses Anomalies*. Saint Blaise.

Levine, A. & Schilder, P. (1940), Motor Phenomena during Nitrogen Inhalation. *Arch. Neurol. & Psychiat.*, 44:1009-1017.

Levy, D. M. (1932), Body Interest in Children and Hypochondriasis. *Am. J. Psychiat.*, 12:295.

————— (1936), *Studies in Sibling Rivalry*. New York: American Orthopsychiatric Association.

Levy-Bruhl, L. (1923), *Primitive Mentality*. London: Allen & Unwin.

Liepmann, H. (1920), Apraxia. *Ergebn. Med.* (Von Bruegsch) 1:516.

Luquet, G. H. (1913), *Les Dessins d'un Enfant*. Paris: J. B. Baillière et Fils.

Magnus, R. (1924), *Koerperstellung*. Berlin: Springer.

————— & DeKleijn, A. (1912), Die Abhaengigkeit des Tonus von der Koepfstellung. *Pfluegers Arch. ges. Physiol.*, 155:455.

Markuszewicz, R. von (1936), Bemerkungen zur phallischen Organisationstute des Sexualtriebes. *Schweizer Arch. Neurol. & Psychiat.*, 38:77-88.

McDermott, J. F. (1935), *Lewis Carroll: "The Russian Journal" and Other Selections*. New York: Dutton.

McGraw, M. B. (1935), *Growth; A Study of Johnny and Jimmy*. New York: Appleton-Century.

Mead, M. (1935), *Sex and Temperament in Three Primitive Societies*. New York: Morrow.

Meyer, A. (1927), Zur Pathologischen Anatomie der epidemischen Metencephalitis des Kindersalters. *Arch. Psychiat.*, 80.

Meyer, P. (1913), Ueber die Reproduktion eingepraegter Figuren und ihrer raumlichen Stellungen bei Kindern und Erwachsenen. *Ztschr. Psychol. & Physiol. Sinnesorgane*, 114:34-91.

Minkowski, M. (1928), Neurobiologischen Studien am menschlichen Foetus. *Abderhaldens Handb. Biol. Arbeitsmet.*, 253:511-618.

Monroe, M. (1932), *Children Who Cannot Read*. Chicago: University of Chicago Press.

Moro, E. (1918), Das erste Trimenon. *Muenchen med. Wochenschr.*, 42:1147.

Moses, B. (1910), *Lewis Carroll in Wonderland and at Home*. New York: Appleton.

Murray, H. A. (1938), *Exploration in Personality*. New York: Oxford University Press.

Neustadt, R. (1928), Die Psychosen der Schwachsinnigen. *Abhandl. Neurol., Psychiat. & Psychol.*, 48:1-188.

Ogden, C. K. (1934), The Magic of Words. *Psyche*, 14:9-18.

————— & Richards, I. A. (1925), *The Meaning of Meaning*. New York: Harper.

Oppenheim, H. (1889), *Die Traumatischen Neurosen*. Berlin: Hirschwald.

Orenstein, L. L. & Schilder, P. (1938), Psychological Consideration of the Insulin Treatment of Schizophrenia. *J. Nerv. & Ment. Dis.*, 88:397-413, 644-660.

Orton, S. T. (1928), "Word Blindness" in School Children. *Arch. Neurol. & Psychiat.*, 14:581-651.

————— (1930), Familial Occurrence of Disorder in the Acquisition of Language. *Eugenics*, 3:1.

————— (1936), *Reading, Writing and Speech Problems in Children*. New York: Norton.

Parker, S. & Schilder, P. (1935), Acoustic Imagination and Acoustic Hallucinations. *Arch. Neurol. & Psychiat.*, 34:744-757.

—————, Schilder, P., & Wortis, H. (1939), A Specific Motility Psychosis in Negro Alcoholics. *J. Nerv. & Ment. Dis.*, 90:1-18.

Pavlov, I. P. (1927), *Conditioned Reflexes*. New York: International Publishers.

————— (1928), *Lectures on Conditioned Reflexes*. New York: International Publishers.

Piaget, J. (1928), *Judgment and Reasoning in the Child*. London: Kegan Paul.

————— (1930), *The Child's Conception of Causality*. New York: Harcourt, Brace.

————— (1932), *The Moral Judgment of the Child*. New York: Harcourt, Brace.

————— (1932a), *The Language and Thought of the Child*. New York: Harcourt, Brace.

Poetzl, O. (1917), Experimentelle erregte Traumbilder. *Ztschr. ges. Neurol. & Psychiat.,* 37:278.

———— (1928), Die Aphasielehre Optisch-agnostische Stoerungen. *Aschapfenbergs Handb. Psychiat.,* Vienna: Springer.

Potter, H. (1933), Schizophrenia in Children. *Am. J. Psychiat.,* 12:1253-1271.

Preyer, W. (1882), *The Mind of the Child.* New York: Appleton, 1889.

Quix, F. H. (1924), L'Examen clinique des symptomes otolithiques. *Soc. Belge D'Otol-Rhinol. & Laryngol.,* 11:24.

Rabiner, A. M. (1935), Significance of Panic and States of Consciousness in Grasping Movements. *Arch. Neurol. & Psychiat.,* 33:976-985.

Rado, S. (1928), Anxious Mother. *Int. J. Psycho-Anal.,* 9:219-226.

———— (1933), Fear of Castration in Women. *Psychoanal. Quart.,* 3:4-17.

Reed, L. (1932), *The Life of Lewis Carroll.* London: Foyle.

Reich, A. (1936), Klinischer Beitrag zum Verstandnis der paranoiden Persoenlichkeit. *Int. Ztschr. Psychoanal.,* 12:315-38.

Richter, K. (1931), The Grasping Reflex in the Newborn Monkey. *Arch. Neurol. & Psychiat.,* 26:784-790.

———— & Bartemier, L. H. (1926), Decerebrate Rigidity of the Sloth. *Brain,* 49:207-225.

Ritterhaus, E. (1921), Die Klinische Stellung des manisch-depressiven Irresein. *Ztschr. Neurol. & Psychiat.,* 72:320-346.

Ross, N. (1936), Hallucinatory Experiences of Changes in Visual Perception. *J. Nerv. & Ment. Dis.,* 83:671-678.

———— & Schilder, P. (1934), Tachistoscopic Experiments on the Perception of the Human Figure. *J. Genet. Psychol.,* 10:152.

Rossel, F. (1925), Das Hilfsschulkind. *Beihefte zur Hilfsschule.* Halle: Niemeyer.

Rotter-Kertesz (1936), Der tiefen psychologische Hintergrund der inzestuoesen Fixierung. *Int. Ztschr. Psychoanal.,* 22:338.

Rubinow, O. & Frankl, L. (1934), Die erste Dingauffassung beim Saeugling. *Ztschr. Psychol.,* 133:1-72.

Russell, B. (1927), *Philosophy.* New York: Norton.

Sanctis, S. de (1909), Dementia Precocissima Catatonica. *Neurolog. Centralbl.,* 28:879.

Saintsbury, G. (1903), *The Short History of English Literature.* Cambridge: Oxford University Press, Vol. 13, p. 186, 3rd edition.

Schilder, P. (1911), Chorea und Athetose. *Ztschr. ges. Neurol. & Psychiat.,* 7:219-261; 11:25-62.

———— (1912) Ueber die Encephalitis periaxialis diffusa. *Dtsch. Ztschr. Nervenheilk.,* 45:1-2.

———— (1912a), *Gesell Schafte Dtsch. Nervenaerzte*, 6(21):192-194.

———— (1913), *Ztschr. ges. Neurol. & Psychiat.*, 15:359-376.

———— (1914), *Dtsch. Ztschr. Nervenheilk.*, 52:419-456.

———— (1921), Ueber die psychischen Stoerungen bei der Encephalitis epidemica des Jahres 1920. *Ztschr. ges. Neurol. & Psychiat.*, 58: 299-340.

———— (1924), *Medizinische Psychologie für Aerzte und Psychologen.* Berlin: Springer. *Medical Psychology* (trans. D. Rapaport). New York: International Universities Press, 1953.

———— (1927), Zentrale Bewegungsstoerungen mit besonderer Beruecksichtigung der Sprache. *Wiener med. Wochenschr.*, 77: 635-668.

———— (1928), *Gedanken zur Naturphilosophie.* Vienna: Springer.

———— (1928a), *Introduction to Psychoanalytic Psychiatry.* New York: International Universities Press, 1951.

———— (1929), Posture and Cerebellum. *Arch. Neurol. & Psychiat.*, 21: 989.

———— (1929a), Conditioned Reflexes. *Arch. Neurol. & Psychiat.*, 22: 425-443.

———— (1931), *Brain and Personality.* New York: International Universities Press, 1951.

———— (1931a), Organic Problems in Child Guidance. *Ment. Hyg.*, 15:480-486.

———— (1933), The Vestibular Apparatus in Neurosis and Psychosis. *J. Nerv. & Ment. Dis.*, 78:1-23, 137-164.

———— (1934), Space, Time and Perception. *Psyche*, 14:124-138.

———— (1934a), Psychiatric Aspects of Chronic Neurological Diseases. Institute on Encephalitis, Birth Injury, Epilepsy, arranged by the Committee on Medical-Social Problems of Chronic Neurological Diseases. Medical Social Service Section, The Welfare Council of New York City, December, 1934 (Mimeographed).

———— (1934b), Somato-Psyche in Psychiatry and Social Psychology. *J. Abn. & Soc. Psychol.*, 29:314-327.

———— (1935), *Image and Appearance of the Human Body: Studies in the Constructive Energies of the Psyche.* New York: International Universities Press, 1950.

———— (1935a), Psychoanalysis of Space. *Psychoanal. Rev.*, 22:36-48.

———— (1935b), Reaction Types Resembling Functional Psychoses in Children on the Basis of an Organic Inferiority of the Brain. *Ment. Hyg.*, 19:439-446.

———— (1936), Language and the Constructive Energies of the Psyche. *Scientia*, 59:149-158, 204-211.

——— (1936a), Analysis of Ideologies as a Psychotherapeutic Method, Especially in Group Treatment. *Am. J. Psychiat.*, 93:601-617.

——— (1937), Psychological Implications in the Motor Development in Children. *Proceed. Fourth Inst. Exceptional Child.* Child Research Clinic of the Woods School, 4:38-59.

——— (1937a), The Relationship Between Social and Personal Disorganization. *Am. J. Sociol.*, 42:832-839.

——— (1937b), Sich-anklammern und Gleichgewicht. *Int. Ztschr. f. Psychoanal.*, 23:313-317.

——— (1938), The Child and the Symbol. *Scientia*, 64:21-26.

——— (1938a), Preface to L. Bender, *Visual Motor Gestalt Test and Its Clinical Use.* New York: American Orthopsychiatric Association.

——— (1938b), Psychoanalytic Remarks on *Alice in Wonderland* and Lewis Carroll. *J. Nerv. & Ment. Dis.*, 87:159-168.

——— (1938c), *Psychotherapy.* New York: Norton, 1951.

——— (1939), Results and Problems of Group Psychotherapy in Severe Neuroses. *Ment. Hyg.*, 23:87-99.

——— (1939a), Relation Between Clinging and Equilibrium. *Int. J. Psycho-Anal.*, 20:58-64.

——— (1939b), The Psychology of Schizophrenia. *Psychoanal. Rev.*, 26:380-398.

——— (1939c), The Concept of Hysteria. *Am. J. Psychiat.*, 95:1389-1413.

——— (1940), Vita and Bibliography of Paul Schilder. *J. Crim. Psychopathol.*, 2:221-234.

——— (1940a), Neuroses Following Head and Brain Injuries. In: *Injuries of the Skull, Brain, and Spinal Cord*, ed., S. Brock. Baltimore: Williams & Wilkins.

——— (1940b), Social Organization and Psychotherapy. *Am. J. Orthopsychiat.*, 10:911-926.

——— (1940c), Cultural Patterns and Constructive Psychology. *Psychoanal. Rev.*, 27:159-176.

——— (1941), Types of Anxiety Neuroses. *Int. J. Psycho-Anal.*, 22:209-228.

——— (1942), *Mind: Perception and Thought in Their Constructive Aspects.* New York: Columbia University Press.

——— (1942a), *Goals and Desires of Man.* New York: Columbia University Press.

——— (1944), Congenital Alexia and Its Relation to Optic Perception. *J. Genet. Psychol.*, 65:67-88.

———— (1951), *Psychoanalysis, Man and Society*. New York: Norton.

———— & Sugar, N. (1926), Zur Lehre von den schizophrenen Sprachstoerungen. *Ztschr. ges. Neurol. & Psychiat.*, 104:689-714.

———— & Wechsler, D. (1934), The Attitudes of Children Toward Death. *J. Genet. Psychol.*, 45:406-451.

———— & ———— (1935), Children's Concept of the Inside of Their Bodies. *Int. J. Psycho-Anal.*, 16:355-360.

Schmidt, G. (1939), Selbstmorderversuche Jugendlicher. *Ztschr. Psychiat. & Ihre Grenzegeliete*, 112:32-43.

Schuster, P. (1923), Zwangsgreifen und Nachgreifen, Zwei Posthemiplegic Bewegungsstoerungen. *Ztschr. Neurol. & Psychiat.*, 83: 586-609.

Schwarz, P. (1924), Erkrankungen des Zentral Nervensystems nach Traumatische Geburtsschaedigung. *Ztschr. ges. Neurol. & Psychiat.*, 90.

Sherrington, C. C. (1911), *The Integrative Action of the Nervous System*. New Haven: Yale University Press.

Spielrein, S. (1923), Die Zeit im Unterschwelligen Seelenleben. *Imago*, 10:300-317.

Staercke, A. (1921), Psychoanalysis and Psychiatry. *Int. J. Psycho-Anal.*, 2:361-415.

Stein, F. (1927), Ueber psychische Zwangsvorgaenge und Angstzustaende bei Blickrampfen. *Arch. Psychiat.*, 81.

Stern, C. & Stern, W. (1922), *Die Kindersprache*. Leipzig: Barth.

Stern, W. (1924), *Psychology of Early Childhood*. London & New York: Holt.

Stransky, E. (1911), *Das Manisch-depressive Irresein*. Leipzig & Vienna: Deuticke.

Strauss, E. (1930), Die Formen des Raeumlichen; ihre Bedeutung fur die Motorik und die Wahnehmung. *Nervenartzeit*, 3:633-656.

Strauss, I. & Savitzky, N. (1934), Head Injury; Neurologic and Psychiatric Aspects. *Arch. Neurol. & Psychiat.*, 31:893.

Stumpf, C. (1900), Zur Methodik der Kinderpsychologie. *Ztschr. paed. Psychol.*, 2:1-21.

Teicher, J. D. (1941), Preliminary Survey of Motility in Children. *J. Nerv. & Ment. Dis.*, 94:277-304.

Troemner, E. (1928), Reflexuntersuchungen an einem Anencephalus. *J. Neurol. & Psychiat.*, 35:194.

Uexkuell, J. von (1927), *Theoretical Biology*. London: International Library of Psychology.

Vogt, C. & Vogt, O. (1920), Zur Lehre von den Erkrankungen des Striopallidaeren Systems. *J. Psychol. & Neurol.*, 25:3.

Volkelt, H. (1914), *Ueber die Vorstellungen dor Tiere*. Leipzig: Engelman.

Walshe, F. M. R & Robertson, G. E. (1933), Observation on Grasping Movements and Tonic Innervation in Cases with Lesions of Frontal Lobes. *Brain*, 56:40-70.

Watson, J. B. (1930), *Behaviorism*. New York: Norton, 1933.

Weaver, E. G. & Bray, C. (1930), The Nature of Acoustic Responses; the Relation Between Sound Frequency and Frequency of Impulses in the Auditory Nerve. *J. Experi. Psychol.*, 13:378-387.

Wechsler, I. S. (1935), Trauma and the Nervous System. *J. Am. Med. Assoc.*, 104:519.

Wernicke, C. (1906), *Grundriss der Psychiatrie*. Leipzig: Barth.

Wertheimer, M. (1923), Untersuchungen zue Lehre von der Gestalt. *Psychol. Forschung*, 4:332-37.

Wheeler, R. H. (1929), *The Science of Psychology*. New York: Crowell.

White, W. A. (1917), Study on the Diagnosis and Treatment of Dementia Praecox. *Psychoanal. Rev.*, 8.

Whitehorn, J. C. (1932), Concerning Emotion as Impulsion and Instinct as Orientation. *Am. J. Psychiat.*, 11:1093-1118.

Wildermuth, H. (1923), Schizophrene Zeichen beim gesunden Kind. *Ztschr. ges. Neurol. & Psychiat.*, 86:119.

Wilson, S. A. K. (1929), *Modern Problems in Neurology*. New York: Williams, Wood.

Winterstein, A. (1921), Der Sammler. *Imago*, 7:180-195.

Wohlwill, F. (1922), Zur Frage der sogenannten Encephalitis Congenita (Virchow). *Ztschr. Neurol. & Psychiat.*, 68:384-415; 73:360-418.

Wundt, M. W. (1904), *Volkerpsychologie, I. Die Sprache*. Leipzig: Deuticke.

———— (1910), *Grundzuge der physiologischen Psychologie*. Leipzig: Deuticke.

Yarnell, H. (1940), Fire Setting in Children. *Am. J. Orthopsychiat.*, 10:272-286.

Yaskin, J. C. (1936), The Psychoneuroses and Neuroses. *Am. J. Psychiat.*, 93:125.

Zilboorg, G. (1936), Differential Diagnosis of Types of Suicides. *Arch. Neurol. & Psychiat.*, 35:270-291.

———— (1937), Consideration of Suicides with Particular Reference to the Young. *Am. J. Orthopsychiat.*, 7:14-31.

Zingerle, H. (1927), Klinische Studie ueber Haltungs und Stellreflexe sowie andere automatische Koerperbewegungen beim Menschen. *Ztschr. ges. Neurol. & Psychiat.*, 107:548-598.

# Index

# Name Index

Abraham, K., 63, 77, 218, 373
Adler, A., 193, 243, 373
Allport, F. H., 107, 373
Amatruda, C. S., 343, 378
Appel, K. E., 189, 374

Bachmann, F., 363-364, 373
Baldwin, J., 14, 373
Balint, M., 83, 373
Bartemier, L. H., 212, 382
Baudouin, C., 295, 373
Bauer, J., 9, 373
Bechtereff, V., 110, 373
Benda, C. E., 182, 373
Bender, L., 2, 3, 11-12, 14-15, 29-41,
    59, 95, 116 ff., 163, 173, 184,
    198, 211, 216, 219, 242, 290,
    301, 339, 340, 373-374
Bernfeld, S., 42, 44, 52, 53, 106, 374
Bettelheim, B., 62, 374
Bieber, I., 183, 214, 374
Blau, A., 328, 374
Bleuler, E., 341, 374
Bond, E. D., 189, 374
Boring, E. G., 9, 374
Bray, C., 107, 386
Breed, F. S., 43, 375
Breuer, J., 98
Briffault, R., 369, 375
Bromberg, W., 55, 136, 195, 287,
    293, 294, 302, 335, 375
Brown, T. G., 9, 375

Buehler, K., 4, 375
Bunzel, B., 320, 376
Byers, R. K., 332, 375

Canestrini, N., 70, 375
Carroll, Lewis, 122-133
Cavan, R. S., 301, 375
Clark, L. P., 196, 375
Coghill, G. E., 214, 375
Cohen-Booth, G., 197, 375
Collingswood, S. D., 122, 375
Corré, A., 301, 375
Cottington, F., 203, 375
Curran, F. J., 1, 10, 376
Currier, F. P. Jr., 363, 376

Darwin, C., 107, 217
Day, C., 371
DeKleijn, A., 166-167, 211-212, 380
de la Mare, W., 122, 376
Delboeuf, A., 106, 376
Deutsch, H., 187, 287, 376
Dewar, M., 363, 376
Dewey, E., 219, 220, 376
Dewey, J., 219, 376
Dix, W. K., 42, 376
Dodgson, C. L., 122
Dorff, G. B., 278, 376
Dublin, L. I., 320, 376

Economo, C. von, 198, 376
Engerth, G., 189, 376

389

# Subject Index

Social adaptation by trial and error, 96-99

Social and personal disorganization, 94 ff.

Social aspect of experience of space, 20-21

Socialization, fundamental form of human experience, 96

Somato-psyche concept of Wernicke, 51

Space and perception, 2-3, 9, 10, 14, 19-21

  action, body image, tone, 211

  and body image, 210

  and erogenous zones, 21

  and play in children, 37, 39

  and time, psychopathology of, 22-29

  distortions of, 125-126

  postural responses in relation to head in space, 212

  psychoanalysis of, 125

  spatial separation from love object in death, 300

Speech and auditory perception, 4

Striopallidar lesion, 169, 176, 182, 189, 198; *see also* Organic brain disease

Subcortical lesions, 202, 204, 208-209, 215; *see also* Organic brain disease

Substantia nigra lesions

  Hallervorden-Spatz disease, 174

  in postencephalitic disorders, 189

  in young children, 172

  *see also* Organic brain disease

Subthalamic lesions, 198-199; *see also* Organic brain disease

Sucking behavior, 7, 9, 40, 162-163, 176, 183, 213-216

Suicidal fantasies in children, 152, 160, 294, 301-326

Suicidal methods of children, 324-325

Suicidal preoccupations in children

  case histories, 301 ff.

  summary of discussion, 321 ff.

Symbol and the child, 117 ff.

  and impulsions, 240

Symbol formation, 102 ff.

Superego formation, 75-76, 78, 81, 82, 242, 244

Sydenham's chorea, 190-191

  case of, 200-201

Synesthesia, 6, 10, 20, 39, 53; *see also* Intersensory perception

Tachistoscope, research with, 12, 38, 358 ff.

Tactual experiences, 9, 10

  in infants, 164

  in newborn, 70

Tactual perception, 6-7, 19-21; *see also* Perception

Taste

  and motility, 40

  and object construction, 40-41

  in newborn, 71 *see also* Perception

Thought, 102-104

  contains within itself a call to action, 61

  processes in children, 335

*Through the Looking Glass*, 122-131

Time and perception, 21-22

  and space, psychopathology of, 22-29

Tone

  activity and perception, 38